Methods in Neurosciences

Volume 1

Gene Probes

Methods in Neurosciences

Edited by

P. Michael Conn

Department of Pharmacology
The University of Iowa
College of Medicine
Iowa City, Iowa

Volume 1
Gene Probes

ACADEMIC PRESS, INC.
Harcourt Brace Jovanovich, Publishers
San Diego New York Boston
London Sydney Tokyo Toronto

COPYRIGHT © 1989 BY ACADEMIC PRESS, INC.
All Rights Reserved.
No part of this publication may be reproduced or transmitted in any form or
by any means, electronic or mechanical, including photocopy, recording, or
any information storage and retrieval system, without permission in writing
from the publisher.

ACADEMIC PRESS, INC.
San Diego, California 92101

United Kingdom Edition published by
ACADEMIC PRESS LIMITED
24-28 Oval Road, London NW1 7DX

INTERNATIONAL STANDARD SERIAL NUMBER: 1043-9471

ISBN 0-12-185251-2 (Hardcover) (alk. paper)
ISBN 0-12-185252-0 (Paperback) (alk. paper)

PRINTED IN THE UNITED STATES OF AMERICA
90 91 92   9 8 7 6 5 4 3 2

Table of Contents

Section III Screening, Sequencing, and Cloning

Section IV Lineage Analysis

Section V Molecular Pathology

Section VI Appendixes

Contributors to Volume 1

Article numbers are in parentheses following the names of contributors. Affiliations listed are current.

MARY ABOOD (15), Department of Psychiatry, Nancy Pritzker Laboratory of Behavioral Neuroscience, Stanford University School of Medicine, Stanford, California 94305

C. ANTHONY ALTAR (15), Pharmacological Sciences, Genentech, Inc., South San Francisco, California 94080

FRANK BALDINO, JR. (16), Cephalon, Inc., West Chester, Pennsylvania 19380

MICHAEL V. L. BENNETT (1), Department of Neuroscience, Albert Einstein College of Medicine of Yeshiva University, Bronx, New York 10461

MARIANN BLUM (17), Dr. Arthur M. Fishberg Research Center in Neurobiology, The Mount Sinai Medical Center, Mount Sinai School of Medicine, The Mount Sinai Hospital, New York, New York 10029

JIM BOULTER (20), Molecular Neurobiology Laboratory, The Salk Institute, San Diego, California 92138

THOMAS O. BROCK (18), Biological Sciences Research Center, The University of North Carolina at Chapel Hill, School of Medicine, Chapel Hill, North Carolina 27599

CONNIE CEPKO (21), Department of Genetics, Harvard Medical School, Boston, Massachusetts 02115

JOHN P. COGHLAN (14), Howard Florey Institute of Experimental Physiology and Medicine, University of Melbourne, Parkville, Victoria 3052, Australia

P. MICHAEL CONN (13), Department of Pharmacology, The University of Iowa, College of Medicine, Iowa City, Iowa 52242

JACK E. DIXON (19), Department of Biochemistry, Purdue University, West Lafayette, Indiana 47907

DANIEL M. DORSA (10), Geriatric Research, Education, and Clinical Center, Veterans Administration Medical Center, Seattle, Washington 98108, and Departments of Medicine and Pharmacology, University of Washington School of Medicine, Seattle, Washington 98195

JAMES H. EBERWINE (15), Department of Psychiatry, Nancy Pritzker Laboratory of Behavioral Neuroscience, Stanford University School of Medicine, Stanford, California 94305

PAUL D. GARDNER (20), Department of Biochemistry, Dartmouth Medical School, Hanover, New Hampshire 03756

CHARLES R. GERFEN (5), Laboratory of Cell Biology, National Institute of Mental Health, National Institutes of Health, Bethesda, Maryland 20892

MARVIN C. GERSHENGORN (3), Division of Endocrinology and Metabolism, Department of Medicine, Cornell University Medical College and The New York Hospital, New York, New York 10021

A. GIAID (9), Department of Histochemistry, Royal Postgraduate Medical School, University of London, Hammersmith Hospital, London W12 ONN, England

S. J. GIBSON (9), Department of Histochemistry, Royal Postgraduate Medical School, University of London, Hammersmith Hospital, London W12 ONN, England

MICHEL GOEDERT (23), Medical Research Council (MRC), Laboratory of Molecular Biology, Cambridge CB2 2QH, England

JIM HARALAMBIDIS (14), Howard Florey Institute of Experimental Physiology and Medicine, University of Melbourne, Parkville, Victoria 3052, Australia

J. FIELDING HEJTMANCIK (13), Institute for Molecular Genetics, Baylor College of Medicine, Houston, Texas 77030

GERALD A. HIGGINS (11), Department of Neurobiology and Anatomy, University of Rochester School of Medicine, Rochester, New York 14642

KEVIN A. KELLEY (22), Dr. Arthur M. Fishberg Research Center in Neurobiology, The Mount Sinai Medical Center, Mount Sinai School of Medicine, The Mount Sinai Hospital, New York, New York 10029

JOHN S. KIZER (18), Departments of Medicine and Pharmacology, Biological Sciences Research Center, The University of North Carolina at Chapel Hill, School of Medicine, Chapel Hill, North Carolina 27599

LESLIE KUSHNER (1), Department of Neuroscience, Albert Einstein College of Medicine of Yeshiva University, Bronx, New York 10461

FERNAND LABRIE (12), MRC Group in Molecular Endocrinology, Laval University Medical Center, Sainte-Foy, Quebec, Canada G1V 4G2

JOHN P. LEONARD (4), Department of Biological Sciences, The University of Illinois at Chicago, Chicago, Illinois 60607

JUAN LERMA (1), Instituto Cajal, Consejo Superior de Investigaciones Cientificas, 28002 Madrid, Spain

MICHAEL E. LEWIS (16), Cephalon, Inc., West Chester, Pennsylvania 19380

JOSEPH T. McCABE (6), Department of Anatomy, Uniformed Services University of the Health Sciences, Department of Defense, Bethesda, Maryland 20814

VEI H. MAH (11), Department of Neurobiology and Anatomy, University of Rochester School of Medicine, Rochester, New York 14642

RICARDO MILEDI (2), Department of Psychobiology, Laboratory of Cellular and Molecular Neurobiology, University of California, Irvine, Irvine, California 92717

MARGARET A. MILLER (10), Geriatric Research, Education, and Clinical Center, Veterans Administration Medical Center, Seattle, Washington 98108, and Department of Medicine, University of Washington School of Medicine, Seattle, Washington 98195

R. NICHOLS (19), Department of Biochemistry, Purdue University, West Lafayette, Indiana 47907

YORAM ORON (3), Department of Psysiology and Pharmacology, Sackler Faculty of Medicine, Tel Aviv University, Ramat Aviv, Tel Aviv 69 978, Israel

IAN PARKER (2), Department of Psychobiology, Laboratory of Cellular and Molecular Neurobiology, University of California, Irvine, Irvine, California 92717

GEORGES PELLETIER (12), MRC Group in Molecular Endocrinology, Laval University Medical Center, Sainte-Foy, Quebec, Canada G1V 4G2

JENNIFER D. PENSCHOW (14), Howard Florey Institute of Experimental Physiology and Medicine, University of Melbourne, Parkville, Victoria 3052, Australia

DONALD W. PFAFF (6, 13), Neurobiology and Behavior Laboratory, The Rockefeller University, New York, New York 10021

J. M. POLAK (9), Department of Histochemistry, Royal Postgraduate Medical School, University of London, Hammersmith Hospital, London W12 ONN, England

SCOTT POWNALL (14), Howard Florey Institute of Experimental Physiology and Medicine, University of Melbourne, Parkville, Victoria 3052, Australia

JAMES L. ROBERTS (17), Dr. Arthur M. Fishberg Research Center in Neurobiology, The Mount Sinai Medical Center, Mount Sinai School of Medicine, The Mount Sinai Hospital, New York, New York 10029

SUSAN RYAN (15), Department of Psychiatry, Nancy Pritzker Laboratory of Behavioral Neuroscience, Stanford University School of Medicine, Stanford, California 94305

RUTH E. SIEGEL (8), Department of Pharmacology, School of Medicine, Case Western Reserve University, Cleveland, Ohio 44106

JACQUES SIMARD (12), MRC Group in Molecular Endocrinology, Laval University Medical Center, Sainte-Foy, Quebec, Canada G1V 4G2

J. H. STEEL (9), Department of Histochemistry, Royal Postgraduate Medical School, University of London, Hammersmith Hospital, London W12 ONN, England

RICHARD E. STRAUB (3), Division of Endocrinology and Metabolism, Department of Medicine, Cornell University Medical College, New York, New York 10021

KATUMI SUMIKAWA (2), Department of Psychobiology, Laboratory of Cellular and Molecular Neurobiology, University of California, Irvine, Irvine, California 92717

LARRY W. SWANSON (7), Neural Systems Laboratory, The Salk Institute, San Diego, California 92138

YIAI TONG (12), MRC Group in Molecular Endocrinology, Laval University Medical Center, Sainte-Foy, Quebec, Canada G1V 4G2

JANICE H. URBAN (10), Geriatric Research, Education, and Clinical Center, Veterans Administration Medical Center, Seattle, Washington 98108, and Department of Pharmacology, University of Washington School of Medicine, Seattle, Washington 98195

ALAN G. WATTS (7), Neural Systems Laboratory, The Salk Institute, San Diego, California 92138

HUI-FEN ZHAO (12), MRC Group in Molecular Endocrinology, Laval University Medical Center, Sainte-Foy, Quebec, Canada G1V 4G2

R. SUZANNE ZUKIN (1), Department of Neuroscience, Albert Einstein College of Medicine of Yeshiva University, Bronx, New York 10461

Preface

The recent increase in knowledge in the neurosciences has been nothing short of explosive. This dramatic growth is reflected by the increased number of published papers in relevant journals and by the increased membership reported by societies catering to this discipline.

The neuroscience discipline is well poised to take advantage of the newest developments in molecular biology, cell biology, electrophysiology, and in other emerging areas. Many world-renowned researchers have been attracted to address the unique challenges and to receive the rewards intrinsic to the understanding of this important area. New methods have been developed and novel model systems identified.

The goal of this volume, as well as of those to follow, is to provide in one source a view of the contemporary techniques significant to a particular branch of neurosciences, information which will prove invaluable not only to the experienced researcher but to the student as well. Of necessity some archival material will be included, but the authors have been encouraged to present information that has not yet been published, to compare (in a way not found in other publications) different approaches to similar problems, and to provide tables that direct the reader, in a systematic fashion, to earlier literature and as an efficient means to summarize data. Flow diagrams and summary charts will guide the reader through the processes described.

The nature of this series permits the presentation of methods in fine detail, revealing "tricks" and short cuts that frequently do not appear in the literature owing to space limitations. Lengthy operating instructions for common equipment will not be included except in cases of unusual application. The contributors have been given wide latitude in nomenclature and usage since they are best able to make judgments consistent with current changes.

I wish to express my appreciation to Mrs. Sue Birely for assisting in the organization and maintenance of records and to the staff of Academic Press for their efficient coordination of production. Appreciation is also expressed to the contributors, particularly for meeting their deadlines for the prompt and timely publication of this volume.

P. MICHAEL CONN

Section I

Gene Expression

[1] Using the *Xenopus* Oocyte System for Expression and Cloning of Neuroreceptors and Channels

Leslie Kushner, Juan Lerma, Michael V. L. Bennett, and R. Suzanne Zukin

Introduction

The *Xenopus* oocyte is a self-contained system that is readily used for expression of proteins encoded by exogenous mRNAs. In 1971, Gurdon *et al.* first demonstrated that injection of foreign mRNA into *Xenopus laevis* oocytes leads to translation (1). Since that time, this system has been used for the translation of a large number of mRNAs into their biologically active products. The oocyte is capable not only of translation of exogenous mRNAs, but also of posttranslational modifications, including processing of precursor molecules (2), phosphorylation (3), and glycosylation (4, 5), as well as assembly of subunits and insertion into the surface membrane with the correct orientation (6, 7). Expressed proteins can be detected for as long as 2 weeks after injection (8) and from as little as 5 pg of mRNA isolated from a tissue (9).

Injection of rat brain mRNA into *Xenopus* oocytes has led to translation and functional expression of voltage-sensitive channels, gap junction proteins, and many neuroreceptors, including receptors for acetylcholine (ACh), serotonin (5-HT), noradrenaline, dopamine, γ-aminobutyric acid (GABA), glycine, and the excitatory amino acids (Table I). The nature of the proteins expressed is dependent on the source tissue from which the RNA is isolated. Differences in proteins expressed, however, may be due not simply to differences in tissue sources, but to peculiarities of the oocyte system; not all mRNAs are equally well expressed and some are not expressed at all (9, 10).

Sucrose density gradient centrifugation (11) and gel electrophoresis (12) have been used to fractionate mRNA by size. Injection of size-selected mRNA has made possible the determination of the size of the mRNA(s) encoding a particular protein of interest (13, 14), as well as separation of mRNAs encoding different polypeptides including receptors and receptor subtypes when the mRNAs are of different sizes (15–17). Recently, the oocyte expression system was used to screen and identify the cDNAs encoding the bovine substance K receptor (18) and the rat brain serotonin 5-HT$_{1c}$ receptor (9). In addition to these studies involving direct expression cloning, the oocyte system was used in conjunction with chromosomal walking to identify the *Shaker* locus of *Drosophila melanogaster* as the gene encoding the "A"-type potassium channel (19). In all three cases there was no direct characterization of protein structure. Previously, cloning of the cDNAs or genes encoding channel and receptor proteins required purification of the protein; the purified protein was used to generate antibodies to screen expression libraries or partially sequenced in order to synthesize oligonucleotide probes to screen cDNA libraries. For proteins whose isolation remains difficult and for which an electrophysiological assay is possible, the oocyte system provides an alternative cloning strategy. For cloned receptors, the oocyte system has been used to validate identification of the cDNA as encoding the protein of interest. In a further application, the oocyte system has been used to express mRNAs transcribed from normal as well as mutationally altered cloned cDNAs in order to study subunit composition and other structure–function relationships (Table II). In several studies, cDNAs have been injected into the oocyte nucleus, resulting in both transcription and translation in the oocyte (20–22).

TABLE I   Neuroreceptors or Ion Channels Expressed in *Xenopus* Oocytes after Injection of Tissue mRNA

Receptor or ion channel	Tissue source	Assay	Reference(s)[a]
Ligand-gated channels			
Nicotinic acetylcholine receptor	*Electrophorus* electric organ	Current clamp	1
	Torpedo electric organ	Voltage clamp	2, 3
		Ligand binding	2
	Cat muscle	Single-channel recording	4
GABA$_A$ receptor	Rat brain	Voltage clamp	5, 6
	Chick brain	Voltage clamp	6–8
	Chick optic lobe	Voltage clamp	9, 10
	Chick optic lobe	Single-channel recording	4
	Human fetal cerebral cortex	Voltage clamp	11
Glycine receptor	Rat brain	Voltage clamp	5, 6, 9
	Rat spinal cord	Voltage clamp	12, 13
	Human fetal cerebral cortex	Voltage clamp	11
	Chick optic lobe	Voltage clamp	9
NMDA receptor	Rat brain	Voltage clamp	14, 15
	NCB-20 cells	Voltage clamp	16

(continued)

TABLE I (*continued*)

Receptor or ion channel	Tissue source	Assay	Reference(s)[a]
Kainate receptor	Rat brain	Voltage clamp	6, 9, 14, 17–20
	Human fetal cerebral cortex	Voltage clamp	21
	Embryonic chick brain	Voltage clamp	6
G-protein-binding receptors			
Adrenergic receptor	Rat brain	Voltage clamp	22
Muscarinic acetylcholine receptor	Rat brain	Voltage clamp	6, 17, 19, 23
Serotonin (5-HT)	Rat brain	Voltage clamp	17, 24–26
		Patch clamp	27
	Rat choroid plexus	Voltage clamp	28
	Human fetal cerebral cortex	Voltage clamp	21
	Mouse brain choroid plexus papilloma	Voltage clamp	29
Dopamine receptor	Rat brain	Voltage clamp	22
Substance K receptor	Bovine stomach	Voltage clamp	30
Substance P receptor	Rat brain	Voltage clamp	19, 30, 31
Neurotensin receptor	Rat brain	Voltage clamp	19, 31
Quisqualate receptor	Rat brain	Voltage clamp	14, 18, 20
Vasopressin receptor	Rat liver	$^{45}Ca^{2+}$ efflux	32
	Rat liver	Voltage clamp	33
Angiotensin II receptor	Rat liver	$^{45}Ca^{2+}$ efflux	32
	Rat liver	Voltage clamp	33
	Bovine adrenal, pituitary	IP_3 production	34
Thyrotropin-releasing hormone receptor	Rat pituitary tumor cells	Voltage clamp	33, 35
	Bovine adrenal, pituitary	IP_3 production	34
Cholecystokinin receptor	Pancreatic AR425J cells	$^{45}Ca^{2+}$ efflux	32
Voltage-gated channels			
Sodium channel	Cat muscle	Voltage clamp	36
	Rat brain	Voltage clamp	9, 36–39
	Human fetal cerebral cortex	Voltage clamp	21
	Chick optic lobe	Voltage clamp	9
	Electrophorus electric organ	Voltage clamp	39
	Torpedo brain	Voltage clamp	40
	Embryonic chick brain	Voltage clamp	6
Potassium channel	Cat muscle	Voltage clamp	36
	Rat brain	Voltage clamp	9, 36, 41, 42
	Torpedo brain	Voltage clamp	40
	Chick optic lobe	Voltage clamp	9
	Embryonic chick brain	Voltage clamp	6
Calcium channel	Rat brain	Voltage clamp	43, 44
	Rat heart	Voltage clamp	43, 44
	Rat skeletal muscle	Voltage clamp	43

(*continued*)

TABLE I (*continued*)

Receptor or ion channel	Tissue source	Assay	Reference(s)[a]
Gap junction proteins			
	Rat liver	Voltage clamp	45
	Rat uterus	Voltage clamp	46

[a] References: (1) S. Kobayashi and H. Aoshima, *Dev. Brain Res.* **24,** 211 (1986); (2) E. A. Barnard, R. Miledi, and K. Sumikawa, *Proc. R. Soc. London B* **215,** 241 (1982); (3) K. Sumikawa, M. Houghton, J. S. Emtage, B. M. Richards, and E. A. Barnard, *Nature (London)* **292,** 862 (1981); (4) R. Miledi, I. Parker, and K. Sumikawa, *Proc. R. Soc. London B* **218,** 481 (1983); (5) K. M. Houamed, G. Bilbe, T. G. Smart, A. Constanti, D. A. Brown, E. A. Barnard, and B. M. Richards, *Nature (London)* **310,** 318 (1984); (6) K. Sumikawa, I. Parker, and R. Miledi, *Proc. Natl. Acad. Sci. U.S.A.* **81,** 7994 (1984); (7) T. G. Smart, A. Constanti, G. Bilbe, D. A. Brown, and E. A. Barnard, *Neurosci. Lett.* **40,** 55 (1983); (8) E. Sigel and R. Bauer, *J. Neurosci.* **8,** 289 (1988); (9) K. Sumikawa, I. Parker, and R. Miledi, *Mol. Brain Res.* **464,** 191 (1988); (10) R. Miledi, I. Parker, and K. Sumikawa, *Proc. R. Soc. London B* **216,** 509 (1982); (11) C. B. Gunderson, R. Miledi, and I. Parker, *Proc. R. Soc. London B* **221,** 235 (1984); (12) S. Berrard, N. F. Biguet, D. Gregoire, F. Blanot, J. Smith, and J. Mallet, *Neurosci. Lett.* **72,** 93 (1986); (13) H. Akagi and R. Miledi, *Science* **242,** 270 (1988); (14) L. Kushner, J. Lerma, R. S. Zukin, and M. V. L. Bennett, *Proc. Natl. Acad. Sci. U.S.A.* **85,** 3250 (1988); (15) T. A. Verdoorn, N. W. Kleckner, and R. Dingledine, *Science* **238,** 1114 (1987); (16) J. Lerma, L. Kushner, D. C. Spray, M. V. L. Bennett, and R. S. Zukin, *Proc. Natl. Acad. Sci. U.S.A.* **86,** 1708 (1989); (17) N. Dascal, C. Ifune, R. Hopkins, T. P. Snutch, H. Lübbert, N. Davidson, M. I. Simon, and H. A. Lester, *Mol. Brain Res.* **1,** 201 (1986); (18) C. B. Gunderson, R. Miledi, and I. Parker, *Proc. R. Soc. London B* **221,** 127 (1984); (19) C. Hironi, I. Ito, and H. Sugiyama, *J. Physiol. (London)* **382,** 523 (1987); (20) H. Sugiyama, I. Ito, and C. Hironi, *Nature (London)* **325,** 531 (1987); (21) C. B. Gunderson, R. Miledi, and I. Parker, *Nature (London)* **308,** 421 (1984); (22) K. Sumikawa, I. Parker, and R. Miledi, *Proc. R. Soc. London B* **223,** 255 (1984); (23) H. Sugiyama, Y. Hisanaga, and C. Hironi, *Brain Res.* **338,** 346 (1985); (24) H. Lübbert, T. P. Snutch, N. Dascal, H. A. Lester, and N. Davidson, *J. Neurosci.* **7,** 1159 (1987); (25) C. B. Gunderson, R. Miledi, and I. Parker, *Proc. R. Soc. London B* **219,** 103 (1983); (26) Y. Sakai, H. Kimura, and K. Okamoto, *Brain Res.* **362,** 199 (1986); (27) T. Takahashi, E. Neher, and B. Sakmann, *Proc. Natl. Acad. Sci. U.S.A.* **84,** 5063 (1987); (28) D. Julius, A. B. MacDermott, R. Axel, and T. M. Jessell, *Science* **241,** 558 (1988); (29) H. Lübbert, B. J. Hoffman, T. P. Snutch, T. van Dyke, A. J. Levine, P. R. Hartig, H. A. Lester, and N. Davidson, *Proc. Natl. Acad. Sci. U.S.A.* **84,** 4332 (1987); (30) Y. Harada, T. Takahashi, M. Kuno, K. Nakayama, Y. Masu, and S. Nakanishi, *J. Neurosci.* **7,** 3265 (1987); (31) I. Parker, K. Sumikawa, and R. Miledi, *Proc. R. Soc. London B* **229,** 151 (1986); (32) J. A. Williams, D. J. McChesney, M. C. Calayag, V. R. Lingappa, and C. D. Logsdon, *Proc. Natl. Acad. Sci. U.S.A.* **85,** 4939 (1988); (33) W. Meyerhof, S. Morley, J. Schwarz, and D. Richter, *Proc. Natl. Acad. Sci. U.S.A.* **85,** 714 (1988); (34) R. P. McIntosh and K. J. Catt, *Proc. Natl. Acad. Sci. U.S.A.* **84,** 9045 (1987); (35) Y. Oron, B. Gillo, and M. C. Gershengorn, *Proc. Natl. Acad. Sci. U.S.A.* **85,** 3820 (1988); (36) C. B. Gundersen, R. Miledi, and I. Parker, *Proc. R. Soc. London B* **220,** 131 (1983); (37) D. S. Krafte, T. P. Snutch, J. P. Leonard, N. Davidson, and H. A. Lester, *J. Neurosci.* **8,** 2859 (1988); (38) A. L. Goldin, T. Snutch, H. Lübbert, A. Dowsett, J. Marshall, V. Auld, W. Downey, L. C. Fritz, H. A. Lester, R. Dunn, W. A. Catterall, and N. Davidson, *Proc. Natl. Acad. Sci. U.S.A.* **83,** 7503 (1986); (39) C. Hirono, S. Yamagishi, R. Ohara, Y. Hisanaga, T. Nakayama, and H. Sugiyama, *Brain Res.* **359,** 57 (1985); (40) C. B. Gunderson, R. Miledi, and I. Parker, *J. Physiol. (London)* **353,** 231 (1984); (41) J. H. Hoger, I. Ahmed, N. Davidson, and H. A. Lester, *Soc. Neurosci. Abstr.* **13,** 177 (1987); (42) B. Rudy, J. H. Hoger, N. Davidson, and H. A. Lester, *Soc. Neurosci. Abstr.* **13,** 178 (1987); (43) N. Dascal, T. P. Snutch, H. Lübbert, N. Davidson, and H. A. Lester, *Science* **231,** 1147 (1986); (44) T. P. Snutch, J. P. Leonard, J. Nargeot, H. Lübbert, N. Davidson, and H. A. Lester, *Soc. Gen. Physiol. Ser.* **42,** 153 (1987); (45) G. Dahl, T. Miller, D. Paul, R. Voellmy, and R. Werner, *Science* **236,** 1290 (1987); (46) R. Werner, T. Miller, R. Azarnia, and G. Dahl, *J. Membr. Biol.* **87,** 253 (1985).

TABLE II   Receptors and Ion Channels Expressed following
          Injection of *in Vitro* Transcribed mRNA

Receptor or ion channel	Tissue source	Reference(s)[a]
Nicotinic acetylcholine receptor	Mouse BC3H-1 cells	1
	Torpedo electric organ	2–5
	Bovine muscle	5
	Rat hypothalamus	6
	Rat PC12 cells	6
GABA$_A$ receptor	Bovine brain	7, 8
Muscarinic acetylcholine receptor	Porcine cerebrum	9
Serotonin (5-HT$_{1C}$) receptor	Rat choroid plexus	10
Substance K receptor	Bovine stomach	11
β-Adrenergic receptor	Human placenta	12
Voltage-gated sodium channels	Rat brain	13–15
Voltage-gated potassium channels	*Drosophila*	16
	Rat hippocampus	17
Gap junction	Rat liver	18, 19
	Rat heart	19
	Xenopus oocyte	20

[a] References: (1) R. J. Leonard, C. G. Labarca, P. Charnet, N. Davidson, and H. A. Lester, *Science* **242**, 1578 (1988); (2) C. Methfessel, V. Witzemann, T. Takahashi, M. Mishina, S. Numa, and B. Sakmann, *Pfluegers Arch.* **407**, 577 (1986); (3) T. Takahashi, M. Kuno, M. Mishina, and S. Numa, *J. Physiol. (Paris)* **80**, 229 (1985); (4) M. Mishina, T. Tobimatsu, K. Imoto, K. Tanaka, Y. Fujita, K. Fukuda, M. Kurasaki, H. Takahashi, Y. Morimoto, T. Hirose, S. Inayama, T. Takahashi, M. Kuno, and S. Numa, *Nature (London)* **313**, 364 (1985); (5) K. Imoto, C. Methfessel, B. Sakmann, M. Mishina, Y. Mori, T. Konno, K. Fukuda, M. Kurasaki, H. Bujo, Y. Fujita, and S. Numa, *Nature (London)* **324**, 670 (1986); (6) J. Boulter, J. Connolly, E. Deneris, D. Goldman, S. Heinemann, and J. Patrick, *Proc. Natl. Acad. Sci. U.S.A.* **84**, 7763 (1987); (7) P. R. Schofield, M. G. Darlison, N. Fujita, D. R. Burt, F. A. Stephenson, H. Rodriguez, L. M. Rhee, J. Ramachandran, V. Reale, T. A. Glencorse, P. H. Seeburg, and E. A. Barnard, *Nature (London)* **328**, 221 (1987); (8) L. A. C. Blair, E. S. Levitan, J. Marshall, V. E. Dionne, and E. A. Barnard, *Science* **242**, 577 (1988); (9) T. Kubo, K. Fukuda, A. Mikami, A. Maeda, H. Takahashi, M. Mishina, T. Haga, K. Haga, A. Ichiyama, K. Kangawa, M. Kojima, H. Matsuo, T. Hirose, and S. Numa, *Nature (London)* **323**, 411 (1986); (10) D. Julius, A. B. MacDermott, R. Axel, and T. M. Jessell, *Science* **241**, 558 (1988); (11) Y. Masu, K. Nakayama, H. Tamaki, Y. Harada, M. Kuno, and S. Nakanishi, *Nature (London)* **329**, 836 (1987); (12) T. Frielle, S. Collins, K. W. Daniel, M. G. Caron, R. J. Lefkowitz, and B. K. Kobilka, *Proc. Natl. Acad. Sci. U.S.A.* **84**, 7920 (1987); (13) V. J. Auld, A. L. Goldon, D. S. Krafte, J. Marshall, J. M. Dunn, W. A. Catterall, H. A. Lester, N. Davidson, and R. J. Dunn, *Neuron* **1**, 449 (1988); (14) W. Stuhmer, C. Methfessel, B. Sakmann, M. Noda, and S. Numa, *Eur. Biophys. J.* **14**, 131 (1987); (15) M. Noda, T. Ikeda, H. Suzuki, H. Takeshima, T. Takahashi, M. Kuno, and S. Numa, *Nature (London)* **322**, 826 (1986); (16) L. C. Timpe, T. L. Schwarz, B. L. Tempel, D. M. Papazian, Y. N. Jan, and L. Y. Jan, *Nature (London)* **331**, 143 (1988); (17) M. J. Christie, J. P. Adelman, J. Douglass, and R. A. North, *Science* **244**, 221 (1989); (18) G. Dahl, T. Miller, D. Paul, R. Voellmy, and R. Werner, *Science* **236**, 1290 (1987); (19) K. I. Swenson, J. R. Jordan, E. C. Beyer, and D. L. Paul, *Cell* **57**, 145 (1989); (20) L. Ebihara, E. C. Beyer, K. I. Swenson, D. L. Paul, and D. A. Goodenough, *Science* **243**, 1194 (1989).

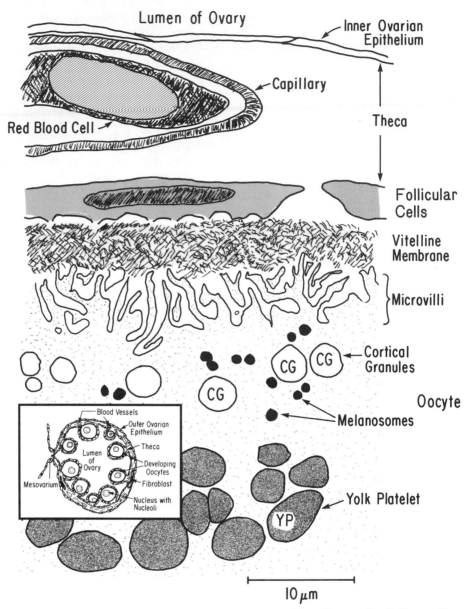

FIG. 1 Surface of the mature oocyte as encountered in a dissected cell. Proceeding from ovarian lumen inward, one passes the inner ovarian membrane, the theca (containing collagen, fibroblasts, and blood vessels), the follicular layer, the transparent vitelline membrane, and the oocyte surface, which has many microvilli. Follicular cells send small processes through the vitelline membrane that form gap

The mature *Xenopus* oocyte is a single cell surrounded by a vitelline membrane, a layer of follicular cells, and the theca, a blood vessel and fibroblast-containing layer (Fig. 1; see Ref. 23 for a description of development). The follicular cells send processes through the vitelline membrane and are electrically coupled to the oocyte by gap junctions formed by these processes (24); follicular cells possess a number of receptors and ion channels not present in the oocyte (25–27). For this reason, oocytes are generally treated with collagenase to remove the follicular layer prior to injection with exogenous mRNA (see below). Removal of the follicular cells eliminates receptors in this layer and the collagenase treatment also destroys some endogenous receptors present on the surface of the oocyte itself (27–29). The oocyte is specialized along its animal–vegetal axis; concentration of the pigment melanin in the animal half of the cell is responsible for its increased coloration. Endogenous mRNAs may be differentially distributed in the cortical cytoplasm of the animal and vegetal poles (30). Endogenous acetylcholine receptors are of highest density at the vegetal pole (31), whereas receptors expressed following injection of rat brain RNA, although differentially distributed, tend to be more concentrated at the animal pole (31, 32).

The *Xenopus* oocyte translation system is particularly useful for the examination of channel proteins, because the oocyte is easily studied with extremely sensitive electrophysiological techniques. We have employed the oocyte to express excitatory amino acid (EAA) and other receptors and channels encoded by rat brain mRNA (32–35). Currents generated by ligand-gated channels upon application of *N*-methyl D-aspartate (NMDA), kainate, and GABA are shown in Fig. 2A. G-protein-linked receptors mediate the responses to carbachol and serotonin shown in Fig. 2B. Application of these drugs appears to liberate inositol phosphates that raise intracellular Ca^{2+}, leading to the opening of Ca^{2+}-activated Cl^- channels. Voltage-activated Na^+ currents are illustrated in Fig. 2C. These inward currents are blocked by tetrodotoxin (TTX). The voltage-clamp technique

---

junctions with the oocyte. There are cortical granules just beneath the oocyte surface, and in the animal hemisphere melanosomes are also found in this region. Yolk platelets give the egg its milky appearance. The oocyte nucleus lies deeper. [Redrawn from J. N. Dumont and A. R. Brummett, *J. Morphol.* **155,** 73 (1978).] (Inset) Cross section of an ovarian lobule. Oocytes develop within the thecal space, which is enclosed by the outer ovarian epithelium abutting the coelom and the inner ovarian epithelium abutting the lumen of the ovary. Oocytes are shed into the coelom by rupture of the outer epithelium. The theca contains fibroblasts, collagen, and blood vessels. [Redrawn from J. N. Dumont and A. R. Brummett, *J. Morphol.* **155,** 73 (1978).]

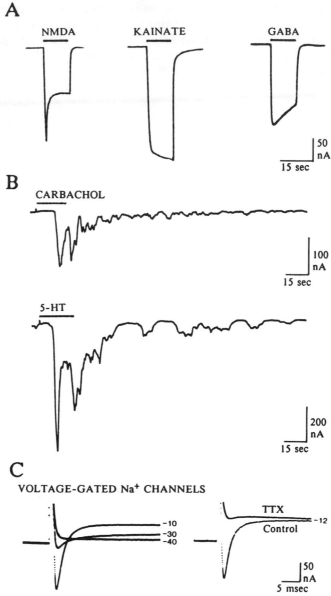

FIG. 2 Responses mediated by receptors and channels expressed in oocytes injected with rat forebrain mRNA. Recordings were carried out under voltage clamp (at a holding potential of −60 mV for A and B) 4–6 days after injection. Inward currents are indicated by a downward deflection. (A) Short latency responses due to activation of ligand-gated channels by NMDA (100 μM), kainate (100 μM), and

can detect currents at the nanoamp (nA) level, which can arise, depending on single-channel conductance, from 100 to 1000 active channels. This number could be provided by a small number of mRNA molecules depending on message stability, translational activity, and subsequent processing and degradation of the protein. Single-channel recording is possible with the patch-clamp technique but requires a much higher level of expression than does whole-cell recording, as there must be a reasonable probability that a patch (less than 1/10,000 of the oocyte's surface) will contain a channel. Amplification appears to be possible for receptors, such as the serotonin 5-HT_{1C} receptor, which are linked to the inositol trisphosphate (IP_3) second messenger system resulting in the opening of the Ca^{2+}-dependent Cl^- channels endogenous to the oocyte (9, 13, 36, 37). It is likely for these receptors that binding of a single ligand molecule leads to opening of many channels. Whatever assay method is employed, the occurrence of similar endogenous proteins should be excluded by comparison of mRNA-injected oocytes with oocytes that are not injected or are injected with water or mRNAs not encoding the protein under study. It is also possible that the exogenous message encodes a factor that induces expression of endogenous genes or messages (see the section *Gap Junctions: Another Channel Family*), but this has never to our knowledge interfered with expression studies.

Ligand-Gated Channels and G-Protein-Linked Receptors: Two Superfamilies

It now appears that all known neurotransmitter receptors belong to one of two receptor superfamilies. One of these comprises the ligand-gated channels and includes the nicotinic ACh, $GABA_A$, and glycine receptors (38, 39). It most probably includes the NMDA, kainate, and channel-forming quisqualate receptors as well. For many years, the nicotinic ACh receptor was the only neuroreceptor for which extensive structural information was

---

GABA (100 μM). The NMDA response (with 10 μM glycine and zero Mg^{2+}) showed a brief initial peak ascribable to desensitization. (B) Responses mediated by G-protein-linked receptors and the endogenous IP_3, Ca^{2+}-activated Cl^- channel system are of longer latency and arise abruptly from the baseline. They consist of multiple phases long outlasting the drug application. (C) Voltage-activated Na^+ currents. The cell was stepped from the holding potential of -80 mV to the indicated value. A transient inward current was evoked by large enough depolarization (left superimposed records). This current was blocked by TTX (right records). [Unpublished records (see Refs. 32–35).]

available. The recent cloning and sequencing of the cDNAs encoding the bovine brain GABA$_A$ (39) and rat spinal cord glycine (40) receptors revealed striking common structural features among all three receptors and led to the proposal that the genes that encode them evolved by duplication of a common ancestral gene and subsequent divergence (38). Each of these receptors is a heterooligomeric glycoprotein of four to five homologous transmembrane polypeptides, sequence similarity being greater among subunits of a single-channel type than between channels. Analysis of hydrophobicity suggest that each subunit contains four or five putative transmembrane-spanning segments, a large N-terminal extracellular domain with several putative glycosylation sites and two cytoplasmic loops, one of which is longer and contains one or more consensus sequences for cAMP-dependent phosphorylation. The common structural features of these receptors reflect their close functional similarity; ligand specificity is presumed to have arisen by minor modifications of a common protein architectural theme.

The second receptor superfamily is that of the G-protein-linked receptors. This group includes rhodopsin (41) and α- and β-adrenergic (42, 43), muscarinic ACh (44, 45), dopamine (46), 5-HT$_{1C}$ (9), and substance K (18) receptors. It most probably includes a number of other neuropeptide receptors as well, such as the opioid, neurotensin, cholecystokinin, GABA$_B$, and substance P receptors, as well as one type of quisqualate receptor. Each of the members of this receptor superfamily comprises a single subunit with significant sequence identity among the members. Sequence identity is most apparent in the transmembrane regions, where it exceeds 80% for some pairs within this group (42, 43, 47). The structure of the β-adrenergic receptor, recently cloned by Lefkowitz and co-workers (43, 47), is typical for these proteins. Predicted features include (1) seven putative transmembrane-spanning domains; (2) a large extracellular N-terminal region which contains several putative glycosylation sites, as well as the presumed transmitter binding site; (3) a very large fourth cytoplasmic loop of varying length, which is essential for binding of G-protein; and (4) a large cytoplasmic C-terminal domain with consensus sequences for cAMP-dependent phosphorylation.

Voltage-Gated Channels: Another Superfamily

In addition to the two receptor superfamilies, voltage-gated sodium and potassium channels and a putative Ca^{2+} channel (identified as a dihydropyridine-binding protein) form a superfamily of structurally related proteins (see Ref. 48). Sodium, potassium, and calcium channels from a variety of tissue sources share common structural motifs. The major subunits of the sodium and calcium channels each have four repeat domains, each of which has six (or four or eight) predicted transmembrane segments. These domains exhibit considerable homology to one another and to the single domain of the potassium channel. It has been suggested that the K^+ channel functions as a tetramer, perhaps heteromeric, and that it may be more like the ancestral, prototypic channel than the other voltage-gated channels that have evolved. These channel molecules are regulated on the millisecond time scale by small changes in voltage across the membrane and on a longer time scale by covalent modification such as phosphorylation which, in the case of the Na^+ channel, affects inactivation. The fourth transmembrane segment (S4) of each repeat domain is thought to play a key role in voltage sensing. It will be of interest to determine the structural basis of voltage sensitivity, selectivity, and modulation of the great diversity of channels and to explore homologies and divergences among them.

Gap Junctions: Another Channel Family

The proteins forming gap junction channels in the rat include a family of three homologous polypeptides termed connexins 26, 32, and 43 from their M_r based on their predicted amino acid sequences; these correspond to 21-, 27-, and 47-kDa proteins, respectively, as determined by SDS-PAGE. Connexins 26 and 32 were originally isolated from rat liver (49, 50) and connexin 43 from rat heart (51), but the tissue distribution is much wider. In addition, there is a homologous protein in lens which may or may not form channels (52, 53). A family of homologous proteins is also found in *Xenopus*, although their detailed relationship to the rat connexins is not yet clear (54, 55).

A single gap junction channel comprises two hexamers (each contributed by a different cell) which form hemichannels (or connexons) in each membrane; the two hemichannels are linked together by juxtaposition of their extracellular faces (for a review, see Ref. 56). Each subunit of the gap junction has four membrane-spanning regions, and both the amino and carboxy termini are cytoplasmic. The carboxy-terminal domain exhibits a high degree of variability in its sequence and may be very small or comprise about half the molecule. It is likely that this region confers much of the specificity in structure and function to a particular gap junction type. In different species and cells, gap junctions are known to be gated by cytoplasmic acidification, high cytoplasmic free Ca^{2+}, voltage, and phosphorylation; in these respects they exhibit properties like those of the ligand-gated and voltage-sensitive channel superfamilies.

Exemplary Studies of Expressed Receptors and Channels

Receptors and channels from each of the four groups have been expressed in the *Xenopus* oocyte in site-directed mutagenesis or expression cloning studies. Perhaps the best characterized in site-directed mutagenesis experiments is the nicotinic acetylcholine receptor (nAChR). Studies in which mRNAs for the α, β, γ, and δ subunits were injected in different combinations have shown that all four are required to produce functional channels (57). The structure of the receptor in relation to gating and permeation through the channel is being studied by site-directed mutagenesis (58, 59). Specific amino acid residues in the α, β, γ, and δ subunits were altered to test the hypothesis that the M2 (or second) membrane-spanning regions of the four subunits line the ion pore and control conductance. As the number of serines (58) or negatively charged residues (59) decreased, there were decreases in the residence time and, consequently, the binding affinity of the putative open channel blocker QX-222, as well as a selective decrease in outward single-channel currents. These findings indicate that clusters of negatively charged and serine residues in M2 and its vicinity determine the rate of ion transport.

In contrast to the nicotinic ACh receptor, a single subunit of the $GABA_A$ receptor can form functional channels in the oocyte (60). The α and β subunits were expressed individually by injection of RNA synthesized from the corresponding cloned cDNAs. Any of three different α RNAs (α_1, α_2, and α_3) and, to a lesser extent, β RNA expressed active channels with the same multiple conductance levels of ~10, 19, 28, and 42 picosiemens (pS). In all cases, channels were potentiated by pentobarbital and inhibited by picrotoxin. The finding that both α and β subunits separately form active channels with several important properties similar to the native receptor suggests that the residues that confer these properties are within the homologous domains shared by the subunits.

Yet another approach to the study of the structural basis of receptor function involves the design and expression of chimeric molecules. Constructs involving portions of the cDNAs encoding the β_1- and β_2-adrenergic receptors were transcribed, and the resulting mRNAs expressed in the *Xenopus* oocyte (61). The pharmacological properties of the expressed chimeric receptors were characterized by both radioligand binding and assays of adenylate cyclase activity with ligands specific for each receptor subtype. General conclusions reached from this study included that agonist binding specificity is conferred primarily by the fourth membrane-spanning region, whereas antagonist specificity resides largely in the sixth and seventh transmembrane regions. It was found, however, that determinants throughout the other transmembrane regions were important in determining specificity for both agonists and antagonists. These observations have lead to a model in which subtype specificity of ligand binding occurs within a pocket formed by the clustering of all seven membrane-spanning helices (61).

The *Drosophila melanogaster Shaker* gene encodes the "A-type" potassium channel or one of its components (62–64). Studies involving the *Xenopus* oocyte were used to demonstrate that a single *Shaker* mRNA suffices to direct the translation of functional A channels (19). There are, however, at least five different proteins that arise from the *Shaker* gene by alternative splicing of the hnRNA. The oocyte system was further used to show that two of the mRNAs each encodes functional channels with properties similar to those of native *Drosophila* muscle "A" channel. As the *Shaker* products resemble individual domains of the sodium channel, it was suggested that the *Shaker* products are subunits of oligomeric channel which, in its native tissue, may be heteromeric.

Expression of cloned gap junction cDNAs in the *Xenopus* oocyte has verified that the putative connexin 32 and 43 cDNAs do each encode proteins that form gap junctions. Encoding of gap junctions by connexin 32 cDNA was shown by injection of mRNA transcribed from cloned connexin 32 cDNA (21, 65). Furthermore, enrichment of liver mRNA by hybrid selection with the cDNA increased expression, and coinjection of liver mRNA with antisense RNA made from the cDNA decreased expression (hybrid arrest) (21). Finally, heat shock promoted expression following injection into the oocyte nucleus of a cDNA construct containing the *Drosophila* heat shock promoter and liver gap junction cDNA (21). A further interesting result with oocyte expression was that cells injected with different RNAs and expressing different connexins can form "heterotypic" junctions in which hemichannels made of different connexin form the channels, and that there is some specificity of formation (65). Oocytes expressing rat connexin 32 will form gap junctions with themselves. However, only oocytes expressing connexin 43 will form junctions with the endogenous connexin in water-injected oocytes; oocytes expressing rat connexin 32 will not. The connexin 43/endogenous junctions have asymmetric properties, i.e., they rectify, as would be predicted from the conventional but until now unsubstantiated view that each membrane provides one hemichannel to complete the coupling pathway. Surprisingly, the conductance of the heterotypic connexin 43/endogenous junctions is much higher than that of the homotypic endogenous junctions and almost as high as that of homotypic connexin 43 junctions. The nature of the regulatory process is unknown, but it is clear that the exogenous RNA leads to much greater expression of endogenous hemichannels in a contacting cell lacking the exogenous RNA.

Recently, the oocyte expression system was combined with electrophysiological assay to isolate a cDNA encoding the bovine neuropeptide substance K receptor (18) and partial (66) as well as full-length cDNAs encoding the serotonin 5-HT$_{1C}$ receptor (9). The substance K and 5-HT$_{1C}$ receptors are single subunit receptors which, in the oocyte, act through the IP$_3$ second messenger system to activate endogenous chloride channels. For each receptor, oocyte expression of agonist-induced receptor-coupled electrophysiological responses was used to screen *in vitro* transcribed RNA from cDNA libraries. In the case of the serotonin 5-HT$_{1C}$ receptor, size-selected RNA from rat choroid plexus was used to generate a cDNA library of 1.2 $\times$ 10^6 independent clones in the cloning vector λZAP (Stratogene). Five pools of 10^5 independent clones were amplified. The DNA from each of these pools of clones was purified and transcribed, and RNA copies of each of the pooled cDNAs were independently microinjected into oocytes. One positive pool was identified which was progressively subdivided into smaller pools through five stages of 10-fold reduction (sib selection) until a single positive clone was found. Interestingly, the 5-HT$_{1C}$ receptor cDNA cloned by this method was only 3 kilobases (kb), although the native mRNA containing this sequence is more than 5 kb (9).

Limitations of Oocyte Expression System

The oocyte does have several shortcomings. Apparently not all channels and receptors are expressed in oocytes; notably, only one type of voltage-gated calcium channel has been detected in oocytes following injection with mRNA from rat brain tissue in which four types have been described (67). In addition, only the 5-HT$_{1C}$ subtype of serotonin receptor has been expressed in oocytes injected with mRNA from rat brain (9), a tissue that has at least five other types of serotonin receptor (68). Thus, there appears to be selective expression in the oocyte, failure at some stage of coupling to channels, or possibly lack of proper posttranslational modification. Not all posttranslational modifications are performed on all exogenous polypeptides in the oocyte. For example, it would appear that, although the voltage-gated sodium channel protein is translated after injection of *Electrophorus* mRNA, it is not inserted as a functional entity in the oocyte membrane due to incorrect processing (10).

The oocyte has a number of endogenous receptors which may interfere with electrophysiological assay of expressed receptors. Receptors endogenous to the denuded oocyte include muscarinic ACh, cholecystokinin, and catecholamine receptors (26–29, 31, 69). The chloride current induced by calcium ions in oocytes can obscure currents through channels encoded by exogenous mRNA (70). However, it is the presence of this current, which can be activated by the IP$_3$ system, that has allowed the detection of many of the G-protein-linked receptors.

Finally, there can be seasonal variations in viability as well as in the degree of expression in *Xenopus* oocytes, with expression being particularly low in late summer or early fall. Variability in the degree of expression is also apparent from oocyte to oocyte, as well as between oocytes derived from different donor frogs. Although the cells are large and readily manipulated and survive for days, each one must be individually injected.

Methods

Preparation of RNA

To use the *Xenopus* oocyte expression system, poly(A)$^+$ mRNA is generally prepared, although total RNA may be adequate for expression of proteins encoded by high-abundance mRNA(s). Total RNA can be isolated by either a modification of the phenol–chloroform extraction method of Bingham and Zachar (71) or a modification of the guanidinium isothiocyanate–CsCl gradient method of Ullrich *et al.* (72). The phenol–chloroform extraction method is particularly suitable for small amounts of tissue. RNA isolated by this method, however, is not very clean of protein and will certainly contain DNA unless it is treated with DNase. The guanidinium isothiocyanate method results in a preparation of RNA which is almost devoid of DNA. However, it requires a larger amount of starting tissue for the RNA band to be visible for aspiration after CsCl density gradient centrifugation. One advantage of this method is that guanidinium isothiocyanate is a powerful RNase inhibitor (73). The tissue of interest must be removed sterilely and as rapidly as possible and frozen in liquid nitrogen. Cells grown in tissue culture are harvested sterilely, and the cell pellet frozen in liquid nitrogen. Tissue may be stored at −76°C indefinitely. In preparing and working with RNA, care must be taken to avoid contamination with RNases. This can be achieved by autoclaving all glassware, autoclaving or filter-sterilizing (using a 0.22-μm membrane filter) all solutions to prevent contamination with bacteria which synthesize RNases, and handling everything with gloves. In addition, all solutions should be treated with the RNase inhibitor diethyl pyrocarbonate (DEPC), 0.1% (i.e., add 0.01 vol of a 10% solution of DEPC in ethanol, let sit overnight, autoclave), unless they contain amines (e.g., Tris) which react with DEPC.

RNA Preparation by Phenol–Chloroform Extraction Method
Tissue is placed in lysis buffer [1 mM EDTA, 350 mM NaCl, 2% sodium dodecyl sulfate (SDS), 7 M urea (Schwarz Mann, MA, ultrapure) 10 mM

Tris-HCl, pH 8.0] (10 vol buffer/wet wt of tissue) and homogenized with a Brinkman Polytron at speed 6. Protease K is added to give a final concentration of 10 μg/ml and the entire lysis solution is incubated at 37°C for 30 min. This preparation is then extracted two times with a solution of one part phenol (saturated with 10 mM Tris/1mM EDTA, pH 8.0) to one part chloroform (4% isoamyl alcohol) and once with chloroform (4% isoamyl alcohol). Nucleic acid is precipitated from the aqueous layer remaining by adding 0.1 vol 3 M sodium acetate, pH 5.0, and 2–3 vol of ice-cold anhydrous ethanol, shaking, and storing at −20°C for at least 2 hr. RNA prepared in this way contains DNA. DNA can be removed by treatment with DNase I or by washing the final precipitate with 3 M sodium acetate, pH 5.0.

RNA Preparation by Guanidinium Isothiocyanate Method

This method is particularly useful for tissues containing high levels of RNase, because guanidinium isothiocyanate is a potent RNase inhibitor. The denaturing solution [4 M guanidinium isothiocyanate (Fluka), 1 M 2-mercaptoethanol, 0.1 M sodium acetate, 0.01 M EDTA] is prepared by first dissolving the guanidinium isothiocyanate by heating at 60–70°C for 10 min, adding the other reagents, and filter-sterilizing through a 0.22-μm membrane filter. Tissue is homogenized in 5 vol of denaturing solution using a Brinkman Polytron. CsCl (1 g per milliliter of solution) is added and dissolved with stirring. This solution is placed in a polyallomer tube, underlaid with one-fourth volume of CsCl cushion solution (0.01 M EDTA, 0.1 M sodium acetate in saturated CsCl), and overlaid with paraffin oil. The tube is centrifuged in a swinging bucket rotor (SW 41) at 45,000 rpm for 16–20 hr at room temperature. Following centrifugation, the band of RNA is clearly visible as a band of white precipitate at the midpoint of the tube that is well-separated from DNA and most protein, which are of lower density and therefore toward the top of the tube. The RNA is removed from the side of the tube with a syringe. This solution is diluted fourfold with extraction buffer (5 mM EDTA, 1% SDS, 10 mM Tris-HCl, pH 7.4). The aqueous solution is extracted with an equal volume of chloroform/n-butanol (4/1, v/v). The aqueous phase is removed and the organic phase is reextracted with an equal volume of extraction buffer. The two aqueous phases are then combined and the RNA is precipitated by mixing with 0.1 vol of 3 M sodium acetate, pH 5.0, and 2–3 vol of ice-cold anhydrous ethanol followed by storage at −20°C for at least 2 hr.

For either method, the precipitated RNA is recovered by centrifugation for 20 min at 8000 rpm at 4°C. The ethanol is removed and the pellet is dried in a Savant Speedvac Concentrator or lyophilized. The pellet is resuspended in water and the concentration may be assessed at this point. The concentration of RNA is determined by measuring the absorbance at 260 nm [$A_{260} = 1$ (1 cm path length) for 40 μg RNA/ml]. An adult rat brain (1.4 g) will yield 1–2 mg RNA. The ratio of A_{260} (λ_{max} for nucleic acid) to A_{280} (λ_{max} for protein), which provides a measure of protein contamination, should be close to 2.0 if contamination is minimal. A ratio of 1.8 is probably sufficient for expression in the oocyte, while RNA with a lower ratio can be used for isolation of mRNA by affinity chromatography. The RNA may be reprecipitated with 0.1 vol of 3 M sodium acetate, pH 5.0, and 2–3 vol of ice-cold ethanol for storage at $-20°C$.

Preparation of mRNA by Oligo(dT) Affinity Chromatography

The mRNA content of most tissue is approximately 2% of the total RNA mass. Most eukaryotic mRNAs contain a polyadenylate [poly(A)] tail at the 3′ end (74). To separate mRNA, total RNA is passed over a column with oligo(dT) chains immobilized to cellulose (75). The poly(A) tail binds, thus separating mRNA from nonpolyadenylated nucleic acids (rRNA, tRNA, and DNA). The partially purified mRNA is then eluted by lowering the ionic strength of the buffer. The capacity of Type 2 oligo(dT)-cellulose (Collaborative Research, Inc., Lexington, MA) is 10 mg of RNA per milliliter of matrix. The column material is prepared by suspension in the elution buffer (10 mM Tris-HCl, pH 7.5), after which it is poured into a plastic minicolumn or a Pasteur pipette plugged with glass wool. The column is equilibrated by washing with 10 bed volumes of loading buffer (0.5 M NaCl, 30 mM EDTA, 0.5% SDS, 0.2% deoxycholate, 10 mM Tris-HCl, pH 7.5). The column exit port is connected to a flow-through spectrophotometer so that A_{260} of the eluate can be monitored. The starting RNA, as an ethanol precipitate, is centrifuged for 20 min at 8000 rpm at 4°C, and the pellet dried in a Savant Speedvac Concentrator. The pellet is resuspended in loading buffer to a concentration of 1 mg/ml, then heated at 65°C for 20 min to disrupt internal base pairing and placed immediately on ice to cool it rapidly to room temperature. The RNA solution is loaded onto the column, and the eluate is collected and applied to the column again to maximize binding. Nonpolyadenylated nucleic acids are washed out of the column with loading buffer until A_{260} is at baseline. Ten column volumes of washing buffer (10 mM Tris-HCl, pH 7.5, 0.5 M NaCl) are passed through the column to remove detergent. Poly(A)$^+$ RNA is eluted with the elution buffer at 46°C and fractions corresponding to the peak absorbance at 260 nm are collected. The poly(A)$^+$ RNA can be assayed, precipitated, and stored as described for total RNA. The column can be regenerated by washing with 0.1 N NaOH, followed by water, and stored at 4°C in 0.2% sodium azide solution to prevent microbial growth.

Size Fractionation of RNA

Prior to oocyte injection, either mRNA or total RNA can be size fractionated by sucrose density gradient sedimentation (11), gel electrophoresis (12), or a combination of the two techniques. With these techniques, information can be gained about the size of the mRNA(s) responsible for expression of the protein and whether subunits encoded by different size mRNAs are required (e.g., 13–17). Also, size fractionation by sucrose density gradient centrifugation has been used to enrich for mRNAs encoding specific receptors and voltage-gated channels (9, 14–16, 76).

Sucrose Density Gradient Centrifugation of RNA

The apparatus is rinsed with 0.1 M NaOH, 95% ethanol, and water prior to use to remove RNases. A linear sucrose gradient [5–25% (w/v) sucrose, 2 mM EDTA, 0.2% lithium dodecyl sulfate, 10 mM HEPES, pH 7.3] is constructed using a gradient mixer and peristaltic pump. The RNA (a concentrated solution in water) is heated for 15 min in a 65°C water bath (to disrupt base pairing), rapidly cooled to room temperature by placing on ice, and applied just below the meniscus of the gradient and against the wall of the test tube with a sterile pipette tip. This tube is centrifuged in a swinging bucket rotor (SW41 or equivalent) at 34,000 rpm, 5°C for 16–20 hr. Fractions are collected (0.5 ml each) using the Beckman fraction recovery system, peristaltic pump, and fraction collector. The location of RNA in the gradient can be monitored as fractions are collected by passing the gradient through an absorbance monitor set to read A_{260}. The linearity of the gradient can be assessed by measuring the refractive index of each sample. The fractions obtained are precipitated at −20°C with 0.1 vol of 3 M sodium acetate, pH 5.0, and 2–3 vol of ice-cold anhydrous ethanol. The precipitate is dried in a Savant Speedvac Concentrator and dissolved in water. The precipitation is repeated several times to remove sucrose and detergent. The size range of each fraction can be assessed in several ways: (1) gel electrophoresis and visualization by ethidium bromide staining or hybridization to ^{32}P-labeled oligo(dT) followed by exposure to X-ray film; (2) including ^{32}P-labeled standards and measuring β-emission of each fraction. mRNA fractions obtained in this way can be injected into *Xenopus* oocytes alone or in combination.

In Vitro Synthesis of mRNA by Transcription of Cloned cDNAs

The *Xenopus* oocyte expression system has been employed in order to verify that cloned cDNAs encode the presumed protein, and to study the structure–function relationships for a receptor or channel by altering subunit composition, by expressing chimeric or construct cDNA(s), or by site-directed mutagenesis. The procedure for transcription is dependent on the vector used for the cDNA. In general, the plasmid is linearized or the phage is cut with a restriction endonuclease to allow unidirectional transcription from the correct promoter region. An RNA polymerase enzyme specific for the promoter in the construct is reacted with a mixture of nucleotides. Transcribed RNA thus obtained can be separated from DNA, free nucleotides, and protein by DNase I treatment followed by phenol–CHCl₃ extraction, then CHCl₃ extraction as for tissue RNA.

Several procedures have been employed in order to enhance expression of transcribed RNA in the oocytes. The most common of these procedures is capping, or addition of either a guanylate or 7-methylguanylate (m^7G) to the 5' end of the transcribed RNA. Either addition is thought to enhance translation of the RNA. Capping can be achieved by including the cap precursor GpppG in the transcription reaction to allow formation of a cap on the 5' end of the transcribed RNA. This procedure has been used to enhance *Xenopus* oocyte expression of gap junction protein (21), nicotinic ACh receptors (77–79), substance K receptors (18), β-adrenergic receptors (80), *Drosophila* K⁺ A channels (19), serotonin receptors (9), and GABA_A receptors (39). To increase expression of GABA_A receptor β subunits, Blair *et al.* (60) polyadenylated β subunit transcripts using *Escherichia coli* polyadenylate polymerase. It has been demonstrated that capping (81, 82) and polyadenylation (81) at the 3' end increase transcript stability following injection into the oocyte. Ebihara *et al.* (54) subcloned their cDNA into the RNA expression vector SP64T to yield a construct containing the cDNA between 5' and 3' noncoding regions of *Xenopus* β-globin. They found that the presence of the β-globin noncoding sequences substantially enhanced expression of gap junction protein in the oocytes. Frielle *et al.* (43) found that RNA transcribed from cDNA for a β-adrenergic receptor that had been truncated by removing a portion of the noncoding region gave increased expression in *Xenopus* oocytes compared to RNA corresponding to the original cDNA.

Preparation and Injection of Oocytes

Removal of Oocytes

An adult *Xenopus laevis* female (Carolina Biologicals, NC; Nasco Inc., Fort Atkinson, WI; or *Xenopus* I, Ann Arbor, MI) is anesthetized by immersion in a tricaine solution (1.5 g/liter) at room temperature for 20–30 min. Successful anesthesia is indicated by lack of response to an abdominal

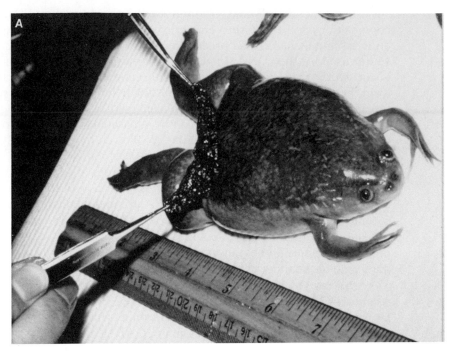

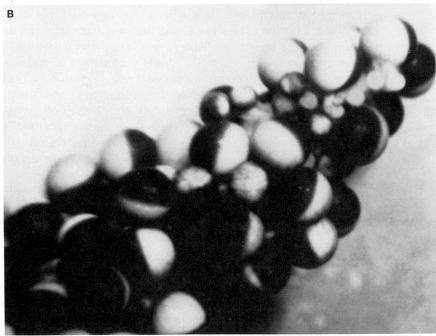

pinch. The anesthetized frog is placed dorsal side up on a wet platform and a small incision (0.5–1 cm) is made in the lower abdomen (Fig. 3A). An ovarian lobe (Fig. 3B) is pulled through the incision, sutured to prevent internal bleeding, and removed into Ca^{2+}-free ND96 (83) (96 mM NaCl, 2 mM KCl, 1 mM MgCl$_2$, 2.5 mM pyruvate, 5 mM HEPES, pH 7.6) at room temperature. The frog is sutured and returned to fresh water. Frogs may be reused and recuperate fully after several weeks.

Removal of Follicular Layer

It may be necessary to remove the follicular layer surrounding the oocyte because it contains receptors and ion channels that may interfere with assay of expressed receptors (25–27). In addition, follicular cells are coupled by gap junctions to the oocyte (24). Removal of the follicular layer may be performed by incubation in collagenase (Type 1A; Sigma, St Louis, MO) followed by manual removal of the partially degraded tissue.

The ovarian lobe is broken up into clumps of 10–20 oocytes, rinsed in Ca^{2+}-free ND96, transferred to a solution of collagenase (2 mg/ml) in Ca^{2+}-free ND96, and incubated at room temperature for 2 hr. The collagenase reaction is stopped by transfer of the oocytes to ND96 (containing 1.8 mM CaCl$_2$). The follicular layer is then removed manually under the dissecting microscope using No. 5 forceps. Oocytes selected should be stage V or VI (which are mature) (23), spherical, with intact membranes, and uniform in coloration within each pole.

Microinjection of Oocytes with RNA

Injection pipettes are constructed by pulling 10-μl glass micropipettes (Drummond Sci. Co., PA, or VWR Sci., PA) in a microelectrode puller to a tip of ~1 μm and, while under microscopic observation, breaking the tip against a glass slide to a diameter of 15 to 20 μm. The pipettes are sterilized by heating in a vacuum oven at 210°C for 2 hr. A small amount of mineral oil (0.5 cm) is injected into the back of a pipette with a sterile needle and syringe. The pipette is secured onto the plunger of a 10-μl micropipettor (Drummond or VWR), which is then dialed down until the oil emerges from the tip; air bubbles should be avoided. The micropipettor is attached to a micromanipulator. The RNA sample to be injected (in 1–5 μl of sterile H$_2$O) is placed on a Parafilm sheet and drawn into the injection needle under observation with a dissecting microscope. The oocytes are injected on a

FIG. 3 (A) Removal of oocytes from an anesthetized *Xenopus*. (B) An ovarian lobule with oocytes at various stages of maturation. The largest are ~1.2 mm in diameter. The animal hemispheres are pigmented with melanin. Capillaries can be seen on the vegetal surface of some cells. (Photographs provided by J. C. Gerhart.)

platform constructed by fixing fiberglass or plastic window screen into a plastic petri dish with silicone glue. The openings of the screen should be the right size to hold an oocyte in place (~1.2 mm square for mature oocytes). The platform should be sterilized by rinsing with 70% (v/v) ethanol and exposure to UV light for 2 hr. Oocytes in sterile ND96 are injected with the appropriate volume (up to 100 nl) and amount (up to 100 ng mRNA or 400 ng total RNA) by dialing down the micropipettor plunger. Movement of the oil/RNA solution interface should be observable. Following injection, the oocytes are incubated for 1 hr in ND 96, washed once with the medium, and transferred to diluted Leibovitz L-15 culture medium [0.7 strength (Sigma), 100 U penicillin, 1 μg/ml streptomycin, 5 mM HEPES, pH 7.6]. The oocytes are incubated at 16–20°C with daily transfer to fresh medium. Oocytes prepared and held in this way can survive for several weeks. Expression of proteins depends on many factors such as health of the donor frog, season of the year, temperature of incubation, and the particular protein. Thus, optimal length of incubation must be determined empirically.

Assay Procedure

An essential requirement for any translation system is a suitable assay for the expressed receptor or ion channel. The *Xenopus* oocyte is particularly amenable to voltage-clamp recording for measurement of expression of receptors and ion channels (Table I). In addition, single-channel recordings by patch clamp (following removal of the vitelline membrane, see below) have been used. Biochemical assays such as ^{125}I-labeled ligand or toxin binding (57, 84) or measurement of the levels of second messengers (43) have also been employed. Measurement of $^{45}Ca^{2+}$ efflux has been used for Ca^{2+}-mobilizing hormone receptors (85). Albino frogs produce oocytes without melanin, which are better for optical techniques. We have employed voltage-clamp recording for the measurement of expression of neurotransmitter receptors in *Xenopus* oocytes (Fig. 2). Clamping amplifiers with high current capacity are required, and settling time after voltage steps may be several milliseconds because of the large membrane capacity. Cells with resting potentials of −50 mV or more and input resistances greater than 0.5 MΩ are preferable. For drug application, the cells are placed in a low-volume (~0.1 ml) trough and perfused with amphibian Ringer's solution containing (mM): NaCl 116, KCl 2, $CaCl_2$ 1, buffered to pH 7.2 with 10 mM HEPES (Mg^{2+} is omitted to record large NMDA responses) (Fig. 4). All drugs are dissolved and applied in this medium. Cells are generally voltage-clamped at a holding potential of −60 mV with two beveled electrodes filled with 1 M KCl (1.0–2.0 MΩ). Pharmacologically active agents are bath-

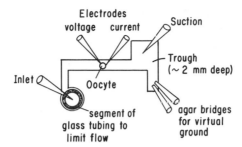

FIG. 4   A practical experimental setup for applying drugs to a voltage-clamped oocyte. The oocyte sits in a shallow trough and is penetrated by two microelectrodes. Fluid is applied in the short segment of tubing on the left that is sitting in the trough. Movement of the fluid is slowed by passing through the narrow space between the tubing and the floor of the trough. Fluid is removed by aspiration on the right. Agar bridges for the ground electrode minimize potential changes associated with changes in fluid composition.

applied with a dead time of <0.4 scc. Solutions are washed out within 2 sec as shown by visual inspection of dye application. Figure 2A and B illustrates typical responses evoked by neurotransmitters and drugs in oocytes injected with rat brain mRNA.

The vitelline membrane is usually left in place; it is permeable to drugs and protects the oocyte from turbulence during perfusion of the cells. For single-channel recording and for gap junction formation the vitelline membrane must be removed. Placing the cells in hypertonic saline (in mM: potassium aspartate 200, KCl 20, MgCl$_2$ 1, EGTA 10, HEPES 10, pH 7.4) for several minutes causes the oocyte to shrink away from the vitelline membrane which can then be removed with fine forceps (86).

Cloning Strategies Involving the Xenopus Oocyte Expression System

cDNAs encoding the bovine substance K receptor (18) and the 5-HT$_{1C}$ receptor (9) have been isolated using the *Xenopus* oocyte for expression. mRNAs are transcribed *in vitro* from pools of cDNA clones and the oocytes injected and evaluated for expression of the protein of interest. The RNA encoding the receptor may first be enriched by size fractionation and this enriched RNA used to construct a cDNA library in order to increase the proportion of clones encoding the receptor (9). In one approach, cDNA is cloned into a vector such as λZAP (Stratogene), in which the cDNA cloning site is bounded by promoters for the T3 and T7 RNA polymerases. A construct of this type allows for the efficient generation of transcripts from the cDNA library for injection into oocytes. If the transcribed library gives a positive result, subdivided mRNA pools (10 or more) are screened for receptor activity using the *Xenopus* oocyte. An active pool is progressively subdivided into smaller pools (sib selection) until a single positive clone is identified (9).

In the event that the receptor of interest is a multisubunit protein whose function requires expression of more than one mRNA, the procedure outlined above would have to be modified. In the course of sib selection, a point would be reached at which all subdivisions of an active pool would be negative. In this case the subdivisions would be recombined in various combinations until activity was regained. This procedure would lead to identification of two or more "necessary" pools. Subdivisions of one of these would be tested in combination with the other pools to identify an active subdivision, which would then be further subdivided until a single active clone was found.

Conceivably, the original necessary pool would encode more than one required subunit. In this case the recombination procedure would have to be repeated. Further subunits could be identified by the same selection method. Alternatively, there might be sufficient homology among subunits that others could be identified by hybridization at low stringency to the cDNA for the first subunit.

References

1. J. B. Gurdon, C. D. Lane, H. R. Woodland, and G. Marbaix, *Nature* (*London*) **233,** 177 (1971).
2. J. Ghysdael, E. Hubert, M. Travnicek, D. P. Bolognesi, A. Burney, Y. Cleuter, G. Huez, R. Kettman, G. Marbaix, D. Portetelle, and H. Chantrenne, *Proc. Natl. Acad. Sci. U.S.A.* **74,** 3230 (1977).
3. L. Gedamu, G. H. Dixon, and J. B. Gurdon, *Exp. Cell Res.* **117,** 325 (1978).
4. A. Colman, C. D. Lane, R. Craig, A. Boulton, T. Mohun, and J. Morser, *Eur. J. Biochem.* **113,** 339 (1981).
5. T. Lund, R. Bravo, H. R. Johansen, J. Zeuthen, and J. Vuust, *FEBS Lett.* **208,** 369 (1986).
6. K. Sumikawa, M. Houghton, J. S. Emtage, B. M. Richards, and E. A. Barnard, *Nature* (*London*) **292,** 862 (1981).
7. I. Parker, C. B. Gundersen, and R. Miledi, *Proc. R. Soc. London B* **226,** 263 (1985).
8. J. Lerma, L. Kushner, R. S. Zukin, and M. V. L. Bennett, unpublished observations (1988).
9. D. Julius, A. B. MacDermott, R. Axel, and T. M. Jessell, *Science* **241,** 558 (1988).

10. W. B. Thornhill and S. R. Levinson, *Biochemistry* **26,** 4381 (1987).
11. O. Mayehas and R. P. Perry, *Cell (Cambridge, Mass.)* **16,** 139 (1979).
12. S. Benoff and B. Nadal-Ginard, *Proc. Natl. Acad. Sci. U.S.A.* **76,** 1853 (1979).
13. H. Lübbert, T. P. Snutch, N. Dascal, H. A. Lester, and N. Davidson, *J. Neurosci.* **7,** 1159 (1987).
14. Y. Harada, T. Takahashi, M. Kuno, K. Nakayama, Y. Masu, and S. Nakanishi, *J. Neurosci.* **7,** 3265 (1987).
15. K. Sumikawa, I. Parker, and R. Miledi, *Proc. Natl. Acad. Sci. U.S.A.* **81,** 7994 (1984).
16. G. St. Laurent, O. Yoshie, G. Floyd-Smith, H. Samanta, and P. B. Sehgal, *Cell* **33,** 95 (1983).
17. T. M. Fong, N. Davidson, and H. A. Lester, *Synapse* **2,** 657 (1988).
18. Y. Masu, K. Nakayama, H. Tamaki, Y. Harada, M. Kuno, and S. Nakanishi, *Nature (London)* **329,** 836 (1987).
19. L. C. Timpe, T. L. Schwarz, B. L. Tempel, D. M. Papazian, Y. N. Jan, and L. Y. Jan, *Nature (London)* **331,** 143 (1988).
20. L. Millstein, P. Eversole-Cire, J. Blanco, and J. M. Gottesfeld, *J. Biol. Chem.* **262,** 17100 (1987).
21. G. Dahl, T. Miller, D. Paul, R. Voellmy, and R. Werner, *Science* **236,** 1290 (1987).
22. G. Spinelli and G. Ciliberto, *Nucleic Acids Res.* **13,** 8065 (1985).
23. J. N. Dumont, *J. Morphol.* **136,** 153 (1972).
24. C. L. Browne, H. S. Wiley, and J. N. Dumont, *Science* **203,** 182 (1979).
25. A. A. Smith, T. Brooker, and G. Brooker, *FASEB J.* **1,** 380 (1987).
26. T. M. Moriarty, B. Gillo, S. Sealfon, and E. M. Landau, *Mol. Brain Res.* **4,** 201 (1988).
27. N. Dascal, *CRC Crit. Rev. Biochem.* **22,** 317 (1987).
28. K. Kusano, R. Miledi, and J. Stinnakre, *J. Physiol. (London)* **328,** 143 (1982).
29. N. Dascal, E. M. Landau, and Y. Lass, *J. Physiol. (London)* **352,** 551 (1984).
30. J. K. Yisraeli and D. A. Melton, *Nature (London)* **336,** 592 (1988).
31. Y. Oron, B. Gillo, and M. C. Gershengorn, *Proc. Natl. Acad. Sci. U.S.A.* **85,** 3820 (1988).
32. J. Lerma, L. Kushner, R. S. Zukin, and M. V. L. Bennett, *J. Cell Biol.* **107,** 766a (1988).
33. L. Kushner, J. Lerma, R. S. Zukin, and M. V. L. Bennett, *Proc. Natl. Acad. Sci. U.S.A.* **85,** 3250 (1988).
34. J. Lerma, L. Kushner, D. C. Spray, M. V. L. Bennett, and R. S. Zukin, *Proc. Natl. Acad. Sci. U.S.A.* **86,** 1708 (1989).
35. J. Lerma, L. Kushner, R. S. Zukin, and M. V. L. Bennett, *Proc. Natl. Acad. Sci. U.S.A.* **86,** 2083 (1989).
36. C. B. Gundersen, R. Miledi, and I. Parker, *Proc. R. Soc. London B* **219,** 103 (1983).
37. T. Takahashi, E. Neher, and B. Sakmann, *Proc. Natl. Acad. Sci. U.S.A.* **84,** 5063 (1987).
38. E. A. Barnard, M. G. Darlison, and P. Seeburg, *Trends NeuroSci. (Pers. Ed.)* **10,** 502 (1987).

39. P. R. Schofield, M. G. Darlison, N. Fujita, D. R. Burt, F. A. Stephenson, H. Rodriguez, L. M. Rhee, J. Ramachandran, V. Reale, T. A. Glencorse, P. H. Seeburg, and E. A. Barnard, *Nature (London)* **328,** 221 (1987).

40. G. Grenningloh, A. Rienitz, B. Schmitt, C. Methfessel, M. Zensen, K. Beyreuther, E. D. Gundelfinger, and H. Betz, *Nature (London)* **328,** 215 (1987).

41. J. Nathans and D. S. Hogness, *Cell* **34,** 807 (1983).

42. H. G. Dohlman, M. G. Caron, and R. J. Lefkowitz, *Biochemistry* **26,** 2657 (1987).

43. T. Frielle, S. Collins, K. W. Daniel, M. G. Caron, R. J. Lefkowitz, and B. K. Kobilka, *Proc. Natl. Acad. Sci. U.S.A.* **84,** 7920 (1987).

44. T. I. Bonner, N. J. Buckley, A. C. Young, and M. R. Brann, *Science* **237,** 527 (1987).

45. T. Kubo, K. Fukuda, A. Mikami, A. Maeda, H. Takahashi, M. Mishina, T. Haga, K. Haga, A. Ichiyama, K. Kangawa, M. Kojima, H. Matsuo, T. Hirose, and S. Numa, *Nature (London)* **323,** 411 (1986).

46. J. R. Bunzow, H. H. M. Van Tol, D. K. Grandy, P. Albert, J. Salon, M. Christie, C. A. Machida, K. A. Neve, and O. Civelli, *Nature (London)* **336,** 783 (1988).

47. B. K. Kobilka, R. A. F. Dixon, T. Frielle, H. G. Dohlman, M. A. Bolanowski, I. S. Sigal, T. L. Yang-Feng, U. Francke, M. G. Caron, and R. J. Lefkowitz, *Proc. Natl. Acad. Sci. U.S.A.* **84,** 46 (1987).

48. W. A. Catterall, *Science* **242,** 50 (1988).

49. D. L. Paul, *J. Cell Biol.* **103,** 123 (1986).

50. B. J. Nicholson, R. Dermietzel, D. Teplow, O. Traub, K. Willecke, and J.-P. Revel, *Nature (London)* **329,** 732 (1987).

51. E. C. Beyer, D. L. Paul, and D. A. Goodenough, *J. Cell Biol.* **105,** 2621 (1987).

52. E. C. Beyer, D. A. Goodenough, and D. L. Paul, *in* "Gap Junctions" (E. L. Hertzberg and R. G. Johnson, eds.), p. 167. Liss, New York, 1988.

53. J. Kistler, D. Christie, and S. Bullivant, *Nature (London)* **331,** 721 (1988).

54. L. Ebihara, E. C. Beyer, K. I. Swenson, D. L. Paul, and D. A. Goodenough, *Science* **243,** 1194 (1989).

55. R. L. Gimlich, N. M. Kumar, and N. B. Gilula, *J. Cell Biol.* **107,** 1065 (1988).

56. E. L. Hertzberg and R. G. Johnson (eds.), "Gap Junctions." Liss, New York, 1988.

57. T. Takahashi, M. Kuno, M. Mishina, and S. Numa, *J. Physiol. (Paris)* **80,** 229 (1985).

58. R. J. Leonard, C. G. Labarca, P. Charnet, N. Davidson, and H. A. Lester, *Science* **242,** 1578 (1988).

59. K. Imoto, C. Busch, B. Sakmann, M. Mishina, T. Konno, J. Nakai, H. Bujo, Y. Mori, K. Fukuda, and S. Numa, *Nature (London)* **335,** 645 (1988).

60. L. A. C. Blair, E. S. Levitan, J. Marshall, V. E. Dionne, and E. A. Barnard, *Science* **242,** 577 (1988).

61. T. Frielle, K. W. Daniel, M. G. Caron, and R. J. Lefkowitz, *Proc. Natl. Acad. Sci. U.S.A.* **85,** 9494 (1988).

62. A. Kamb, L. E. Iverson, and M. A. Tanouye, *Cell* **50,** 405 (1987).

63. D. M. Papazian, T. L. Schwarz, B. L. Tempel, Y. N. Jan, and L. Y. Jan, *Science* **237,** 749 (1987).

64. B. L. Tempel, D. M. Papazian, T. L. Schwarz, Y. N. Jan, and L. Y. Jan, *Science* **237,** 770 (1987).

65. K. I. Swenson, J. R. Jordan, E. C. Beyer, and D. L. Paul, *Cell,* in press (1989).

66. H. Lübbert, B. J. Hoffman, T. P. Snutch, T. van Dyke, A. J. Levine, P. R. Hartig, H. A. Lester, and N. Davidson, *Proc. Natl. Acad. Sci. U.S.A.* **84,** 4332 (1987).

67. T. P. Snutch, J. P. Leonard, J. Nargeot, H. Lübbert, N. Davidson, and H. A. Lester, *Soc. Gen. Physiol. Ser.* **42,** 153 (1987).

68. R. E. Heuring and S. J. Peroutka, *J. Neurosci.* **7,** 894 (1987).

69. N. Dascal, I. Lotan, B. Gillo, H. A. Lester, and Y. Lass, *Proc. Natl. Acad. Sci. U.S.A.* **82,** 6001 (1985).

70. R. Miledi and I. Parker, *J. Physiol.* (*London*) **357,** 173 (1984).

71. P. M. Bingham and Z. Zachar, *Cell* (*Cambridge, Mass.*) **40,** 819 (1985).

72. A. Ullrich, J. Shine, J. Chirgwin, R. Pictet, E. Tischer, W. J. Rutter, and H. M. Goodman, *Science* **196,** 1313 (1977).

73. J. J. Chirgwin, A. E. Przbyla, R. J. MacDonald, and W. J. Rutter, *Biochemistry* **18,** 5294 (1979).

74. G. Brawerman, *Prog. Nucleic Acid Res. Mol. Biol.* **17,** 117 (1976).

75. H. Aviv and P. Leder, *Proc. Natl. Acad. Sci. U.S.A.* **69,** 1408 (1972).

76. A. L. Goldin, T. Snutch, H. Lübbert, A. Dowsett, J. Marshall, V. Auld, W. Downey, L. C. Fritz, H. A. Lester, R. Dunn, W. A. Catterall, and N. Davidson, *Proc. Natl. Acad. Sci. U.S.A.* **83,** 7503 (1986).

77. J. Boulter, J. Connolly, E. Deneris, D. Goldman, S. Heinemann, and J. Patrick, *Proc. Natl. Acad. Sci. U.S.A.* **84,** 7763 (1987).

78. K. Imoto, C. Methfessel, B. Sakmann, M. Mishina, Y. Mori, T. Konno, K. Fukuda, M. Kurasaki, H. Bujo, Y. Fujita, and S. Numa, *Nature* (*London*) **324,** 670 (1986).

79. K. Sumikawa and R. Miledi, *Proc. Natl. Acad. Sci. U.S.A.* **85,** 1302 (1988).

80. B. K. Kobilka, T. S. Kobilka, K. Daniel, J. W. Regan, M. G. Caron, and R. J. Lefkowitz, *Science* **240,** 1310 (1988).

81. D. R. Drummond, J. Armstrong, and A. Colman, *Nucleic Acids Res.* **13,** 7375 (1985).

82. Y. Furuichi, A. LaFiandra, and A. J. Shatkin, *Nature* (*London*) **266,** 235 (1977).

83. N. Dascal, T. P. Snutch, H. Lübbert, N. Davidson, and H. A. Lester, *Science* **231,** 1147 (1986).

84. M. Mishina, T. Tobimatsu, K. Imoto, K. Tanaka, Y. Fujita, K. Fukuda, M. Kurasaki, H. Takahashi, Y. Morimoto, T. Hirose, S. Inayama, T. Takahashi, M. Kuno, and S. Numa, *Nature* (*London*) **313,** 364 (1985).

85. J. A. Williams, D. J. McChesney, M. C. Calayag, V. R. Lingappa, and C. D. Logsdon, *Proc. Natl. Acad. Sci. U.S.A.* **85,** 4939 (1988).

86. C. Methfessel, V. Witzemann, T. Takahashi, M. Mishina, S. Numa, and B. Sakmann, *Pfluegers Arch.* **407,** 577 (1986).

[2] Expression of Neurotransmitter Receptors and Voltage-Activated Channels from Brain mRNA in *Xenopus* Oocytes

Katumi Sumikawa, Ian Parker, and Ricardo Miledi

The small size and inaccessibility of neurons in the brain greatly complicate the study of the neurotransmitter receptors and voltage-activated channels of the brain. A way around many of the difficulties encountered when studying these molecules in the brain cells has recently become available, with the finding that functional neurotransmitter receptors can be "transplanted" from the brain into the membrane of frog oocytes. This is done by injecting *Xenopus* oocytes with mRNA extracted from the brain. The mRNA is translated by the oocyte, and functional receptors and channels are inserted in the plasma membrane. Because of the large size of the oocyte (over 1 mm diameter), the receptor and channel molecules can then be studied by electrophysiological and biochemical techniques with much greater ease than is possible when they are present in their "native" neuronal cells (for reviews, see Refs. 1 and 2). Using this method, we have transplanted into oocytes most of the known receptors to neurotransmitters [acetylcholine (ACh), serotonin, γ-aminobutyric acid (GABA), glycine, glutamate, N-methyl-D-aspartate (NMDA), aspartate, noradrenaline, dopamine, β-alanine, etc.), as well as the voltage-operated channels (Na$^+$, K$^+$, Ca^{2+}, Cl$^-$). This chapter describes the use of *Xenopus* oocytes for the study of brain neurotransmitter receptors and ion channels.

Procedures used for the transplantation of neurontransmitter receptors and voltage-activated ion channels are shown diagrammatically in Fig. 1 and each stage is described in more detail below.

Extraction and Purification of mRNA

Extraction of Total RNA from the Brain

Extraction of total RNA is the most important step in the transplantation, because the quality of the mRNA dictates the type and number of neurotransmitter receptors and voltage-operated ion channels which are expressed in the oocyte membrane. Several techniques are available for

Methods in Neurosciences, Volume 1

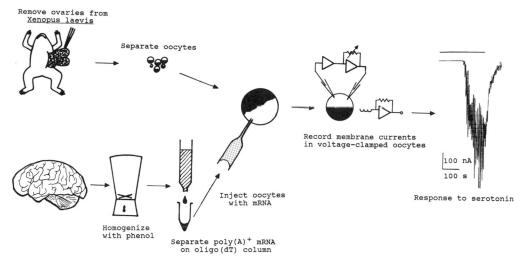

FIG. 1   Stages in the transplantation of receptors and channels from brain to oocyte.

isolating intact RNA from fresh and frozen tissues (3, 4). Among them, the guanidinium thiocyanate method (5) is the most widespread, because it is a more efficient protein denaturant (i.e., more efficient ribonuclease inactivator) than other denaturants. However, in our hands the RNA extracted from the brain with this method is generally less effective in expressing functional receptors and ion channels in the oocyte as compared with RNA extracted by the phenol–chloroform method. Therefore, we describe here a protocol for the extraction of RNA using phenol–chloroform as a protein denaturant and a means of separating the proteins from the nucleic acids, which consistently provides us with active mRNA coding for many brain neurotransmitter receptors and voltage-activated ion channels.

For safety, goggles and disposable plastic gloves should be worn during the following procedure. Disposable plastic gloves also protect RNA solutions from ribonucleases present on the skin. Always use sterile solutions, glassware, and plasticware. Water and all buffer solutions are sterilized by autoclaving for 1 hr. All glassware is baked for at least 4 hr at 250°C (or for at least 8 hr at 180°C). Plastic centrifuge tubes [Sepcor polypropylene centrifuge tubes with fluorocarbon O ring (Fisher, Pittsburgh, PA) or its equivalent] are placed in 1 N HCl overnight and rinsed thoroughly with distilled water and autoclaved for 0.5 hr. Individually wrapped, sterile disposable glass pipettes and sterile disposable tips for pipettors are used for handling solutions.

1. Place homogenizer probe (Polytron or its equivalent) in 0.1% (v/v)

diethyl pyrocarbonate (DPC; Sigma, St. Louis, MO) for 0.5 hr at room temperature and rinse thoroughly with autoclaved water.

2. Dissolve 100 g phenol [white loose crystals (Fisher, Mallinckrodt, Paris, KY; Baker, Phillipsburg, NJ)] in 11 ml of homogenization buffer [200 mM Tris-HCl, pH 9.0/50 mM NaCl/10 mM EDTA/0.5% (w/v) SDS] at 37°C just before use and add 0.11 g 8-hydroxyquinoline.

3. Pipette 10 ml of homogenization buffer into a sterile 50-ml cylinder (Pyrex). Add 0.01 g heparin (Sigma) and 10 ml phenol presaturated with homogenization buffer.

4. Place homogenizer probe into the 50-ml cylinder and start mixing the solution. Drop 1 g of brain tissue into the mixing solution and homogenize for 2–3 min at a setting of 5–6 at room temperature (for more RNA, 10 g of brain tissue can be processed with a 10-fold scale up).

5. Transfer homogenate into a 50-ml Sepcor centrifuge tube and shake vigorously for 5 min at room temperature.

6. Centrifuge in a swinging bucket rotor (Beckman JS 13.1 rotor or its equivalent) at 11,000 rpm for 10 min at about 15°C.

7. Use a glass pipette to remove the bottom phenol layer and discard this. Save the top layer and fluffy white material.

8. Add 10 ml chloroform and shake vigorously for 5 min at room temperature. Centrifuge as before.

9. Remove and discard the bottom chloroform layer. Save the top layer including the fluffy white material.

10. Repeat step 8.

11. If the fluffy white material is packed into a narrow band forming a small interface layer, collect upper aqueous layer (avoiding taking the interface layer) into a fresh 50-ml centrifuge tube (Sepcor) containing 10 ml phenol/chloroform (1:1). Shake vigorously for 5 min at room temperature.

If there is a large interface layer, remove the chloroform layer, and repeat step 8 before collecting the aqueous layer.

12. Centrifuge as before.

13. Remove upper aqueous layer, avoiding white interface material, and collect into a fresh 50-ml centrifuge tube (Sepcor) containing 10 ml phenol/chloroform (1:1). Shake hard for 5 min at room temperature and centrifuge as before.

14. Repeat step 13 until the interface is gone (generally 2–3 extractions).

15. Then collect the upper aqueous layer into a fresh 50-ml centrifuge tube (Sepcor) containing 10 ml chloroform. Shake hard and centrifuge as before.

16. Collect the upper aqueous layer, measuring its volume with a pipette, and transfer into a fresh 50-ml centrifuge tube (Sepcor) kept on an ice. Add 4 M NaCl solution to make a final concentration of 0.2 M (i.e., add 50 μl NaCl solution per milliliter collected), and then add 2.5 vol of cold (−20°C)

absolute ethanol. Allow the DNA and RNA to precipitate at −20°C for at least 2 hr or at −80°C for at least 0.5 hr (it is possible to leave the preparation indefinitely at this stage).

17. Centrifuge to collect DNA and RNA in a swinging bucket rotor (Beckman JS 13.1 or its equivalent) at 11,000 rpm for 30 min at 4°C.

18. Remove the ethanol supernatant as much as possible and discard. Dissolve the DNA and RNA pellet (it is not necessary to first dry the pellet) in 5 ml of cold 20 mM HEPES–NaOH, pH 7.5. With the solution on ice, slowly add 0.9 g of NaCl (use a baked spatula) to bring solution to 3 M. Leave overnight at −15°C or on ice. This step precipitates RNA, leaving most of the DNA in solution.

19. Centrifuge as in step 17 and discard the supernatant, saving the pellet. Wash the pellet with 10 ml of cold 3 M sodium acetate, pH 6.0. For this purpose, the pellet is first ground well with a baked glass rod, and then sodium acetate is added and vortexed.

20. Centrifuge as in step 17 for 5 min and discard the supernatant. Wash the pellet as in step 19.

21. Repeat step 20.

22. Centrifuge as in step 17 for 5 min and remove most of the supernatant. Wash the pellet with cold (−20°C) 75% ethanol as in step 19.

23. Repeat step 22.

24. Centrifuge as in step 17 for 5 min and discard supernatant. (If the RNA is not used immediately, store the RNA in 75% ethanol at −80°C.)

25. Dry the pellet in vacuum and dissolve the pellet (i.e., RNA) in 400 μl cold 20 mM HEPES–NaOH, pH 7.5. The concentration of RNA can be determined by measuring the OD$_{260}$ of a 10 μl RNA solution. An OD$_{260}$ of 1 corresponds to approximately 40 μg/ml RNA. About 1 mg of total RNA should be recovered. The OD$_{260}$/OD$_{280}$ ratio, which reflects the degree of contamination by protein and phenol, should be 2.0. The RNA solution can be stored in sterile microcentrifuge tubes at −80°C or used for isolation of poly(A)$^+$ mRNA as described below.

Purification of Poly(A)$^+$ mRNA by Chromatography on Oligo(dT)-Cellulose

To date, the great variety of receptors and channels expressed by brain mRNA in oocytes have all been induced by poly(A)$^+$ mRNA. A few preliminary experiments showed that oocytes injected with poly(A)$^-$ mRNA did not respond to the various neurotransmitters tested. Therefore, the next stage is the removal of unwanted RNA species from the poly(A)$^+$ mRNA.

All these manipulations are carried out at room temperature.

1. Autoclave a column (Econo-column 0.7 × 10 cm; Bio-Rad or its equivalent) and connect it to a UV monitor (Pharmacia or its equivalent) via autoclaved silicone tubing.

2. Suspend 0.2 g oligo(dT)-cellulose (Sigma or its equivalent) in autoclaved water and pour into the column.

3. Wash the column and all connecting system successively with
(a) 20 ml of 0.1 N NaOH,
(b) 20 ml of autoclaved water,
(c) 20 ml of 0.5 M KCl/5 mM HEPES–NaOH, pH 7.5.

4. Add an equal volume of 1 M KCl to the RNA solution to bring to 0.5 M KCl and slowly apply the RNA solution onto the column.

5. Collect the unbound RNA, which elutes, and reapply it to the column.

6. Wash the column with 0.5 M KCl/5 mM HEPES–NaOH, pH 7.5, until the OD_{260} returns to close to zero. The flow rate can be increased to save time.

7. Wash the column with 0.1 M KCl/5 mM HEPES–NaOH, pH 7.5, until the OD_{260} returns to close to zero.

8. Elute poly(A)$^+$ mRNA with warm (30–40°C) 5 mM HEPES–NaOH, pH 7.5, and collect the poly(A)$^+$ mRNA peak into a 15-ml sterile (baked), siliconized Corex tube on ice. The volume of the mRNA solution should be minimized to ensure good recovery of the mRNA in step 9.

9. Add 4 M NaCl to the mRNA solution to make to 0.2 M final concentration and precipitate the mRNA with 2.5 vol of absolute ethanol at −20°C overnight.

10. Collect the mRNA by centrifugation in a swinging bucket rotor (Beckman JS 13.1 or its equivalent) at 10,000 rpm for at least 0.5 hr at 4°C. Discard the supernatant and rinse the pellet (mRNA) carefully with 5 ml of cold (−20°C) 75% ethanol. Discard the ethanol. The mRNA can be stored in 75% ethanol at −80°C indefinitely, or it can be dried and dissolved in 50 μl of sterile water. The OD_{260} of a small sample should be measured to determine recovery. The yield of mRNA is normally 2–5% of the RNA applied to the column. The mRNA solution should be divided into small aliquots in sterile microcentrifuge tubes and stored at −80°C. Avoid repeated freezing and thawing of the mRNA solution.

Preparation and Injection of Oocytes

Preparation of Xenopus Oocytes for Microinjection

Female *Xenopus laevis* are obtained from commercial suppliers (e.g., Nasco Inc, Fort Atkinson, WI; *Xenopus* I, Ann Arbor, MI), and sacrificed by decapitation. Pieces of ovary are dissected out, and individual oocytes at

Dumont stages V and VI (6) are manually stripped from the ovary using watchmaker's forceps under a dissecting microscope. These oocytes are maintained in culture at 16°C, in Barth's solution [88 mM NaCl, 1 mM KCl, 2.4 mM NaHCO$_3$, 0.82 mM MgSO$_4$, 0.33 mM Ca(NO$_3$)$_2$, 0.41 mM CaCl$_2$, 7.5 mM Tris-HCl at pH 7.6] containing 50 units (U)/ml nystatin (Sigma) and 0.1 mg/ml gentamycin (Sigma). The dissected oocytes are cultured overnight and healthy oocytes are selected for injection. It is not advisable to use oocytes immediately after manual dissection, because some oocytes may be damaged. After incubation overnight the damaged oocytes can be easily identified. For more details, see Ref. 6.

Injection of mRNA into Xenopus Oocytes

This subject has been described in detail (6) and is mentioned only briefly here. *Xenopus* oocytes are injected with about 50 nl of poly(A)$^+$ mRNA solution (routinely 1 mg/ml), using hydraulic pressure ejection from a calibrated glass micropipette. Avoid injection into the pigmented region and do not allow the oocytes to dry out during injection. The RNA solution should be centrifuged briefly before use for injection. This helps remove particles which may otherwise be present in the RNA solution and might block the injection micropipette. The number of functional receptors or ion channels expressed in the plasma membrane of the oocyte varies with the amount of mRNA injected and, in the cases of voltage-activated sodium channel and kainate receptor (7), is directly proportional to the amount of mRNA injected over a large range. However, the expression of some other types of receptors varies nonlinearly with the amount of mRNA injected (M. Carpenter, unpublished observations), so it is advisable to determine empirically the optimal amount of mRNA to be injected for any particular receptor or ion channel of interest.

After injection, the oocytes are cultured at 16°C in sterile Barth's solution. Culturing at 16°C, instead of 18–21°C (normal incubation temperature), the oocytes survive for longer periods (some oocytes survived for >2 months). Before doing detailed electrophysiological experiments on oocytes injected with mRNA, it is necessary to assess the time course of expression of receptor interested in oocyte's membrane. This is because different receptor proteins and/or the corresponding mRNAs have different stabilities in the oocytes (Table I). We usually examine the oocytes 2 to 7 days after injection.

Preparation of Oocytes for Recording

Electrophysiological recordings may be made from intact follicular oocytes as they are obtained from the ovary, i.e., the oocyte proper, surrounded by

TABLE I   Time-Dependent Expression of GABA and
Kainate Receptors in Oocytes[a]

Receptor	Current (nA)	
	3–5 days after injection	11–15 days after injection
GABA	634 ± 136 ($n = 8$)	192 ± 112 ($n = 4$)
Kainate	284 ± 58 ($n = 8$)	853 ± 165 ($n = 4$)

[a] Data are given as means $\pm$ SEM. Oocytes were injected with chick brain mRNA and were tested with GABA (1 mM) and kainate (0.1 mM).

enveloping follicular, epithelial, and other layers. However, the presence of additional layers makes the oocytes more difficult to penetrate with microelectrodes. Furthermore, the follicular cells are electrically coupled to the oocyte, and possess a variety of neurotransmitter receptors (8, 9), which may complicate recordings. It is often helpful, therefore, to treat oocytes with collagenase so as to remove the follicular and other cell layers before recording (10).

A few tens of oocytes are placed in small vials containing 0.5–1 mg collagenase (type 1, Sigma) dissolved in 1 ml of Ringer's solution (composition in mM; NaCl, 120; KCl, 2; CaCl$_2$, 1.8; HEPES, 5, at pH about 7.0). The vials are gently rotated for about 1 hr at room temperature, and the oocytes are then washed with several changes of Ringer's solution. Gentle shaking will often detach the enveloping cell layers, producing ghosts, which can readily be seen by eye. If the envelopes do not detach with shaking, they can be peeled off using fine forceps under a dissecting microscope. Prolonged treatment with collagenase at higher concentrations removes or destroys some of the induced channels and receptors in the oocyte membrane.

Shortly after collagenase treatment, the oocytes have low resting potential and input resistance. Thus, treatment is best done a day or more before recording starts, and the oocytes are returned to culture in Barth's medium in the meantime. We normally treat oocytes with collagenase about 2 days after they have been injected with mRNA, but it is also possible to treat the oocytes prior to injection. After they recover from the collagenase treatment, the oocytes have a higher resting potential (around −100 mV), a higher input resistance (1 MΩ or more), and a reduced capacitance.

It is also possible, though more laborious, to remove the follicular cells mechanically without the use of collagenase. The first step is to "pop out" the oocytes from their epithelia when removing them from the ovary. The oocytes are then rolled over the surface of a polylysine-coated microscope slide, in the bottom of a dish filled with Ringer's solution (9). The follicular cells stick tightly to the slide, and detach, forming a ribbon which is visible by eye.

Electrophysiological Recording from mRNA-Injected Oocytes

Recordings of membrane currents in mRNA-injected oocytes provide a highly sensitive and selective assay for the expression of ion channels gated by voltage or ligands, and allow the functional properties of the channels to be explored. Voltage clamping of the oocyte using a two-electrode clamp is the most simple and straightforward technique, and the following sections describe our methods in detail. The sensitivity of the oocyte expression and recording system is so high that it is possible to detect the translation of just a few copies of a particular message. For example, the limit of resolution with the voltage clamp is about 1 nA, so that it is possible to detect the opening of less than 1000 channel molecules, if the current passing through each is 1 pA or more.

An alternative approach is to use patch-clamp techniques to record from single channels. This allows a more detailed characterization of single-channel properties, but is not so useful for assaying the ability of mRNA preparations to induce particular receptors of channels. The application of patch-clamp recording to the oocyte is described in Ref. 11.

Several recent reviews (1, 2) deal with the types of electrical responses which may be induced in the oocyte by foreign mRNA, and with those receptors and channels which are native to the oocyte.

Voltage-Clamp System

Oocytes are clamped using a conventional two-electrode clamp, in which one electrode serves to monitor the membrane potential, while the other is used to inject current so as to maintain the potential at any desired value.

Both electrodes are made from standard glass micropipettes, pulled from glass capillary tubing including an internal filament (World Precision Instruments, New Haven, CT; A-M Systems, Everett, WA; and many other suppliers) for ease of filling. The voltage recording pipette is filled with 3 M KCl, and the current electrode with 3 M potassium acetate or KCl (potassium acetate is better if large outward currents are to be clamped). An important point is that both electrodes must be of low resistance, a few megaohms or less. This can be achieved by gently breaking the tips of the pipettes against the base of the recording chamber, or against each other, while monitoring the resistance. In the case of the recording pipette, a low resistance minimizes the noise introduced into the clamp. For the current electrode, a low resistance is needed so that large currents may be injected into the oocyte. Currents of tens of microamperes are sometimes required to charge rapidly the membrane capacitance when stepping the membrane potential to activate voltage-gated channels, and similarly large ligand-gated currents may be induced by potent mRNA preparations. In practice, the tip size of the pipettes is a matter of compromise; the electrical properties of the pipettes improve with increasing size, but more damage is done to the oocyte on impalement. Some donors yield oocytes which can withstand the use of large pipettes, while other oocytes may be very fragile.

The voltage-clamp circuit must be able to produce quite large ($>10\ \mu$A) output currents. Some commercial designs use a series resistor in the current path, which may produce an unacceptable limitation in maximum current. We use a homemade design (Fig. 2), in which the output is driven by a high-voltage op-amp, to allow greater currents to be injected through an electrode of given resistance.

The clamp current is monitored through a virtual ground circuit, connected to the fluid in the recording chamber. It is helpful to use two switched feedback resistors in this circuit, with values of 100 KΩ and 1MΩ. The higher value gives a higher recording gain (1 mV per nanoampere) for use when examining small currents, while the lower value avoids overload during large responses or capacitative spikes. A range of switched capacitors across the feedback resistors provide a simple low pass filter, with cut-off frequencies between 100 Hz and 5 KHz.

Chlorided silver wires establish electrical contact with the micropipettes, and with the fluid in the recording chamber. The bath electrodes are connected via glass tubes filled with agar in Ringer solution, so that the ionic composition of the bathing solution may be changed without altering the junction potential of the electrodes. Separate electrodes, and agar brides, are used to connect the current monitor and the indifferent side of the voltage recording amplifier to the bath, since a common electrode may introduce errors in measurement of the potential when large currents are clamped.

The function of the current-passing electrode is controlled by a reed switch, mounted in a head-stage close to the electrode. This allows the electrode to be connected either to the clamp output, or to a voltage-recording amplifier. It is convenient to monitor the potential while inserting the electrode into the oocyte, and after insertion of both electrodes the clamp can be activated by switching the electrode to the current-passing mode.

Immediately after inserting the microelectrodes, the resting potential and

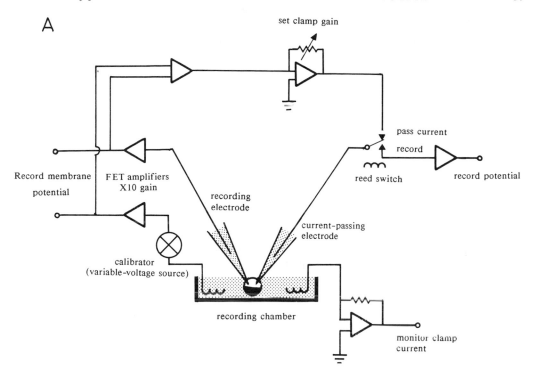

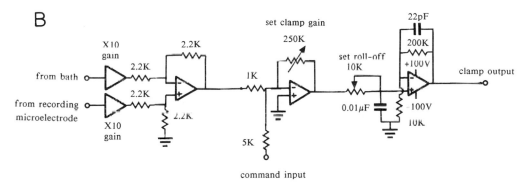

FIG. 2   Two-electrode voltage clamp for recording membrane currents in oocytes. (A) Schematic of complete clamp system. (B) Circuit diagram of high-voltage clamp. The output op-amp is type 3582J (Burr-Brown), and other op-amps are type OF 720 (Computing Techniques), or equivalent high-quality FET op-amps.

input resistance of the oocyte are usually low, and spontaneous oscillations in membrane current may be evoked. Allowing the oocyte to recover for a few minutes will often give an improvement in potential and a more stable baseline.

Recording Chamber

Recordings are made while the oocyte is continuously superfused with frog Ringer's solution in a small (0.5 ml or less) plexiglass chamber. Solution flows into the chamber by gravity from a reservoir placed on a shelf about 50 cm above the chamber. An inverted U tube of glass is connected to the inflow of the chamber by a length of silicone rubber tubing containing the perfusate, and the end of the U tube dipped into a beaker or flask. Air is first removed from the tube, and the solution then flows continuously by siphon action, at a rate which is adjusted by a clamp on the rubber tube. Changes in the perfusate are made by pinching the rubber tube (to stop the introduction of air bubbles), and transferring the U tube to a different flask. For most purposes, this extremely simple system works well, and its only major disadvantage is the dead time of several seconds introduced by the column of fluid in the tubing.

Solution is removed from the chamber through an outflow pipe, which is connected to a vacuum line (or water pump) via a series of two side-arm flasks. The flasks serve as a reservoir to collect the fluid, and as an air gap to electrically isolate the fluid in the recording chamber from ground. The second flask serves as a backup in case the first accidentally overflows, and increases the electrical isolation. A flask with a capacity of 2 liters is sufficient to allow several hours recording without emptying. Some care is needed in selecting the type of tubing used to connect the chamber outflow to the side-arm flask, since many tubes (especially silicone rubber) produce electrical artifacts in the current monitor circuit when fluid and air bubbles pass along the tube. The length of both the inflow and exit tubes should be kept as short as is convenient, and they should be arranged to minimize vibration or movement, as this can introduce electrical artifacts.

Since the oocyte is spherical, it must be held in position in the chamber. We use either of two methods to do this. In the first, the oocyte is placed in a conical hole (~1 mm diameter) in a small stainless steel disk (the egg cup) placed on the floor of the chamber. The second method involves forming a ring of petroleum jelly (Vaseline) on the chamber floor, to make a central depression into which the oocyte fits. This is done by extruding Vaseline through a hypodermic syringe using a blunted needle. In both cases, the oocyte is dropped into place in the chamber, after transfering it with a Pasteur pipette.

A dissecting microscope with a magnification of ×10 to ×40 gives adequate visibility to position and insert the microelctrodes. The oocyte is illuminated from above by a microscope lamp or fiber optic illuminator. Because of the large size of the oocyte, almost any type micromanipulator is adequate to position the electrodes, and it is unnecessary to take great precautions to isolate the recording system from vibrations.

Microinjection into Oocyte While Recording

In some experiments it is convenient to be able to inject substances into the oocyte while recording; for example, EGTA may be injected to block the oscillatory chloride currents mediated by several neurotransmitters (12), or calcium may be injected to activate chloride channels (10). Electrically charged molecules and ions may be injected by iontophoresis, but it is generally preferable to use pressure ejection. A micropipette is filled with the solution to be injected and, if sufficient quantities are available, this should be passed through a 0.22-μm Millipore filter to remove particles which might block the pipette. The micropipette is then mounted in the recording setup, and connected to a device which can apply brief (10–1000 msec) pneumatic pulses of variable (0–200 KPa) pressure. Commercial instruments are available for this purpose (e.g., Picopump, World Precision Instruments, New Haven, CT), or they can be easily made from a solenoid valve and a pressure regulator. As pulled, the micropipettes are too fine to eject fluid, and the tip should be gently broken to a diameter of a few micrometers. The ability of the pipette to eject fluid can be monitored by applying pneumatic pulses with the tip raised into the air. With newly made pipettes the expelled fluid usually runs up the side of the pipette, making quantitation difficult. However, after a pipette has been inserted in an oocyte, pneumatic pulses applied with the pipette in the air usually produce a discrete droplet of fluid at the tip. The diameter of the droplet can be measured by a calibrated micrometer in the microscope eyepiece, and used to estimate the volume. It is convenient, for this purpose, to draw a calibration curve on double-log axes, of droplet diameter versus volume.

Insertion of the injection pipette into an oocyte can be monitored by recording membrane current while clamping at a potential of −60 mV. The injection pipette is gradually advanced toward the oocyte, and its penetration is signaled by a rapid, transient inward deflection at the current trace. We sometimes also monitor insertion of the recording pipette by recording the potential from this pipette.

Volumes of a few nanoliters may be safely injected without causing damage. However, it is important to avoid contamination by calcium in the injection solution, since concentrations of only a few picomolar are sufficient to activate chloride currents. Thus, the solution for injection should usually include about 50 μM EDTA, to chelate any contaminating calcium. Furthermore, a few pressure pulses are applied just before inserting the pipette, to flush out fluid in the tip of the pipette which becomes contaminated by calcium from the bathing solution.

Other Applications

Use of Size-Fractionated mRNA

The use of fractionated rather than whole poly(A)$^+$ mRNA offers many important advantages for the study of receptors and ion channels expressed in the oocyte (13). For instance, specific mRNAs are more concentrated, so that larger responses are obtained. More importantly, by injecting the appropriate fraction, it becomes possible to incorporate only a desired receptor or ion channel type. For example, if one wants to study the characteristics of Na$^+$ and K$^+$ channels in the brain, it is normally necessary to use pharmacological agents to block one type of channel. However, this is not necessary in oocytes because the Na$^+$ and K$^+$ channel mRNAs can be separated, and injected into the oocytes to express only one type of channel (13). Another example is that the two mRNA species coding for glutamate receptors can be separated and used to characterize the two glutamate receptor subtypes encoded (13). A further advantage of fractionation is that it may disclose heterogeneity among mRNAs encoding a particular receptor (14). The mRNA size fractionation is also useful to examine the presence of other mRNA species with different sizes encoding a second subunit or a factor, such as an enzymatic activity that modulates the properties of the channels (15, 16).

Partial purification of mRNA can be achieved either by sucrose density gradient centrifugation (13) or by gel electrophoresis (4, 17). However, we usually found that the mRNAs fractionated by agarose gel electrophoresis do not translate well in *Xenopus* oocyte. An important advantage of sucrose gradient centrifugation is that fractionated mRNA can be recovered easily and efficiently and is still translationally active. However, the resolving power of this technique is much less than that of gel electrophoresis. We describe here the procedure for partial purification of mRNA by sucrose gradient centrifugation. For further purification of mRNA by gel electrophoresis, see Ref. 17.

1. Treat centrifuge tubes for the Beckman SW 40 Ti (or its equivalent) and

gradient maker with 0.2% (v/v) DPC overnight, and rinse thoroughly with autoclaved water before use.

2. Prepare 10% (w/w) and 31% (w/w) sucrose solutions in 10 mM HEPES–NaOH, pH 7.5/1 mM EDTA/0.1% (w/v) lithium dodecyl sulfate and treat with 0.05% (v/v) DPC overnight. Autoclave the DPC-treated sucrose solutions for 15 min. Autoclaving can ensure complete removal of DPC.

3. Make 10–31% linear sucrose gradients in centrifuge tubes and keep on ice for 30 min. The gradients may be prepared with a gradient maker or using frozen step gradients by the method of Luthe (18). [The latter method is easier, reproducible, and provides equally good fractionation (M. M. Panicker and A. Morales, unpublished results).]

4. Heat the poly(A)$^+$ mRNA solution (100–200 μg in 100–200 μl of 5 mM HEPES-NaOH, pH 7.5) at 65°C for 5 min, cool on ice, and load onto the sucrose gradient.

5. Centrifuge immediately for 19 hr at 2°C on a Beckman SW 40 Ti rotor at 39,000 rpm.

6. Collect fractions (about 0.4 ml) in sterile microcentrifuge tubes. Add 20 μl of 4 M NaCl and 2.5 vol of cold (−20°C) absolute ethanol. Allow the mRNA to precipitate at −20°C overnight.

7. Centrifuge in a swinging bucket rotor (Beckman JS 13.1 or its equivalent) at 11,000 rpm for 1 hr at 2°C. Discard supernatant and rinse the RNA pellets twice with 1 ml of cold (−20°C) 75% ethanol.

8. Dry the RNA pellets in vacuum and dissolve in 10–20 μl of autoclaved water. Store at −80°C until used for injection.

Use of Antisense RNAs and Oligonucleotides

Gene expression in various cells, including *Xenopus* oocytes and mammalian cells, can be selectively inhibited by antisense RNA (RNA that is complementary to mRNA) (for a review, see Ref. 19). This inhibition sometimes involves hybridization between an antisense RNA and its counterpart mRNA, which results in an inhibition of mRNA translation (20). Synthetic oligonucleotides, which are complementary to mRNA, can also be used to inhibit translation of corresponding mRNA. Complementary oligonucleotides appears to promote target mRNA degradation by an RNase H-like activity (21, 22). Since many receptor and ion-channel cDNAs have been isolated and their mRNA sequences are available, antisense RNA and complementary oligonucleotides to a particular receptor or ion-channel mRNA can be synthesized. These molecules can be injected into oocytes together with total brain mRNA to block the translation of complementary mRNA. This approach is useful to examine receptor or ion-channel heterogeneity, blocking expression of one receptor (or ion channel) subtype with a specific oligonucleotide and studying another subtype encoded by a similar, but not identical, mRNA. Use of antisense RNA and complementary oligonucleotides to inhibit the expression of functional receptors in *Xenopus* oocytes has been described (23) and, therefore, will be only briefly summarized here. For more details, see Refs. 23 and 24.

1. Synthesize antisense RNA or complementary oligonucleotide (20-mers work well). For a detailed procedure for the synthesis of antisense RNA, see Refs. 23 and 25. Custom syntheses of oligonucleotides of specific sequences are now readily available from commercial sources.

2. To ensure absence of ribonuclease activity, extract the antisense RNA or complementary oligonucleotide solution with an equal volume of phenol/chloroform (1:1) in a microcentrifuge tube. Centrifuge briefly and collect the upper aqueous solution into a siliconized, sterile microcentrifuge tube. Add 4 M NaCl solution to a final concentration of 0.2 M and precipitate the antisense RNA, or complementary oligonucleotide, with 2.5 vol of absolute ethanol overnight at $-20°C$.

3. Centrifuge in a swinging bucket rotor (Beckman JS 13.1 or its equivalent) at 11,000 rpm for 1 hr at 4°C. Discard supernatant and rinse the pellet carefully with 1 ml of cold ($-20°C$) 75% ethanol. Dry the pellet under vacuum and dissolve in a small volume of sterile water.

4. Measure the absorbance of a diluted sample at 260 nm to estimate the concentration of antisense RNA, or complementary oligonucleotide. An OD_{260} of 1 corresponds to approximately 20 μg oligonucleotide/ml. Adjust concentration of 1 μg/μl and store at $-80°C$ until use.

5. For injection into oocytes, mix 1 μl of mRNA solution (2 mg/ml) with 0.1–1 μg of antisense RNA, or complementary oligonucleotide, in 1 μl of water on a sterile tissue culture dish (35 × 10 mm; Falcon) on ice. Since overinjection of these molecules results in nonspecific inhibition of expression of all receptors and ion channels, an optimal concentration for each antisense molecule must be determined. Five to fifty nanograms per oocyte is a good concentration to try first.

6. The above mixture can then be injected into oocytes to study the effect of antisense RNA or complementary oligonucleotide on the expression of functional receptors or ion channels.

Acknowledgments

Work in the authors' laboratories is supported by grants NS 23284, GM 39831, and NS 25928 from the U.S. Public Health Services.

References

1. N. Dascal, *CRC Crit. Rev. Biochem.* **22,** 317 (1987).
2. R. Miledi, L. Parker, and K. Sumikawa, *in* "Fidia Award Lecture Series" (J. Smith, ed.). Raven, New York, 1989.
3. M. J. Clemens, *in* "Transcription and Translation: A Practical Approach" (B. D. Hames and S. J. Higgins, eds.), p. 211. IRL Press, Oxford, 1984.
4. T. Maniatis, E. F. Fritsch, and J. Sambrook, "Molecular Cloning: A Laboratory Manual." Cold Spring Harbor Laboratory, Cold Spring Harbor, New York, 1982.
5. R. J. MacDonald, G. H. Swift, A. E. Przybyla, and J. M. Chirgwin, *in* "Methods in Enzymology" (S. L. Berger and A. R. Kimmel, eds.), Vol. 152, p. 219. Academic Press, Orlando, Florida, 1987.
6. A. Colman, *in* "Transcription and Translation: A Practical Approach" (B. D. Hames and S. J. Higgins, eds.), p. 271. IRL Press, Oxford, 1984.
7. K. Sumikawa, I. Parker, and R. Miledi, *Prog. Zool.* **33,** 127 (1986).
8. R. M. Woodward and R. Miledi, *Proc. Natl. Acad. Sci. U.S.A.* **84,** 4135 (1987).
9. R. Miledi and R. M. Woodward, *J. Physiol.* (*London*) in press (1989).
10. R. Miledi and I. Parker, *J. Physiol.* (*London*) **357,** 173 (1984).
11. C. Methfessel, V. Witzeman, T. Takahashi, M. Mishina, S. Numa, and B. Sakmann, *Pfluegers Arch.* **407,** 577 (1986).
12. I. Parker, C. B. Gundersen, and R. Miledi, *Neurosci. Res.* **2,** 491 (1985).
13. K. Sumikawa, I. Parker, and R. Miledi, *Proc. Natl. Acad. Sci. U.S.A.* **81,** 7994 (1984).
14. H. Akagi and R. Miledi, *Science* **242,** 270 (1988).
15. B. Rudy, J. H. Hoger, H. A. Lester, and N. Davidson, *Neuron* **1,** 649 (1988).
16. V. J. Auld, A. L. Goldin, D. S. Krafte, J. Marshall, J. M. Dunn, W. A. Caterall, H. A. Lester, N. Davidson, and R. J. Dunn, *Neuron* **1,** 449 (1988).
17. H. Lübbert, T. P. Snutch, N. Dascal, H. A. Lester, and N. Davidson, *J. Neurosci.* **4,** 1159 (1987).
18. D. S. Luthe, *Anal. Biochem.* **135,** 230 (1983).
19. P. J. Green, O. Pines, and M. Inouye, *Annu. Rev. Biochem.* **55,** 569 (1986).
20. D. Melton, *Proc. Natl. Acad. Sci. U.S.A.* **82,** 144 (1985).
21. P. Dash, I. Lotan, M. Knapp, E. R. Kandel, and P. Goelet, *Proc. Natl. Acad. Sci. U.S.A.* **84,** 7896 (1987).
22. J. Shuttleworth and A. Colman, *EMBO J.* **7,** 427 (1988).
23. K. Sumikawa and R. Miledi, *Proc. Natl. Acad. Sci. U.S.A.* **85,** 1302 (1988).
24. H. Akagi, D. Patton, and R. Miledi, *Proc. Natl. Acad. Sci. U.S.A.,* in press (1989).
25. D. A. Melton, *in* "Methods in Enzymology" (S. L. Berger and A. R. Kimmel, eds.), Vol. 152, p. 288. Academic Press, Orlando, Florida, 1987.

[3] Expression of Mammalian Plasma Membrane Receptors in *Xenopus* Oocytes: Studies of Thyrotropin-Releasing Hormone Action

Richard E. Straub, Yoram Oron, and Marvin C. Gershengorn

Introduction

Oocytes from the African frog *Xenopus laevis* have become a widely used and important tool in the study of mammalian receptors, ion channels, and transporters (for reviews, see Refs. 1–6). Microinjection of exogenous messenger RNA from a variety of sources, including tissues, cell lines, and *in vitro* transcriptions, leads to production of new proteins. *Xenopus* oocytes will then with high fidelity modify, process, sort, and assemble even multisubunit membrane proteins. Acquired receptors retain many of their native functional characteristics, including ligand binding, agonist rank order and efficacy, desensitization, and signal pathway identity. For example, oocytes injected with messenger RNA coding for adrenergic receptor chimeras were employed to delineate the functional domains involved in ligand-binding specificity and effector coupling of adrenergic receptors (7). Messenger RNA coding for mutant LDL receptors was injected into oocytes and receptor-mediated endocytosis was studied directly in the oocyte (8). Oocytes have also been used as a bioassay for mRNA activity when probes were unavailable (9, 10). Recently, *Xenopus* oocytes have been used as the primary tool in the expression cloning of cDNA coding for proteins for which there was no sequence information or antibodies available. These include interleukin 4 (11), the lymphocyte IgE receptor (12), substance K receptor (13), Na^+/glucose transporter (14), and the serotonin 1c receptor (15, 16). Here we describe the methods we have used and the results obtained in characterizing the thyrotropin-releasing hormone (TRH) receptor expressed in oocytes and in the use of the oocyte as a bioassay of receptor messenger RNA activity.

Methods in Neurosciences, Volume 1

Methods

A number of articles on the methods for microinjection of *Xenopus* oocytes have been published (1, 17–21). The methods described below were developed in collaboration with Dr. Boaz Gillo.

Purchase and Maintenance of Xenopus laevis

We purchase oocyte-positive females, HCG tested for functioning ovaries, from Nasco (Fort Atkinson, WI, cat. no. IM535MV). The frogs are kept in tanks of tap water which have been allowed to stand for 24 hr to allow chlorine to evaporate. Optimum water temperature is 18–20°C. Tanks should be filled with water, 2–3 liters per frog, to a height of 15–20 cm to allow the frogs to come to the surface easily to breathe. Securely fastened, ventilated soft plastic covers keep the frogs from escaping or damaging themselves. A fixed 12-hr light–dark cycle is maintained, with light from 9 AM to 9 PM. Each frog receives 2 g of Nasco frog brittle (cat. no. SA 5961IMMV) twice a week, and the water is changed a few hours after feeding and whenever it becomes cloudy. Frogs are transferred using a large aquarium net. We maintain a sufficient number of frogs to permit a given frog to recover for at least 10 weeks after surgery before reuse.

Removal and Preparation of Oocytes

Preparation

Surgery and subsequent manipulations of the oocytes are done under sterile conditions, using a hood, filtered solutions, sterile 2-ml plastic pipettes, and ethanol-treated and flamed dissection instruments. The instruments needed are two pairs of fine forceps, one pair of blunt forceps, scissors, scalpel, and surgical needle. Also required are filter-sterilized OR-2, OR-2E (see Table I), distilled water, and OR-2 without Ca^{2+}. Make 15 ml of 2 mg/ml collagenase [type Ia, Sigma (St. Louis, MO), cat. no. C-9891] in OR-2 without Ca^{2+} and filter sterilize.

Anesthesia

Place the frog in 500 ml of dechlorinated tap water containing 0.2% of MS-222 [3-aminobenzoic acid ethyl ester, methane sulfonate salt (Sigma, cat. no. A5040)]. Wear gloves, as this compound is a potential carcinogen. Wait 20 min and check for responsiveness. If the frog responds to touch, continue to observe at 10-min intervals until fully anesthetized, but no longer than 50 min overall.

TABLE I   Composition of OR-2 Solutions

OR-2 (pH 7.5)		OR-2E (pH 7.5)	
NaCl	82 mM	OR-2 plus:	
KCl	2.5 mM	Sodium pyruvate	2.5 mM
NaOH	3.8 mM	Na_2HPO_4	0.5 mM
Na_2HPO_4	1 mM	Theophylline	0.5 mM
$CaCl_2$	2 mM		
$MgCl_2$	1 mM		

Surgery

Place the frog on its back on a wet laboratory pad in the hood, and wet the abdomen with sterile water. Prevent the skin from drying out during surgery. With an alcohol pad, swab a small area just above the leg to the left or right of the midline. Lift the skin with forceps and make a 1-cm incision through both skin and body wall with the scalpel. Using blunt forceps, gently tease out a section of ovary containing clumps of oocytes and, using a scalpel, separate it from the remaining ovarian tissue. Place the clumps of oocytes into sterile OR-2 without Ca^{2+}. Continue until a sufficient number of oocytes has been removed. Push any remaining tissue back into the abdominal opening and sew the incision with a silk cutting needle [Ethicon (Somerville, NJ) cat. no. 681H] held in forceps, performing 2–3 stitches of three knots each. During recovery from the anesthetic, place the frog in shallow tap water for a few hours, with her head out of water. After recovery, the frog is placed in its own tank marked with the date of surgery for 1 month before being returned to the communal tank.

Collagenase Treatment (Defolliculation)

With forceps, gently separate the oocytes into clumps of about 5 cm in diameter. Wash each clump three times by immersion and swirling in fresh OR-2 without Ca^{2+}. Place the clumps in two sterile 15-ml conical flasks, each containing 6 ml of filter-sterilized collagenase solution, and incubate with constant rolling or gentle agitation for 2–3 hr at 20°C, changing the collagenase solution after 1 hr. After the oocytes have completely separated, wash three times with OR-2 and transfer into a 100-mm petri dish containing OR-2. Under a low-power microscope, using a 2-ml plastic pipette, select and remove to another dish containing OR-2E the largest undamaged oocytes which have the most distinct hemispheric coloration, i.e., a pale yellow vegetal hemisphere and a dark brown or black animal hemisphere. Avoid small, irregular, or mottled oocytes and oocytes with remaining attached cells or blood vessels. Allow at least 1 hr in OR-2E at 20°C before injection. One advantage of allowing overnight equilibration in OR-2E before injection is that it allows unhealthy oocytes to die and then be excluded from the experiment.

Injections

Preparation of RNA

Cytosolic and poly(A)$^+$ RNA is prepared as described (9) and should be spun for 1 min in the cold immediately before injection to pellet debris which might clog the injection pipette.

Preparation and Loading of the Pipette

Microinjection pipettes are prepared by pulling 10-μl microdispenser replacement tubes [VWR (Piscataway, NJ) cat. no. 53508-400] on a vertical pipette puller [David Kopf Instruments (Tuga, CA) model 720] at setting 14.5 with the solenoid set to 5. Wear gloves when handling the pipettes and locate the heating element as close to the end of the tube as possible to maximize the length of the finished pipette. Under a microscope, break the tip of the pipette against the edge of a fire-cracked glass slide such that the external diameter of the tip is about 20 μm. Pipettes with tips of less than 15 μm diameter clog easily with cytoplasm or debris, and pipettes greater than 25 μm cause excessive damage to the oocyte. With a 1-ml syringe fill the pipette with mineral oil, ejecting oil through the tip and continually adding oil while removing the syringe so that there are no bubbles and the pipette is completely filled. The microinjector (10 μl VWR Digital Microdispenser, cat. no. 53506-100) is attached with two hose clamps to a micromanipulator [Narishige (Tokyo, Japan) cat. no. MM-333] which is screwed to a lead brick for stability. Rotate the plunger on the microinjector counterclockwise until the dials reads 000. Gently and slowly slide the pipette over the metal plunger, forcing oil through the tip until the flat end of the pipette meets the flat part of the microinjector. Carefully but firmly tighten the nut. Rotate the plunger very slowly until the dial reads 700: this will allow 3 μl of solution to be taken up into the pipette to inject at least 30 oocytes at 50 nl each. When the pipette is in air, always leave a drop of oil (or RNA solution) on the tip to keep air from traveling into the body of the pipette. Place 3.5 μl of the RNA solution on Parafilm which has been stretched over a small lead block and put the block under a low-power microscope so that the drop occupies about one-quarter of the field. Lower the pipette tip, which still has a drop of oil on it, down to just above the level of the Parafilm, in the field but safely away from the drop. Move the tip down and let the Parafilm remove the oil drop; oil is now conveniently flush with the tip. Retract the tip slightly and move the pipette laterally so that the tip moves into the drop. Very slowly rotate the plunger counterclockwise, taking the RNA into the pipette and moving the block as necessary to avoid debris and inclusion of air. Continue until most of the drop is taken up, leaving some behind and ejecting a small amount while removing the pipette from the drop.

Injections

The oocyte injection bath consists of a 35-mm petri dish which has been scored in a grid pattern with a heavy guage needle and filled with sterile OR-2. The bath can be reused many times if scrubbed and rinsed with distilled water, ethanol, and sterile OR-2 after each use. The accuracy and reproducibility of the injections at several injection volumes should be determined first, by injecting a radioactively labeled trace and then counting the oocyte. The effectiveness of the injection technique can also be monitored by observing the fate of injected dye. The dye can be observed to spread quickly through the cytoplasm; if the injection is too shallow, the dye will be extruded back into the bath. The point of injection should be either in the vegetal hemisphere or at the equator, but in either case the animal hemisphere should be avoided to minimize damage to the nucleus which increases the mortality rate. The point of injection should be the same for all oocytes, and the injection pipette may be used to carefully roll the oocyte over to provide the proper orientation.

Arrange three lines of 10 oocytes each in the bath, and move the bath stage so that the first oocyte in the first line is in the center of the microscope field. It is advisable to arrange the oocytes the same and to follow the same injection order each time to keep track accurately of injected versus uninjected oocytes as well as RNA usage. Lower the injection pipette tip toward the first oocyte to be injected and, while still in the air, eject a small amount to confirm that the pipette is indeed working. Lower the pipette further until the tip makes contact with the oocyte, slowly creating a dimple. Continue very slowly until the oocyte membrane pops back, then continue until the pipette tip is about one-fourth (250 μm) of the way into the oocyte. Note the position of the dial on the microinjector, and slowly rotate the plunger clockwise until the dial has moved five small notches, corresponding to 50 nl. Large oocytes can be injected with up to 100 nl, but 50 nl is a good compromise, allowing for accurate delivery and minimizing the effects of injection on oocyte health. During injection, each oocyte will actually inflate slightly. If this is not observed, the pipette may be clogged, and this can be checked by raising the tip out of the bath and ejecting a drop into the air. Keep the injection pipette stand stationary and move the oocyte bath stage to bring the next oocyte into position for injection. Between oocytes, inspect the pipette tip frequently, ejecting RNA as necessary to keep cytoplasm from clogging the pipette. After all of the oocytes have been injected, remove them to a multiwell cell culture dish containing OR-2E and, if multiple sets are to be done, replace the bath OR-2 between each set.

Incubation

The time between injection and assay depends on the kinetics of expression and the particular protein function being observed. For receptor expression, we have found that the response to TRH is first evident between 8 and 12 hr, and is maximal from 30 to 72 hr after injection. Incubate at 20°C for 2–3 days. Each day, visually inspect both injected and uninjected oocytes with the microscope, removing dead and damaged oocytes and replacing the OR-2E.

Electrophysiological Assay

A single oocyte is placed in the bottom of a 0.4-ml capacity Lucite perfusion chamber which has a conical interior that causes the oocyte to come to rest by gravity at the same place each time. To avoid shear forces, oocytes are gently transferred using large-bore short Pasteur pipettes. Allow oocytes to roll out of the pipette rather than squeezing the pipette bulb. Drugs are added in the perfusate, which has a flow rate of 5 ml/min. Electrodes are pulled from glass capillaries without filament [World Precision Instruments (New Haven, CT) cat. no TW150-6] on a vertical pipette puller at setting 13.5 with the solenoid set to zero. Electrodes are filled with filtered 3 M KCl and a small amount of paraffin oil is placed at the open end to prevent drying out. In most experiments, current is monitored with oocytes maintained under voltage clamp at -70 V using a Dagan (Minneapolis, MN) 8500 intracellular preamp clamp. Tracings are recorded on a flat-bed two-pen recorder [Houston Instrument (Austin, TX) Microscribe Series 4500 strip chart recorder]. Electrode resistance and impedance are measured with a dual-trace oscilloscope [Leader (Hauppaugue, NY) model LBO-522]. Resistances of 0.5–3 $M\Omega$ are acceptable. Reversal potentials were determined from intersects of V–I curves obtained by voltage ramp (1.0 sec duration) applied to the oocyte at rest and during a response to TRH (22). Chloride concentration in the bath was varied by exchanging sodium acetate for an equivalent amount of sodium chloride.

Results

In pituitary cells, the TRH receptor is coupled to the phosphoinositide/ calcium signal transduction pathway (23, 24). Stimulation of the TRH receptor (TRH-R) causes activation of a guanine nucleotide-binding protein which activates phospholipase C to generate inositol trisphosphate and diacylglycerol, leading to the elevation of intracellular calcium and to secretion. Previous work characterizing the pathway used by endogenous oocyte muscarinic receptors (22, 25–28) and muscarinic and serotonin receptors acquired by the oocyte after injection of rat brain mRNA (29, 30) had shown that the acquired receptors, which in their native tissue were coupled to the phosphoinositide/calcium pathway, could also utilize the same signaling pathway in the oocyte. Stimulation of injected oocytes by acetylcholine (ACH) or serotonin caused inositol trisphosphate-mediated release of intracellular calcium which, in the oocyte, opens plasma membrane chloride channels, resulting in membrane depolarization. We thought that this may also be possible for the TRH receptor, and therefore we isolated and injected cytosolic RNA from a cloned pituitary cell line (GH$_3$), and monitored the membrane electrical activity of the oocyte upon application of TRH.

We found that uninjected oocytes had no response to TRH, but that oocytes injected with cytosolic RNA from GH$_3$ pituitary cells showed a robust membrane depolarization upon stimulation by TRH. We characterized the acquired response to TRH by varying the amount and source of RNA injected and by analyzing in detail the features of the response. The response to TRH was often observed by 8 to 12 hr and was maximal between 30 and 72 hr after injection. A typical response to 1 μM TRH (Fig. 1A) (9) consisted of a rapid, transient depolarizing current that developed 20 to 30 sec after exposure to TRH (denoted as D1$_T$ by analogy to the D1 response caused by ACH). This response was followed by prolonged depolarizing current of much smaller amplitude, often accompanied by very large superimposed current fluctuations. Because the second depolarizing current was variable and was often obscured by current fluctuations, all quantitation was performed on the D1$_T$ component of the response. The magnitude of the response was dependent on the amount of RNA injected. Threshold responses (approximately 10 to 20 nA) were obtained when 20 ng of RNA was injected (Fig. 1B). Progressively larger responses were observed when the amount of RNA injected was increased from 20 to 320 ng. Responses similar to those observed in oocytes injected with total cytosolic RNA were observed in oocytes injected with RNA enriched for the polyadenylated [poly(A)$^+$] species from GH$_3$ cells (Fig. 1C). We also tested a variant GH$_3$ cell clone (GH-Y) (31) that had no detectable TRH-Rs. In oocytes injected

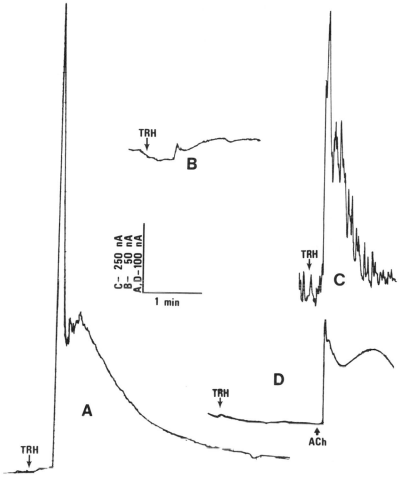

FIG. 1   Current responses to TRH in *Xenopus* oocytes injected with RNA from GH₃ or GH-Y cells. The upward deflection represents an inward depolarizing current. (A) Oocyte injected with 320 ng of GH₃ cell cytosolic RNA. (B) Oocyte injected with 20 ng of GH₃ cell cytosolic RNA. (C) Oocyte injected with 20 ng of poly(A)⁺-enriched GH₃ cell RNA and 100 ng of carrier tRNA (*Escherichia coli,* Boehringer-Mannheim). (D) Oocyte injected with 140 ng of cytosolic RNA from GH-Y cells. Assays were performed 48 hr after injection. TRH (1 μM, large arrows) or 0.1 μM ACh (small arrow) was added for 1.5 min. [Reproduced with permission from Y. Oron, R. E. Straub, P. Traktman, and M. C. Gershengorn, *Science* **238,** 1406 (1987).]

with either cytosolic or poly(A)$^+$ RNA from GH-Y cells, there was no response to TRH even though they still showed a response to ACH (Fig. 1D). These data suggest that GH-Y cells lack TRH-Rs because they are deficient in mRNA activity that encodes a functional TRH-R. Taken together, we conclude that the oocyte is a valid assay for the bioactivity of the messenger RNA for the TRH receptor.

While the complex depolarizing current caused by TRH has the same general form in each oocyte, there are a number of variations. The typical response to 0.1 to 1 μM TRH applied for 1–2 min consists of three components. (1) A rapid, transient large depolarizing current appeared usually within 25 sec of exposure and peaked 1–3 sec later. The decay of this component was slower than its onset (Fig. 2A–C) (32). (2) A slow prolonged depolarizing current that sometimes exhibited a distinct peak 3–5 min after the beginning of exposure to TRH, particularly at lower concentrations of TRH (Fig. 2A and B), but was often fused with the descending limb of the rapid response (Fig. 2C). This component often continued for 10 min or more after washout of TRH. (3) Rapid, large current fluctuations appeared after the peak of the first component and continued for a prolonged time (Fig. 2A and B). The fluctuations broadened and became less frequent with time (Fig. 2A and B). The three components could also be identified in voltage recordings, resulting in depolarization to -25 to -18 mV (Fig. 3) (32). In order to resolve which ions carried the current in the TRH response, we measured the reversal potential (V_{rs}) for the rapid (r) and slow (s) components of the response. Representative $V-I$ curves are shown in Fig. 4a and b (32). The values obtained for both components were close to the calculated V_r of Cl$^-$ (22). Further, manipulations of Cl$^-$ and K$^+$ in the bath indicate that the TRH-stimulated current was carried predominantly by Cl$^-$, and that K$^+$ did not participate in the response.

To define further the acquired TRH response, we compared it to the endogenous muscarinic response and the muscarinic response acquired after injection of rat brain RNA (32). A comparison of these three responses is shown in Fig. 5 (33). Figure 5A exemplifies a typical response to TRH in a defolliculated oocyte injected with an optimal amount of GH$_3$ cell RNA. Figure 5B shows the response to ACH in uninjected follicles, native oocytes surrounded by follicular cells. Figure 5C represents the acquired muscarinic response in defolliculated oocytes injected with an optimal amount of rat brain total RNA. The acquired responses were similar whether they were monitored in denuded (defolliculated by collagenase treatment) oocytes or in follicles, whereas the intrinsic ACH response was consistently observed only in oocytes in follicles. All three responses had the usual rapid, transient depolarizing current which generally contains superimposed current fluctuations. First, the amplitude of the rapid depolarizing current (D1) of the

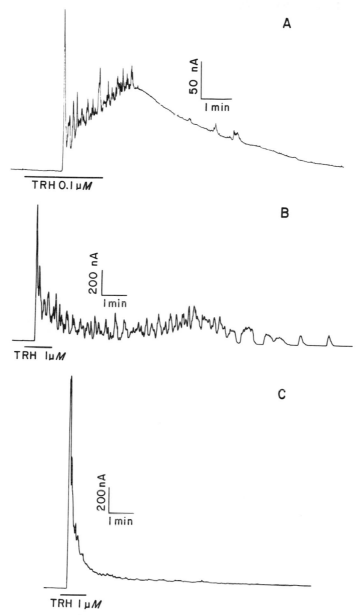

FIG. 2 (A–C) Variation in membrane current responses to TRH in oocytes injected with GH₃ cell cytosolic RNA. Three representative responses to TRH in oocytes from different donors. Oocytes were injected with 200 ng each of total cytosolic RNA and responses were tested 48 hr later. Oocytes were clamped at −80 mV. [Reproduced with permission from Y. Oron, B. Gillo, R. E. Straub, and M. C. Gershengorn, *Mol. Endocrinol.* **1**, 918 (1988).]

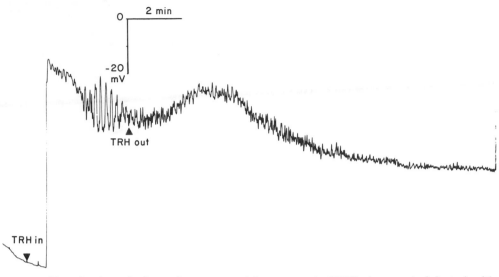

FIG. 3   A typical membrane potential response to TRH. An oocyte injected with 240 ng total cytosolic RNA was assayed 48 hr later. TRH (1 μM) was present for the interval delimited by the arrows. Note the typical second phase ($D2_T$), with a peak at approximately 5 min after the beginning of the response and exhibiting large voltage fluctuations. [Reproduced with permission from Y. Oron, B. Gillo, R. E. Straub, and M. C. Gershengorn, *Mol. Endocrinol.* **1,** 918 (1988).]

acquired responses was greater than the amplitude of the intrinsic ACH response. Second, the patterns of the prolonged depolarizing currents were similar for the acquired TRH and ACH responses but these were different from that of the intrinsic ACH response. Third, in the acquired responses, the prolonged depolarizing currents were usually smaller in amplitude than the rapid depolarizing currents and did not attain distinct peak values. In the intrinsic ACH response, the prolonged depolarizing current showed a distinct, broad peak of variable duration (Fig. 5B). We also analyzed the latency period between addition of a maximally effective concentration of each agonist and the onset of activation of the rapid depolarizing current, and found that the duration of this period was characteristic for each response. The latency period for the acquired TRH response was 16.6 ± 1.4 sec (n = 29), for the intrinsic ACH response 2.3 ± 2.9 sec (n = 45), and for the acquired ACH response it was 6.9 ± 0.8 sec (n = 16). Using other techniques, including intracellular injection and inhibition of the response by a competitive antagonist, we have recently found that the latency of the TRH response appears to vary inversely with the number of occupied TRH receptors (34).

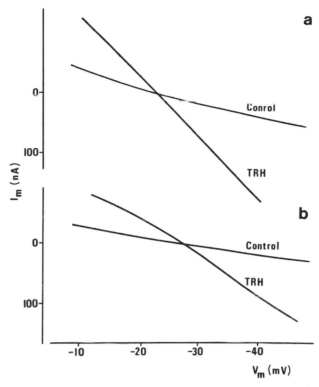

FIG. 4   *V–I* relationship of the TRH response. Oocytes were injected with 240 ng of total cytosolic RNA and tested 48 hr later. Two oocytes from the same donor were clamped at −50 mV. The *V–I* curve in the unstimulated oocytes was obtained (control), then the cells were challenged with 0.1 μM TRH and the *V–I* curve was obtained again during the (a) $D1_T$ and (b) $D2_T$ response. A lower TRH concentration was used to prevent the interference of the large response current with the *V–I* curve throughout the duration of the clamp. [Reproduced with permission from Y. Oron, B. Gillo, R. E. Straub, and M. C. Gershengorn, *Mol. Endocrinol.* **1,** 918 (1988).]

Next, we compared the three responses when agonists were added by pressure injection in a small volume (10–20 nl) directly to the animal or vegetal hemisphere, instead of being included in the perfusate. As expected, the responses were markedly smaller with local application of agonists than with global application, but in addition there were significant differences in the response elicited by application at the animal versus the vegetal hemisphere. For the acquired TRH and the acquired ACH responses, application of the agonist at the animal hemisphere elicited a much larger rapid depolarizing current than application at the vegetal hemisphere. In

A   B   C

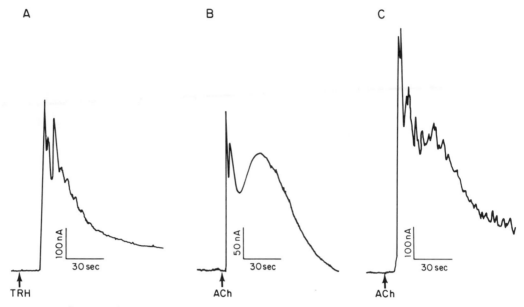

FIG. 5   Comparison of three different response types. Typical membrane current responses in *Xenopus* oocytes during perfusion. (A) Acquired response to TRH (1 μM). The response was obtained in a defolliculated oocyte, clamped at -60 mV, 42 hr after injection of 300 ng of GH$_3$ cell cytosolic RNA. (B) Intrinsic response to ACh (10 μM). The response was obtained in an uninjected follicle clamped at -80 mV. (C) Acquired response to ACh (100 μM). The response was obtained in a defolliculated oocyte, clamped at -60 mV, 48 hr after injection of 250 ng of rat brain total RNA. The arrows indicate the beginning of 1 min addition of agonist to the perfusion medium. The dead time of the perfusion system (5.5 sec) was subtracted. Note the differences in the current calibration scales. [Reproduced with permission from Y. Oron, B. Gillo, and M. C. Gershengorn, *Proc. Natl. Acad. Sci. U.S.A.* **85,** 3820 (1988).]

contrast to these acquired responses, the intrinsic response to ACH was greater when ACH was applied at the vegetal hemisphere than when it was applied to the animal hemisphere. We suggest that this asymmetry may reflect the density and distribution of functional TRH and muscarinic receptors.

Since we had demonstrated that the magnitude of the TRH response in oocytes reflects the amount of receptor mRNA injected, we thought that, with the appropriate controls, the oocyte might be used as a bioassay for TRH-R message. It had been known for some time that the TRH receptor exhibits homologous down-regulation of receptor number (35, 36). It ap-

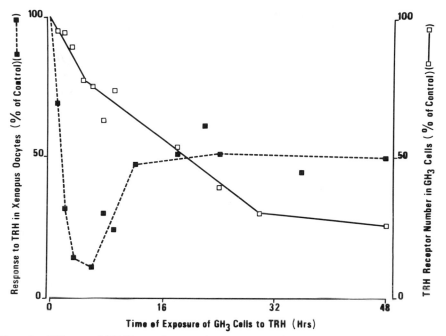

FIG. 6   Effects of TRH on the number of TRH receptors on GH₃ cells and on receptor mRNA activity assayed in *Xenopus* oocytes. For incubation of GH₃ cells, cells (1.8×10^8) from the same passage were distributed equally into six flasks. TRH ($1 \mu M$) was added for the indicated times before harvesting. For measurement of TRH receptor number, 10^6 cells were used and the binding assay was performed with 1 nM [³H]methyl-His-TRH (New England Nuclear) (35). Nonspecific binding, less than 5% of total, was determined with 0.5 μM unlabeled TRH. Assays for the measurement of mRNA activity were performed 48 to 72 hr after injection of 130 to 150 ng of GH₃ cell cytosolic RNA. Results from four binding and eight receptor mRNA activity assay experiments were pooled and are presented as percentage of control. The mean SEMs for the measurement of receptor binding and receptor mRNA activity were 3.2 ± 0.67% and 12 ± 1.6%, respectively. [Reproduced with permission from Y. Oron, R. E. Straub, P. Traktman, and M. C. Gershengorn, *Science* **238,** 1406 (1987).]

pears that rapid internalization is not involved (31), but the mechanism of down-regulation had not been investigated further since neither an antibody to the receptor or a probe for the mRNA was available. In order to study the process of down-regulation, GH₃ cells were grown for 1 to 48 hr in the presence or absence of 1 μM TRH. The TRH-R number was measured in GH₃ cells, and TRH-R mRNA activity was assayed in parallel in oocytes. For this set of experiments, 130 to 150 ng of cytosolic RNA was injected into oocytes of the same batch to monitor changes in mRNA activity most sensitively. TRH caused a time-dependent decrease in the number of receptors that was half-maximal after 12 hr and reached a new steady state (approximately 30% of control) after 30 hr (Fig. 6) (9). In contrast to the continuous decrease in receptor number, the effect on TRH-R mRNA activity was complex (Fig. 6). TRH caused a rapid decrease in receptor mRNA activity which reached a minimum of approximately 15% of control between 3 and 6 hr. This was followed by an increase to approximately 50% of control mRNA activity by 12 hr, and this level was maintained for at least 48 hr. The initial decrease in mRNA activity was rapid and preceded the decline in receptor number, and therefore may be a cause of the net loss of cell surface receptors. We have not pursued the rebound and stabilization aspects of the mRNA activity curve. To determine whether this initial decrease in receptor mRNA activity was due to inhibition of transcription, we compared the effect of actinomycin D with that of exposure to TRH. At both 3 and 6 hr, TRH was much more effective in causing the rapid decrease in mRNA activity than was actinomycin D (data now shown). In addition, the actinomycin D data provide an estimate of the half-life of the TRH-R mRNA activity of about 3 hr. Hence, because virtually complete arrest of transcription did not mimic the effect of TRH, the rapid decrease in receptor mRNA activity appears at least in part to be posttranscriptional.

References

1. J. B. Gurdon and M. P. Wickens, *in* "Methods in Enzymology" (R. Wu, L. Grossman, and K. Moldave, eds.), Vol. 101, p. 370. Academic Press, New York, 1983.
2. C. D. Lane, *Curr. Top. Dev. Biol.* **18,** 89 (1983).
3. E. A. Barnard, D. Beeson, G. Bilbe, *et al., J. Recept. Res.* **4,** 681 (1984).
4. H. Soreq, *CRC Crit. Rev. Biochem.* **18,** 199 (1985).
5. N. Dascal, *CRC Crit. Rev. Biochem.* **22,** 317 (1987).
6. T. P. Snutch, *Trends Neuro Sci.* (*Pers. Ed.*) **11,** 250 (1988).
7. B. K. Kobilka, T. S. Kobilka, K. Daniel, J. W. Regan, M. G. Caron, and R. J. Lefkowitz, *Science* **240,** 1310 (1988).
8. S. L. Peacock, M. P. Bates, D. W. Russell, M. S. Brown, and J. L. Goldstein, *J. Biol. Chem.* **263,** 7838 (1988).
9. Y. Oron, R. E. Straub, P. Traktman, and M. C. Gershengorn, *Science* **238,** 1406 (1987).
10. M. B. Boyle, N. J. MacLusky, F. Naftolin, and L. K. Kaczmarek, *Nature* (*London*) **330,** 373 (1987).
11. Y. Noma, P. Sideras, T. Naito, *et al., Nature* (*London*) **319,** 640 (1986).
12. C. Ludin, H. Hofstetter, M. Sarfati, *et al., EMBO J.* **6,** 109 (1987).

13. Y. Masu, K. Nakayama, H. Tamaki, Y. Harada, M. Kuno, and S. Nakanishi, *Nature (London)* **329,** 836 (1987).
14. M. A. Hediger, M. J. Coady, T. S. Ikeda, and E. M. Wright, *Nature (London)* **330,** 379 (1987).
15. H. Lübbert, B. J. Hoffman, T. P. Snutch, *et al., Proc. Natl. Acad. Sci. U.S.A.* **84,** 4332 (1987).
16. D. Julius, A. B. MacDermott, R. Axel, and T. M. Jessell, *Science* **241,** 558 (1988).
17. A. Sloma, R. McCandliss, and S. Pestka, *in* "Methods in Enzymology" (S. Pestka, ed.), Vol. 79, p. 68. Academic Press, New York, 1981.
18. A. Colman, *in* "Transcription and Translation: A Practical Approach" (B. D. Hames and S. J. Higgins, eds.), pp. 271–302. IRL Press, Oxford, 1984.
19. M. J. Hitchcock, E. I. Ginns, and C. J. Marcus Sekura, *in* "Methods in Enzymology" (S. L. Berger and A. R. Kimmel, eds.), Vol. 152, p. 276. Academic Press, Orlando, Florida, 1987.
20. C. J. Marcus Sekura and M. J. Hitchcock, *in* "Methods in Enzymology" (S. L. Berger and A. R. Kimmel, eds.), Vol. 152, p. 284. Academic Press, Orlando, Florida, 1987.
21. D. A. Melton, *in* "Methods in Enzymology" (S. L. Berger and A. R. Kimmel, eds.), Vol. 152, p. 288. Academic Press, Orlando, Florida, 1987.
22. N. Dascal, E. M. Landau, and Y. Lass, *J. Physiol. (London)* **352,** 551 (1984).
23. M. C. Gershengorn, *Recent Prog. Horm. Res.* **41,** 607 (1985).
24. M. C. Gershengorn, *Annu. Rev. Physiol.* **48,** 515 (1986).
25. Y. Oron, N. Dascal, E. Nadler, and M. Lupu, *Nature (London)* **313,** 141 (1985).
26. N. Dascal, B. Gillo, and Y. Lass, *J. Physiol. (London)* **366,** 299 (1985).
27. E. Nadler, B. Gillo, Y. Lass, and Y. Oron, *FEBS Lett.* **199,** 208 (1986).
28. B. Gillo, Y. Lass, E. Nadler, and Y. Oron, *J. Physiol. (London)* **392,** 349 (1987).
29. C. B. Gundersen, R. Miledi, and I. Parker, *Nature (London)* **308,** 421 (1984).
30. N. Dascal, C. Ifune, R. Hopkins, *et al., Mol. Brain Res.* **1,** 201 (1986).
31. J. Halpern and P. M. Hinkle, *Proc. Natl. Acad. Sci. U.S.A.* **78,** 587 (1981).
32. Y. Oron, B. Gillo, R. E. Straub, and M. C. Gershengorn, *Mol. Endocrinol.* **1,** 918 (1988).
33. Y. Oron, B. Gillo, and M. C. Gershengorn, *Proc. Natl. Acad. Sci. U.S.A.* **85,** 3820 (1988).
34. Submitted for publication.
35. P. M. Hinkle and A. H. Tashjian, Jr., *Biochemistry* **14,** 3845 (1975).
36. M. C. Gershengorn, *J. Clin. Invest.* **62,** 937 (1978).

[4] Expression of Exogenous Voltage-Gated Calcium Channels in *Xenopus* Oocytes

John P. Leonard

With the advent of the *Xenopus* oocyte system, it has become possible to study a variety of Ca^{2+} channels in a standard test environment removed from the potential difficulties associated with the voltage clamping of fine neuronal processes. The oocyte mRNA expression system should ultimately allow examination of a multitude of questions about the structural basis for the functional heterogeneity of Ca^{2+} channels. Of course, the expression of voltage-dependent calcium channels in *Xenopus* oocytes is subject to the same constraints that hold for expression of other voltage-dependent ion channels and neurotransmitter receptors (see Chapters [1]–[3], this volume). These constraints include the need for (1) intact mRNA encoding a functional channel, (2) proper care and injection of oocytes, and (3) electrophysiological methods tailored to reveal the channel of interest. This chapter will focus on each of these three key elements in turn, particularly as they relate to the expression of Ca^{2+} channels. The general approach outlined below is precisely as diagrammed in Fig. 1 of Chapter [2] in this volume.

Intact mRNA is one absolute requirement for the successful expression of exogenous Ca^{2+} channels in oocytes. The requirement for intact mRNA encoding ion channels is not difficult to meet when the RNA is produced by *in vitro* transcription from cDNA clones. When cDNA clones for complete Ca^{2+} channels become available, these will presumably provide the best source of mRNA for expression in oocytes. At present, RNA must be isolated directly from the tissue of interest. The presence of RNases in tissues can make the procedure difficult and is the primary reason that the various RNA isolation procedures are tissue specific. The following section is a description of reliable methods for isolating RNA from rat brain and from rat heart that will produce functional Ca^{2+} channels in oocytes.

RNA Isolation Procedures

The techniques involve cell/tissue disruption, inactivation of RNases, and separation of RNA from DNA, proteins, and polysaccharide. For good quality, high-molecular-weight RNA one must avoid the following: inactiva-

Methods in Neurosciences, Volume 1

tion of RNA by RNases, strong shearing forces, high temperature, high alkalinity, high acidity, and high ionic strength. For best results, use highest quality reagents, i.e., ultrapure urea, guanidine from Schwarz/Mann (Cleveland, OH). Either redistill the phenol or buy redistilled phenol from BRL [molecular biology grade (Gaithersburg, MD)]. Degradation of RNA is most likely to occur during the initial breakage of the cells when nucleases are released. This step is best done with cold solutions and on ice. Bake the glassware to be used at 150–200°C for 3–12 hr. RNases are present in the sweat on the fingers, so wear gloves at all times when working with RNA.

Urea/SDS/LiCl Procedure for Rat Brain

This method is from Ref. 1 as modified by Terry P. Snutch (Biotechnology Laboratory, University of British Columbia, Vancouver, British Columbia, Canada).

This method has two advantages in that it gives high-molecular-weight RNA that translates efficiently in *Xenopus* oocytes and does not involve any lengthy centrifugation through CsCl. Three potential disadvantages should also be noted. (1) Be careful not to precipitate DNA along with the RNA. Even if you plan to isolate poly(A)$^+$ RNA, contaminating DNA will clog up the oligo(dT) column and make life difficult. (2) Urea is not a great RNase inhibitor, so this method does not work well for tissues with significant amounts of RNase. (3) The method is also not great for RNA isolation from tissue culture cells since lots of DNA coprecipitates with the RNA. This method works especially well for brain RNA preparations.

Solutions

A. 6 M urea
   3 M LiCl
   10 mM sodium acetate, pH 5.0
   0.1% SDS—added just prior to use

When the SDS is added to the urea/LiCl, some of it precipitates. This does not affect the results but it looks rather messy. This can be avoided if 0.1% sarkosyl is used instead of SDS.

B. 10 mM Tris-HCl, pH 7.5
   1 mM EDTA
   0.5% SDS

C. Sevag—is chloroform : isoamyl alcohol (24 : 1)
D. Phenol—must be equilibrated prior to use. Add a stir bar and about 100 ml of autoclaved water to a 100-g bottle of redistilled phenol (BRL) and let them mix at room temperature for 20 min (first melt the phenol at 50–60°C). As they mix, add about 30 ml of 2 M Tris-HCl, pH 7.5, and 1 ml of 5 M NaOH. After letting the two phases separate, check the pH of a sample of the aqueous layer; it should be between pH 7.0 and 7.5. If not, adjust accordingly. Use what you need and store the rest at −20°C. If the phenol becomes pink or yellow, discard the solution, as the oxidation products formed will degrade RNA.
E. 2.5 M sodium acetate, pH 5.2
F. Autoclaved water
G. 95% (v/v) ethanol

Procedure

1. Homogenize the tissue with 10–15 strokes of a 7.5-ml Dounce homogenizer using 7 ml of solution A per gram of tissue (a 2-week-old rat brain is approximately 1 g). Styrofoam shipping lids make convenient disposable dissection platforms. An oval weighing spatula is useful for transferring brains to the homogenizer.

2. The mixture is left overnight on ice in the cold room to precipitate the RNA.

3. Mix each tube thoroughly by inverting. Pellet the RNA in a Sorvall (SS-34) centrifuge at 10,000 rpm for 25 min (or similar high-speed centrifuge) at 4°C.

4. Discard the supernatant and dissolve the pellet in 1–2 ml of solution B per gram of tissue. Pipetting the solution up and down is usually sufficient to dissolve the pellet.

5. Extract the solution three times with 1 vol of a phenol : Sevag solution [phenol : chloroform : isoamyl alcohol = 25 : 24 : 1 (v/v)]. Do each of these extractions on a shaker in the cold room for 15 min for large-scale RNA preparations. For small-scale preparations, it is sufficient to use cold phenol : Sevag and mix by hand for 1 or 2 min. The organic and aqueous layers are separated by a 5-min spin in a desktop centrifuge in the cold room. Keep the aqueous layer for all organic extractions.

6. Extract the solution twice with 1 vol of Sevag as in step 5.

7. Add 0.1 vol of 2.5 M sodium acetate, pH 5.2; add 2.5 vol of 95% ethanol; leave at −20°C for 3–12 hr.

8. Pellet the RNA in a Sorvall (SS-34) at 10,000 rpm for 10 min. Wash the pellet once in 80% ethanol, then repellet. Dry and dissolve the RNA in

sterile water (about 1 ml per gram of tissue). At this point the RNA is clean enough for Northern blots and to isolate poly(A)$^+$ RNA.

9. For *in vitro* translations or injections into *Xenopus* oocytes of total RNA, it should first be reprecipitated as in step 7.

10. Wash the RNA pellet twice in 80% ethanol, dry, and take up in sterile water at 1–2 mg/ml.

11. Store at −80°C.

RNA can be injected into oocytes as either total RNA or with a poly(A)$^+$ selection first. Yield of total RNA: a 14-day-old rat brain should give 1.2–1.4 mg RNA per brain.

Guanidine Hydrochloride Procedure

This method is from Refs. 2 and 3 as modified by Terry P. Snutch.

The advantages of this isolation method are as follows. (1) It yields high-molecular-weight RNA that translates efficiently in *Xenopus* oocytes. (2) There is little or no contamination of protein or genomic DNA. (3) It does not involve any lengthy centrifugation through CsCl. (4) The method works equally well on soft tissues (e.g., brain) and fibrous tissues (e.g., heart) and on tissue culture cell lines. Two potential disadvantages should be considered. (1) This procedure is not efficient for the purification of small-molecular-weight RNAs (less than 120 bases). (2) A small amount of closed circular DNA, if present in the tissues of interest (i.e., extrachromosomal transposon DNA), will copurify with the RNA, but this is not a major problem (4).

Solutions

A. 6 *M* guanidine hydrochloride
   200 m*M* sodium acetate, pH 5.0
   100 m*M* 2-mercaptoethanol
B. 7.5 *M* guanidine hydrochloride
   25 m*M* sodium citrate, pH 7.0
   50 m*M* 2-mercaptoethanol
C. Sevag—is chloroform : isoamyl alcohol (24 : 1)
D. Phenol—must be equilibrated prior to use. Follow exact method described in the section above for the urea/SDS/LiCl procedure.
E. 2.5 *M* sodium acetate, pH 5.2
F. Autoclaved water
G. 95% (v/v) ethanol

Procedure

1. Homogenize tissues with either a Dounce homogenizer (soft tissues, tissue culture cells) or a Polytron (fibrous tissues) in about 8–10 ml of ice-cold solution A per gram of tissue (a 2-week-old rat brain weighs approximately 1 g) or about 15–20 ml of solution A per milliliter of packed cells for tissue culture cells. If the tissue is fibrous (heart, muscle), spin in a Sorvall (SS-34) at 10,000 rpm for 5 min to remove unhomogenized material before going to step 2. This is not necessary for tissue culture cells.

2. Add 0.65 vol of 95% ethanol and leave at −20°C overnight.

3. Pellet RNA in Sorvall (SS-34) (or similar high-speed centrifuge) at 10,000 rpm (4°C) for 10 min, discard supernatant. If a low yield is expected, it is best to do all centrifugations in a swinging bucket rotor instead of a fixed angle rotor.

4. Dissolve pellet in ice-cold solution B (about 1–2 ml per gram of tissue). Pipette solution up and down or lightly vortex to help it go into solution, but never heat to dissolve (RNA is very sensitive to heat in 7.5 M GuHCl). If the material does not dissolve, it is not RNA. Spin briefly, discard the pellet, and take the supernatant to the next step. Step 4 can be ignored for tissue culture RNA preparations; simply proceed from step 3 to step 7.

5. Add 0.025 vol of 1 M acetic acid (to lower pH and facilitate RNA precipitation) and then add 0.5 vol of 95% ethanol; keep at −20°C for 3–12 hr.

6. Pellet RNA as in step 3.

7. Take up pellet in sterile, autoclaved water (about 0.5 ml per gram of tissue or 5 ml per milliliter of packed cells).

8. Extract the solution three times with 1 vol of a phenol : Sevag solution [phenol : chloroform : isoamyl alcohol = 25 : 24 : 1 (v/v)]. Do each of these extractions on a shaker for 15 min in the cold room for large-scale RNA preparations. For small-scale and tissue culture cells, just use cold phenol : Sevag and mix by hand for 1–2 min. The organic and aqueous layers are separated by a 5-min spin in a desktop centrifuge in the cold room. Keep the aqueous layer for all organic extractions.

9. Extract twice with 1 vol of Sevag as in step 8.

10. Add 0.1 vol of 2.5 M sodium acetate, pH 5.0; add 2.5 vol 95% ethanol; leave at −20°C for 3–12 hr.

11. Pellet RNA as in step 3. Wash the RNA once in 80% ethanol. Dry and take up the pellet in sterile water at a concentration of 1–2 mg/ml. At this point the total RNA is clean enough for Northern blots and to isolate poly(A)$^+$ RNA.

12. For *in vitro* translations or injections into *Xenopus* oocytes of total RNA, it should first be reprecipitated as in step 10.

13. Pellet the RNA as in step 3, wash twice with 80% ethanol, and take up RNA in sterile water at a concentration of 1–2 mg/ml.

14. Store at −80°C.

RNA can be injected into oocytes either as total RNA or with a poly(A)$^+$ selection first. Yields of total RNA: a 2-day-old rat brain will give 600–900 μg/g tissue, a 2-day-old rat heart will give 600–700 μg/g tissue, and tissue culture cells will give 1–2 mg/ml packed cells.

If one is using a small source of tissue, such as cultured cells, it may not be advisable to attempt oligo(dT) purification, as this often causes a further loss of activity. Total RNA will suffice for injection as long as it has been cleaned by 2–3 extra 80% ethanol washes. Of course, for many molecular procedures polyadenylated mRNA must be used. Standard oligo(dT) procedures for the isolation of polyadenylated mRNA are widely available and will not be repeated here.

Preparation and Injection of Oocytes

Xenopus Frogs and Oocytes

Xenopus laevis can be reliably obtained from several commercial sources including *Xenopus* I, Inc. (Ann Arbor, MI) and Nasco Biologicals, Inc. (Fort Atkinson, WI). It is convenient to use mature females that have previously been injected with human chorionic gonadotropin to show that the ovaries are functioning and to induce a fresh cycle of oocyte development. Female frogs usually produce healthy oocytes if certain measures are taken (5). *Xenopus* are kept at 17–19°C, on a 12 hr off/12 hr on dark/light cycle. The frogs are fed beef heart or liver twice a week (about 8 g/frog). The tanks are washed with water twice per week. Even when the frogs are properly tended, there are times when healthy oocytes are not being produced. A new shipment of frogs may be required.

All frog surgery is done under anesthesia induced by 0.2% 3-aminobenzoic acid ethyl ester (tricaine methane sulfonate or MS-222). A 1–2 cm incision is made in the abdomen and several ovarian lobes removed (6). Sterile, 70% ethanol-treated surgical instruments are used for all procedures. The frog's skin is kept moist during surgery to prevent acidification. The incision is sutured with surgical silk and the frog is placed in shallow water in a small tank to allow it to recover from anesthesia before placing it in a special tank for postoperative frogs. The wounds heal very quickly, perhaps due to the presence of novel antibiotics in the skin (7). Every ovary contains hundreds of oocytes so only a fraction are removed at any one time. The ovarian lobes are pulled apart by blunt dissection with fine forceps and small clumps of oocytes are isolated.

The oocytes are then denuded of overlying follicle cells by treatment with 2 mg/ml collagenase (Sigma type I-A), in Ca^{2+}-free solution of the following composition (mM): NaCl, 82.5; KCl, 2.0; MgCl$_2$, 1.0; HEPES, 5.0 (pH 7.4). This procedure does not affect the electrophysiological responses of the oocytes (measured at least 36 hr later) or in any way alter its ability to translate ion channel mRNA (reviewed in Ref. 8). The collagenase treatment should be terminated when about 50% of the oocytes are stripped of overlying follicle cells (1.5–3 hr). This helps to avoid overdigestion and, often, many of the nondenuded cells will become defolliculated later as the sack of follicle cells sticks to the bottom of the culture dish. The oocytes are then thoroughly washed in normal oocyte saline containing (in mM): NaCl, 96; KCl, 2; CaCl$_2$, 1.8; MgCl$_2$, 1; and HEPES–NaOH, pH 7.5, and supplemented with 100 U/ml penicillin and 100 μg/ml streptomycin and 2.5 mM sodium pyruvate. If healthy oocytes die quickly after only 1 day, it may help to switch antibiotics and use 0.1 mg/ml gentamycin. Oocytes are not used for injection of mRNA for at least 2 hr after defolliculation.

Selection of oocytes is an often-overlooked important step. If many of the initially isolated oocytes lyse, spilling yoke out, then this may be a "bad frog" whose oocytes may die before they are of any use. Selection of the healthier oocytes should be done immediately after defolliculation. The search-image is essentially a uniform pigmentation of the animal pole of stage V and VI oocytes (9). Cells to be avoided include those with diffuse lightening at the tip of the animal pole. Such cells are undergoing spontaneous maturation. Other cells to avoid are any cells with dark spots, splotches, or marbling. If the wash solution around the defolliculated oocytes is very cloudy even after several rinses and becomes even more cloudy after 30 min in culture, then the oocytes are probably unusable.

Injection and Culture of Oocytes

After selection of healthy stage V and VI oocytes (based on morphology at a magnification of 25×), the oocytes are usually injected with 70-nl aqueous samples of mRNA (1 mg/ml). A 35-mm Falcon tissue culture dish can be used to construct an injection chamber. Use 0.5 mm^2 nylon monofilament mesh (Small Parts, Inc., Miami, FL) to prevent the oocytes from rolling around. This mesh can be cemented into the chamber with Sylgard. Squirt a large drop of water into the central area of the mesh to keep the Sylgard out of this region during curing. Injection is accomplished under a dissecting microscope with a Drummond 10-μl microdispensor mounted on a micromanipulator (Brinkmann or Narashige). A simple plexiglass collar can be

constructed to attach the Drummond microdispenser to the micromanipulator. It is essential to order extra metal rods for the microdispenser as only
straight rods will work. If one becomes bent, it will auger out a large hole as
it is advanced down the glass capillary tube.

Glass microdispensor needles with very gradual shanks are pulled with a
microelectrode puller and then broken to a 20-μm tip opening with a
fire-polished Pasteur pipette or sterile forceps. During each injection session
one group of oocytes (positive control) is injected with a previously
characterized RNA sample of known effectiveness. In this way, the blame
for any failure of oocytes injected with new mRNA samples to express
ion channels can be assigned to the RNA sample and not to a general translational failure of oocytes from a particular frog. After injection, oocytes are incubated at 20°C in sterile penicillin/streptomycin-
or gentamycin-supplemented normal oocyte saline as listed above. The
dishes are kept in a humid atmosphere and the solution is replaced at least
once a day. Under these conditions the oocytes can be maintained in good
health for up to 10 days. Calcium channels are usually observable 3–6 days
after injection.

Electrophysiology of Ca^{2+} Channels Expressed in Oocytes

Two-Electrode Voltage Clamping

The round shape of the oocyte is ideal for two-electrode voltage clamping
and the large size is convenient. On the other hand, large size means that
there is an extensive membrane capacitance to charge (0.5 μF), which limits
clamp speed. Reasonable two-electrode voltage clamping has been performed using various commercial clamp systems including the ±80 V Dagan
8500 and 8800 and the ±30 V Axoclamp 2-A. There is also a new (±130 V)
instrument designed for oocytes (Dagan) that should be somewhat faster. As
usual for two-electrode voltage clamps, operator-controlled factors that limit
speed are electrode resistance and capacitive coupling between the current
and voltage electrodes. One generally uses 3 M KCl-filled electrodes with
resistances of <1 MΩ and either large KCl/agar bridges or Ag/AgCl pellets.
The bridges are essential when Cl$^-$-free salines are used because of the
junction potentials created on the Ag/AgCl pellets. Capacitive coupling is
reduced by placing an insulated metal foil ground shield in the bath between
the current and the voltage electrode. When all these precautions are taken
and the bath level is kept as low as possible to decrease pipette capacitance,
one sees settling times of the capacitive current of 1–3 msec at room
temperature. This clamp speed is adequate for most of the currents
examined but slight improvements can be made by lowering electrode

resistance even further (to 0.2 MΩ) by pulling borosilicate glass in two stages as for patch pipettes and then filling the leaky pipettes with an intracellular-like saline (10). Clamp speed can be significantly improved by using small stage II oocytes that have a surface area roughly 10% of that of stage V and VI oocytes. However, RNA injection of such small oocytes requires special apparatus such as a Nanopump (World Precision Instruments, New Haven, CT) or other ultrastable device. Activation time course and tail currents are often too fast for routine two-electrode clamping. For such cases, one can perform "big patch" recordings as described below.

Patch Clamping

The patch-clamp technique can be used on oocytes both to record macroscopic currents with improved time resolution following a voltage step (11, 12) and to make traditional single-channel recordings (10, 12–15). In order to obtain gigaohm seals on the oocyte surface, it is essential to remove the vitelline membrane which surrounds the cell. Oocytes are placed in a hypertonic solution containing normal saline plus 60–100 mM extra NaCl (some oocytes shrink more than others). This treatment causes a gap to form between the plasma membrane and the vitelline membrane, allowing the vitelline membrane to be stripped away with forceps under a dissecting microscope. Such naked oocytes must not be exposed to an air–water interface because they will burst. Gigaohm seal formation for both big and small patches is achieved in a manner basically the same as for other cells (16). Patch pipettes are pulled in two stages and then coated with Sylgard to within 100 μm of the tip and finally fire-polished. It is more difficult to obtain gigaohm seals with the larger-diameter patch pipettes.

"Big Patches"

Soft glass capillaries (e.g., Kimble #73811) are pulled in two stages (16 and 11 A), producing pipette tip diameters of 25–30 μm. The resistance of such a pipette in normal oocyte saline is about 200 KΩ. Seal formation can occur quite abruptly but usually develops over a few tens of seconds. Gentle suction is mandatory with such a large opening, so use a micrometer syringe (2 ml Gilmont) after the pipette has touched the membrane. In good circumstances 20% of the attempts result in 1–3 GΩ seals. Typical pipettes enclose a geometric membrane surface area (assuming a hemispherical shape) of about 400 μm^2. However, due to the extensive folding of the oocyte surface, the actual membrane area enclosed is greater than 2000 μm^2.

Thus, the typical big patch pipette encloses about one ten-thousandth of the total oocyte membrane surface area. We would therefore expect to record on average 30 pA from such a patch when the whole-cell current is 300 nA. Although a 30-pA current was resolvable during a study of Na^+ currents (11), a 100-pA current is preferable. For this reason, when one needs to measure macroscopic I_{Ba} with the higher time resolution of patch recording, the oocytes must be injected with mRNA which is 3–5 times more concentrated than the usual 70-ng sample. This boosting procedure has been effective for I_{Na} (14,17), as the currents increase linearly with mRNA in this concentration range. Once cDNA clones are available, one will be able to titrate the density of channels on the surface membrane to any desired level. When sufficient channel density has been achieved, it will be possible to use the more convenient smaller-diameter patch pipette (12) to record macroscopic I_{Ba} with excellent time resolution.

Single-Channel Recording

In contrast to pipettes for big patch recording, for small patches I use hard glass [e.g., KG-33 from Garner Glass Co. (Claremont, CA)]. The oocyte is a very good preparation to study single-channel properties, except for the occasional interference of "stretch-activated channels" in the cell-attached mode. The outside-out patch configuration is preferred because, in this case, interference from "stretch" channels is rare (10, 18, 19). Seal resistance of most patches is >20 GΩ and remains so for 10–45 min. An advantage of the oocyte expression system for single-channel recording is that, by varying the amount of mRNA injected, one can control the amount of expression of the channel. One could then find an expression level where a typical 10–20 MΩ pipette generally does not enclose more than one ion channel, thus facilitating analysis. Traces without channel openings are averaged and subtracted from each individual trace to eliminate uncompensated capacitance and leak. This method is often slightly better than use of a scaling procedure.

Isolation of Exogenous Ca^{2+} Currents

Endogenous Activity

One constraint on any *in vivo* expression system is the need to control for any endogenous ion channel activity that may be present. There is, in fact, a small endogenous activity of voltage-dependent calcium channels in oocytes (13, 20–23). Levels of endogenous channels vary from frog to frog, but not between oocytes of the same stage from a given frog. While channels may be undetectable from many frogs, an exceptional frog may produce oocytes that show a 50 nA peak barium current. This phenomenon is not restricted to calcium channels. For example, oocytes from approximately 2% of frogs show bona fide tetrodotoxin-sensitive Na^+ currents. One solution to this problem is to increase the signal-to-noise ratio by overwhelming the small endogenous Ca^{2+} channel activity with the exogenous Ca^{2+} channels of interest. In addition, it is quite helpful if there are clear differences in the properties of the endogenous channel and the exogenously induced channel. This allows one to dissect out the current of interest either pharmacologically or by using particular voltage-clamp pulse protocols.

Inhibition of Other Contaminating Currents

In normal oocyte saline, depolarization of a noninjected oocyte by a standard two-electrode voltage clamp from a holding potential of -100 to 0 mV elicits a small, slow transient outward current. This current is a calcium-dependent chloride current turned on by the entry of calcium through endogenous voltage-activated channels (24, 25). In the Cl-containing oocyte salines used, E_{Cl} is about -25 mV. Therefore, outward ICl_{Ca} is elicited by Ca^{2+} channel activity at voltages more depolarized than -25 mV (E_{Cl}), and inward ICl_{Ca} is elicited by Ca^{2+} channel activity at voltages more hyperpolarized than -25 mV. In contrast to noninjected cells, oocytes injected with rat brain mRNA show much larger calcium-dependent chloride currents due to the translation of new populations of calcium channels with properties distinct from the endogenous channels (13, 20–23). Although this activation of endogenous calcium-dependent Cl channels by Ca^{2+} influx provides an amplified, sensitive assay for the presence of Ca^{2+} channels, the outward Cl^- current obscures the much smaller inward Ca^{2+} current, making direct analysis of the Ca^{2+} current impossible.

While the Ca^{2+} current is difficult to observe directly, Ba^{2+} currents through Ca^{2+} channels are measurable (13, 20–23, 26). We use Ba^{2+} instead of Ca^{2+} because Ba^{2+} often permeates Ca^{2+} channels better than Ca^{2+} and especially because Ba^{2+} substitutes poorly for Ca^{2+} in the activation of the ICl_{Ca} (25). However, barium can cause some activation of ICl_{Ca} (27). The Ba^{2+}-activated ICl_{Ca} can be substantially inhibited but not completely eliminated by Cl^- channel blockers of the anthracene carboxylate or stilbene classes (1 mM of 9-anthracene carboxylate, or 4,4'-dinitrostilbene-2,2'-disulfonic acid, or 4,4'-diisothiocyanatostilbene-2,2'-disulfonic acid; sonication helps dissolve these drugs). Niflumic acid or flufenamic acid (Sigma) may block these Cl^- channels more completely (M. M. White, personal communication). Ba^{2+} currents are measured in $BaCl_2$ saline of the following composition (mM): $BaCl_2$, 40; NaCl, 50; KCl, 2; HEPES–NaOH, 5 (pH 7.5) or, for comparison, Cl^--free barium methanesulfonate (BaMS) saline of the same cationic composition (mM): Ba(OH)$_2$, 40; NaOH, 50; KOH, 2; HEPES, 5 (pH 7.4 with methanesulfonic acid). The latter saline is only nominally 40 mM Ba, as a certain amount always precipitates out. It looks cloudy but will settle out overnight and can be decanted or filtered. Also, N-methyl-D-glucamine is a useful Na$^+$ substitute to check suspected Na$^+$ currents.

Use of Cl$^-$-free saline does not eliminate possible interference from Ba^{2+}-activated ICl_{Ca}. In Cl$^-$-free saline, E_{Cl} is quite positive and any Ba^{2+}-activated ICl_{Ca} would be an inward current (since Cl$^-$ is negatively charged, this is an efflux of internal Cl$^-$). Indeed, such inward ICl_{Ca} is clearly seen in Ca^{2+}-containing saline if methanesulfonate is substituted for Cl$^-$. Similarly, when large amounts of Ba^{2+} are pressure-injected into an oocyte voltage-clamped at -60 mV, a very small inward ICl_{Ca} is activated (27). Inward ICl_{Ca} is apparently less prominent than outward ICl_{Ca} in BaCl$_2$ saline. Because of solubility problems with high barium methanesulfonate saline, for routine purposes it is easier to use BaCl$_2$ saline with K$^+$ and Cl$^-$ channel blockers. Again, because the Cl$^-$-channel blockers are not entirely effective, it is necessary to demonstrate that the electrophysiological parameters measured are independent of external Cl$^-$.

As expected after injection of whole brain or heart mRNA from a rat into *Xenopus* oocytes, a variety of neurotransmitter receptors and ion channels are expressed. These include voltage-activated Na$^+$ and K$^+$ channels as well as the Ca^{2+} channels of interest (reviewed in Refs. 8 and 28). In order to reduce K$^+$ conductance to facilitate measurement of I_{Ba}, two strategies are useful. Oocytes can be exposed to incubation medium in which the K$^+$ had been replaced by Cs$^+$ for at least 24 hr before voltage clamping. This procedure reduces I_K, measured as the outward current at $+50$ mV in the presence of Cd$^+$, on average by 70% and in favorable cases by >95%. This lengthy pretreatment is a drawback, as is the slight Na$^+$ loading after exposure to K$^+$-free saline. On return to K$^+$-containing saline there is a significant Na/K pump-mediated hyperpolarization (21). The more usual way to block K$^+$ conductances is by replacement of external Na$^+$ with 20–50 mM tetraethylammonium and 5 mM 4-aminopyridine.

Complete Na$^+$ replacement has the added advantage that one does not need TTX to prevent voltage-dependent Na$^+$ currents. Otherwise, all Ba^{2+} currents should be measured in the presence of 1 μM TTX to block voltage-dependent Na$^+$ currents. Any remaining contaminating K$^+$ currents are isolated from Cd^{2+}-inhibitable Ba^{2+} current by subtracting currents recorded in the presence of 100 μM Cd^{2+} from prior records of total current. The Cd^{2+} subtraction method is satisfactory only when contaminating currents are small relative to I_{Ba} and will, of course, not eliminate currents activated by Ba^{2+} influx. Therefore, Cd^{2+} subtraction will not eliminate any ICl_{Ca} activated by barium.

Acknowledgments

I thank Terry P. Snutch of the University of British Columbia, Vancouver, British Columbia, Canada, for the RNA isolation protocols and numerous collaborations. I also thank my colleagues in the Henry Lester and Norman Davidson laboratories at Caltech, and in the Biology Department at The University of Illinois at Chicago. Work in the author's laboratory is supported by NIH Grant #NS 26432-01.

References

1. C. Aufray and F. Rougeon, *Eur. J. Biochem.* **107,** 303 (1980).
2. J. M. Chirgwin, A. E. Przybyla, R. J. MacDonald, and W. J. Rutter, *Biochemistry* **18,** 5294 (1979).
3. R. A. Cox, *in* "Methods in Enzymology" (L. Grossman and K. Moldave, eds.), Vol. 12, p. 120. Academic Press, New York, 1968.
4. A. M. Rose and T. P. Snutch, *Nature* (*London*) **311,** 485 (1984).
5. A. L. Brown, "The African Clawed Toad, *Xenopus laevis:* A Guide for Laboratory Practical Work," 140 pp. Butterworth, London, 1970.
6. A. Colman, *in* "Transcription and Translation: A Practical Approach" (B. D. Hames and S. J. Higgins, eds.), p. 271. IRL Press, Oxford, 1984.
7. L. D. Fricker, *Einstein Q. J. Biol. Med.* **6,** 36 (1988).
8. N. Dascal, *CRC Crit. Rev. Biochem.* **22,** 317 (1987).
9. J. N. Dumont, *J. Morphol.* **136,** 153 (1972).
10. C. Methfessel, V. Witzeman, T. Takahashi, M. Mishina, S. Numa, and B. Sakmann, *Pfluegers Arch.* **407,** 577 (1986).
11. J. P. Leonard, T. P. Snutch, H. Lübbert, N. Davidson, and H. A. Lester, *Biophys. J.* **49,** 386a (1986).
12. W. Stuhmer, C. Methfessel, B. Sakmann, M. Noda, and S. Numa, *Eur. Biophys. J.* **14,** 131 (1987).
13. J. R. Moorman, Z. Zhau, G. E. Kirsch, A. E. Lacerda, J. M. Caffrey, D. M. K. Lam, R. H. Joho, and A. M. Brown, *Am. J. Physiol.* **253,** H985 (1987).
14. D. S. Krafte, T. P. Snutch, J. P. Leonard, N. Davidson, and H. A. Lester, *J. Neurosci.* **8,** 2859 (1988).
15. V. J. Auld, A. L. Goldin, D. S. Krafte, J. Marshall, J. M. Dunn, W. A. Caterall, H. A. Lester, N. Davidson, and R. J. Dunn, *Neuron* **1,** 449 (1988).
16. O. P. Hamill, A. Marty, E. Neher, B. Sakmann, and F. J. Sigworth, *Pfluegers Arch.* **391,** 85 (1981).
17. K. Sumikawa, I. Parker, and R. Miledi, *Prog. Zool.* **33,** 127 (1986).
18. F. Guhary and F. Sachs, *J. Physiol.* (*London*) **352,** 685 (1984).
19. X. C. Yang and F. Sachs, *Biophys. J.* **53,** 412A (1988).
20. N. Dascal, T. P. Snutch, H. Lübbert, N. Davidson, and H. A. Lester, *Science* **213,** 1147 (1986).
21. J. P. Leonard, J. Nargeot, T. P. Snutch, N. Davidson, and H. A. Lester, *J. Neurosci.* **7,** 875 (1987).

22. T. P. Snutch, J. P. Leonard, J. Nargeot, H. Lübbert, N. Davidson, and H. A. Lester, *Soc. Gen. Physiol. Ser.* **42,** 154 (1987).
23. J. Umbach and C. Gundersen, *Proc. Natl. Acad. Sci. U.S.A.* **84,** 5464 (1987).
24. R. Miledi, *Proc. R. Soc. London B* **215,** 491 (1982).
25. M. E. Barish, *J. Physiol. (London)* **342,** 309 (1983).
26. E. Sigel and R. Baur, *Proc. Natl. Acad. Sci. U.S.A.* **85,** 6192 (1988).
27. R. Miledi and I. Parker, *J. Physiol. (London)* **357,** 173 (1984).
28. T. P. Snutch, *Trends NeuroSci. (Pers. Ed.)* **11,** 250 (1988).

Section II

In Situ and Solution Hybridization

[5] Quantification of *in Situ* Hybridization Histochemistry for Analysis of Brain Function

Charles R. Gerfen

Introduction

Applications of *in situ* hybridization histochemistry (ISHH) to localize the expression of messenger RNAs (mRNAs) in the brain has provided a relatively recent analytical method for studies in neuroscience (1, 2). Histochemical localization of mRNAs is accomplished by application to tissue sections of radioactively labeled probes that contain complementary DNA (or RNA) sequences to the mRNA that is to be localized. This technique complements immunohistochemical techniques for describing the organization of neural systems in terms of the complex repertoires of chemical phenotypes of which they are composed. Both techniques have specific merits, for example, immunohistochemical techniques provide morphological data about labeled cells, whereas the ISHH technique is localized only to the cell perikarya and so does not provide such information. On the other hand, ISHH does, in some instances, provide a more reliable means of determining the neurochemical capabilities of neurons. For example, in the striatum the distribution of certain opiate peptides in neurons could be inferred from immunohistochemical localization of the terminal distribution of these peptides, but a clear mapping of the cells of origin was difficult. ISHH techniques have provided a clear mapping of the striatal neurons expressing the mRNA for these peptides, which confirmed the inferred distribution (3). Immunohistochemical techniques, while extremely powerful for analysis of static conditions of the phenotypic expression of neurochemicals, have not been readily adapted for quantitative measure of changes in expression. There are a number of reasons contributing to this inadequacy related to the histochemical signal; i.e., the variability of the parameters of tissue fixation affect the antigenicity of the specific molecule that is to be localized. ISHH techniques offer many attributes that make quantitative assessment of changes in mRNA levels possible. This chapter provides a method by which ISHH may be used to analyze quantitatively changes in mRNA expression in individual cells in experiments that provide the means to determine how components of neural systems interact to alter the function of those neural systems.

The methodological approach described here involves four components. First is the basic oligonucleotide probe ISHH method, which is a straight adaptation of that described by Young *et al.* (2, 4). Second is a procedure for generating standards to measure known relative quantities of labeled mRNA expression. Third, image analysis techniques enable the relative quantities of mRNA expression localized with ISHH to be analyzed on an average per cell basis. Fourth is the design of the experiment to incorporate appropriate controls to serve as the basis for quantitating changes in mRNA expression across experimental conditions. Considerations of the ISHH technique that will not be covered in this chapter are related to the general basis and design of the ISHH methods themselves. Comprehensive reviews of these matters are provided elsewhere (5, 6).

Oligonucleotide Probes for ISHH

The methods described here use relatively short synthetic complementary DNA (cDNA) oligonucleotides as probes, which are labeled by the addition of [^{35}S]dATP tails. However, these methods could be easily adapted to the use of ribonucleotide probes as well. It is not within the scope of this chapter to compare in detail the two types of methods. While in theory the ribonucleotide probes offer greater sensitivity, the oligonucleotide ISHH technique has proved in practice to provide great sensitivity for localization of the mRNAs for most of the neurochemicals that we have examined. Substantive reviews of the rationale and verification of the reliability of this technique have been provided elsewhere. The basic rationale for using the oligonucleotide technique for quantitative analysis is 2-fold. First, by using synthetic cDNA oligonucleotides of a standard length, 48 bases, the conditions for the histochemical procedure may be applied in a standard fashion. Thus, parameters of the hybridization steps and wash conditions of this technique, which must be varied when probes of different lengths are used, may be kept constant. Second, the use of relatively short oligonucleotide probes provides the means of specifically localizing mRNAs that code for peptides or proteins that may have close sequence homology with other peptides or proteins. For example, many of the enzymes in the brain are members of families of enzymes that have common regions of sequence homology. Synthetic oligonucleotides, when selected for unique coding regions, allow the localization of specific isozymes, without the problems attending cross hybridization with mRNAs coding for related isozymes. The method for using oligonucleotide probes for ISHH has been detailed previously (2–4).

Tissue Preparation

Either unfixed or perfusion fixed brains may be used for this procedure. Unfixed brains are cut frozen in a cryostat to a thickness of 12 μm and adhered to glass slides that have been coated twice with gelatin. Sections are dried to the slide on a warm plate for 2 min and stored desiccated at $-20°$C until processed further. When processed further, the sections are first warmed to room temperature for 10 min, fixed in a 4% formaldehyde solution in phosphate-buffered saline (PBS) for 10 min, rinsed, and incubated in a fresh solution of 0.25% acetic anhydride in 0.1 M triethanolamine and 0.9% saline (pH 8.0) for 10 min. Next the slide-mounted sections are dehydrated in a series of ascending concentrations of ethanol and defatted for 2 × 5 min in chloroform, rehydrated, and air dried. These sections are then ready for the hybridization procedure.

Tailing Procedure

Purified oligonucleotides (48-base cDNAs) are stored at a concentration of 5 μM. These probes are end labeled for hybridization with the following protocol.

1. React the following mixture at 37°C for 5 min:
   Distilled water   29.6 μl
   Oligonucleotide (5 μM)   1 μl
   5× tailing buffer   10 μl
   [^{35}S]dATP   About 5 μl
      (final concentration is 1 μM of 1350 Ci/mM [^{35}S]dATP)
   Terminal deoxynucleotidyltransferase: (20 U/μl, Bethesda Research Labs, MD)   5 μl
2. Stop reaction with addition of 1 μl tRNA and 400 μl Tris–EDTA (TE).
3. Extract with phenol/chloroform/isoamyl alcohol (IAA) (50 : 49 : 1) and save aqueous phase.
4. Extract with chloroform/IAA and save aqueous phase.
5. Add 0.05 vol of 4 M NaCl and 1 ml ethanol and allow to cool in dry ice for 30 min.
6. Spin mixture slush for 30 min at 4°C to pellet tailed oligonucleotide.
7. Wash pellet with ice-cold ethanol, draw off all liquid, and resuspend in 50 μl TE.
8. Count the disintegrations per minute (dpm) of 1 μl (generally dpm are on the order of 1,000,000–2,000,000/μl).

The tailing procedure adds a poly(dATP) tail of approximately 15–25 bases in length. The tail length is checked by polyacrylamide gel electrophoresis.

Hybridization

Tailed probes are added to the following hybridization buffer to reach a concentration of 1,000,000 dpm per 25 μl of buffer (25 μl of buffer is the volume added to each rat brain section).

Hybridization buffer
4× SSC (1× SSC = 150 mM NaCl/15 mM sodium citrate, pH 7.2)
50% formamide
0.02% Ficoll
0.02% 360K poly(vinylpyrrolidone) (360 kDa)
0.02% bovine serum albumin
250 μg/ml yeast tRNA and 500 μg/ml single-stranded salmon DNA
10% dextran (500 kDa)
100 mM dithiothreitol (DTT, added just prior to hybridization)

The hybridization buffer may be made up as a stock solution and stored at −20°C until used.

Labeled probes are added to the hybridization buffer and then added to the slide-mounted prepared brain sections in a volume of 25 μl per section which are then covered with Parafilm and incubated at 37°C for 18 hr. After this incubation the Parafilm coverslips are floated off in 1× SSC and the slide-mounted sections rinsed in three washes of 1× SSC. The slides are then washed four times for 15 min each in 2× SSC and 50% formamide, followed by two 30-min washes in 1× SSC and a brief water rinse before the sections are rapidly dried. The slide are then dipped in NTB emulsion (diluted 1:1 with water) and exposed for 4–12 weeks, after which they are developed in D-19 developer for 2 min, fixed, rinsed, counterstained with thionin, dehydrated, and coverslipped out of xylene.

Standards for ISHH

Standards for ISHH are generated by diluting [^{35}S]dATP-tailed oligonucleotide probes with nonradioactive dATP-tailed oligonucleotides. For each oligonucleotide used in a given experiment, two end-labeling tailing reactions are run in tandem, using identical reagents but containing equimolar concentrations of [^{35}S]dATP and nonradioactive dATP, respectively. It is assumed that if all the parameters of the reaction have been kept constant, the two reactions will generate similar length tails added to the oligonucleotides, which may be checked by running the products of the reactions on gels to determine the length of the tails. Standards are then generated by combining the products of the two tailing reactions in ratios that produce probes that contain 0, 25, 50, 75, and 100% radioactive tailed probe diluted with unlabeled probe to keep the total molar ratio of probe constant for each hybridization. These mixtures of equimolar concentrations of probes are added to the hybridization buffer and applied to sections that serve as standards for each experiment. The experimental sections are hybridized with the normal concentration of probes containing 100% radioactive tails. The hybridization and subsequent processing of the tissue is done concurrently to sections containing the standards and the experimental probes.

This procedure for the generation of standards is used for the following reasons. First, standards for quantitative measure are required to be able to assign relative quantities of generated silver grains to varying amounts of radioactive probe. Simple standards that contain varying amounts of radioactivity applied to glass slides may accomplish this goal. However, these do not control the parameters of hybridization of the probes in tissue, such as the penetration of the probes into the tissue, and the dynamics of diffusion of the probes and radioactive emission particles out of the tissue. Second, it is preferable to use standards in which the molar concentration of oligonucleotide is the same as that used for the experimental hybridization. This rationale controls for the possibility that the concentration of oligonucleotide in the hybridization reaction may affect the amount of subsequent ISHH labeling. Thus, this procedure is theoretically superior to that in which varying concentrations of radioactive oligonucleotides (in increasing molar concentrations) are added to generate standards. Third, the standards measure relative labeling that occurs in individual cells. This is an important consideration in that, with the application of image analysis routines described below, it is possible to determine relative changes in mRNA expression on an average per cell basis.

Figure 1 shows individual neurons from sections labeled with a cDNA probe complementary to the messenger RNA for rat enkephalin that contained 25% (Fig. 1A), 50% (Fig. 1B), 75% (Fig. 1C), and 100% (Fig. 1D) radioactive probes. There is a linear relationship in the average numbers of grains per labeled cell and the amount of radioactivity in the probe standards used (see below).

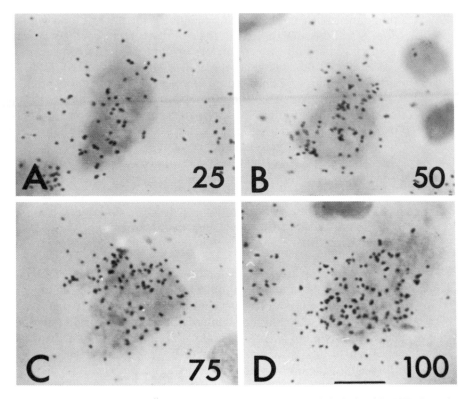

FIG. 1   Computer display of neurons that have been labeled with ISHH probe standards containing varying concentrations of radioactivity at a magnification (original: ×400) that displays individual grains. The ratios of radioactive to nonradioactive probe applied to sections from which these neurons were located are (A) 25 : 75%, (B) 50 : 50%, (C) 75 : 25%, (D) 100 : 0%. Bar, 10 μm.

Image Analysis of ISHH

With the generation of standards as described above it is possible to use the ISHH method to measure changes in relative expression of mRNA following functional changes in neuronal systems. Obtaining the full utility of this procedure requires not only that the standards provide a means of equating the density of label produced in the tissue to the amount of radioactivity applied in each probe standard, but also the determination that the same number of cells are labeled across the range of standard probes used. This type of analysis provides information concerning whether changes in the amount of mRNA expression as measured with ISHH occur as a result of a change in the number of cells expressing a given mRNA or as a change in the amount of expression per cell.

The ability to quantify ISHH at the cellular level depends on two processes. First, the ability to relate a measure of the number of grains generated in individual cells to the standards. Second, the ability to detect cells that contain varying amounts of label as labeled cells. While this is a straightforward proposition, in practice it is rather difficult to program a computer to detect cells that are densely labeled and those that contain only 25% of that label both as labeled objects. One factor is the magnification that one is willing to work with. At relatively high magnification, for example, at a magnification that shows one to five cells per field, it is possible to count the number of grains over each cell. At this magnification the image analysis problem is relatively trivial. However, to optimize the utility of the ISHH technique for quantitative analysis working at high magnification is cumbersome. For this reason, a microscopic magnification has been chosen that allows the analysis of a field of some 200 cells. At this magnification, individual silver grains may not be resolved, rather the density of the aggregate of silver grains over a given cell visualized with dark-field illumination (measured as transmission) is used as the measure of label. With the calibration routines described below, it is possible to correlate transmission levels measured per cell at a relatively low magnification to actual grains per cell.

From an image analysis point of view, the task of quantifying ISHH label is broken into three parts. (1) The total number of neurons in a field is counted. (2) The total number of labeled cells, regardless of their level of label, is counted. (3) The relative density of label per labeled cell is determined. To accomplish these tasks with an image analysis system requires the ability to modify the original digitized images into a form from which the appropriate data may be extracted and to be able to redirect sampling of that data from three aligned images. The routines used for these procedures will be discussed below. The image analysis system used in these studies was developed by Loats Associates, Inc. (LAI, Westminister, MD). This system utilizes a Dage nuvicom video camera that produces a digitized image with 256×256 pixel resolution. Additional features of this system are the ability to compose strings of image modification routines into macros that are used to modify an image into one that may be analyzed for both object numbers and density of label. Sampling routines give the ability to analyze matched areas from three separate images simultaneously (redirected analysis). While the LAI system is specifically designed to accomplish these tasks, other image analysis systems contain most of the requisite functions to enable this analysis.

Image Capture

Sections are prepared as described above, with Nissl staining of cell bodies. Each area to be analyzed is digitized twice, once in bright-field for the Nissl staining and a second time in dark-field for the ISHH labeling. The contrast and lighting parameters are optimized for the particular lighting to obtain the widest range of gray scales for each. These parameters, once established, are used throughout the digitizations for a single experiment, which holds constant the lighting to enable the relative intensity of label from separate brains to be analyzed. It is important that the bright-field and dark-field digitization of a sampled area be done without moving the sample relative to the camera; thus the two images remain aligned for the subsequent analysis routines. In the description below, the calibration of dark-field transmission levels as a measure of label per cell is discussed first, and then the image analysis requirements for cell counting are discussed.

Calibration of ISHH Standards

As an example, we have analyzed the expression of enkephalin messenger RNA in the striatum of normal adult rats. The probe used in this experiment is a 48-oligonucleotide-long cDNA probe that is complementary to the messenger RNA for rat enkephalin. To adjacent brain sections through the striatum the tailed probe is added in equimolar concentrations, which contain ^{35}S- and cold-tailed probes in ratios of 100:0, 75:25, 50:50, and 25:75 ([^{35}S]dATP-tailed oligo:cold dATP-tailed oligo). Before application of the probe standards, the dpm of the mixtures are measured to determine if the proper ratios of radioactive and cold probes have been mixed. Areas from the same region of adjacent sections that have been hybridized with the different dilution standards are used for image analysis quantification. For the purposes of analysis of the level of label per cell, the only image modification that is done to the dark-field image (from which transmission levels are used as a measure of label) is to threshold the image to display only that part of the image that is produced by the silver grains. For the purposes of quantification it is essential that the same threshold is used for all images.

The first stage of image analysis involves calibrating the analysis routines to correlate the actual number of grains per cell with the level of light transmission per cell measured at low microscopic magnification. This calibration procedure is perhaps the most crucial in the quantification procedure because it establishes the limits of resolution for measuring relative differences in mRNA expression per cell. In order to eliminate several sources of error that may result from image modification routines, much of the calibration routine demands manual counting. First, five areas from comparable regions of the striatum of five animals for each standard level (25, 50, 75, and 100%) are digitized at a microscopic magnification of ×100, which is a field containing approximately 200 neurons. For each of these regions, each of the labeled neurons is then examined at a magnification of ×400, which allows the individual grains to be counted. The grains counted manually for each neuron at high magnification are then charted against the integrated transmission level for each neuron (the sum of transmission for the pixels over each neuron) measured at ×100 magnification with dark-field illumination. Figure 2 shows a photograph of the image

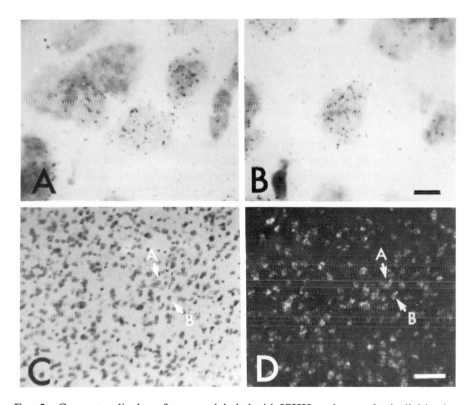

FIG. 2   Computer display of neurons labeled with ISHH probe standards digitized at high magnification (A and B) and at low magnification (×100) under bright-field (C) and dark-field (D) illumination. Grains over cells (three cells in A and one in B) are counted at high magnification and located at low magnification (C and D). Integrated transmission levels (sum of transmission/cell) are determined for each cell by selecting the cell in D. Bars, 10 μm for A and B and 100 μm for C and D.

analysis screen in which neurons at ×400 are displayed (Fig. 2A and B). At this magnification each grain over the labeled cells is counted manually. These neurons are then located in the field at ×100 magnification (Fig. 2C), and the transmission for each cell measured under dark-field illumination (Fig. 2D). First, there is a linear relation between the average number of grains per cell and the percentage of radioactivity in the applied standard probes (see Fig. 5). Figure 3 provides a graph of the number of grains per cell versus the integrated transmission per cell measured at low magnification for 40 cells for each standard (25, 50, 75, and 100%). As can be seen from Fig. 3, the relationship is nonlinear. For the standards used, the relationship between transmission and grain number is best fit with a second-order polynomial equation.

This exercise, though extremely tedious, provides the means of determining the confidence level for measuring relative expression of mRNA in a population of neurons. Several points should be stressed. (1) The calibration curve generated is then used as a means of determining the average relative label per cell. Thus, it is essential that the standards used encompass the widest range of label per cell for each experiment. If an experiment is analyzed in which a particular treatment results in a marked increase in label per cell, then the standards must be applied to sections from that animal. (2) This exercise demonstrates that, for a given probe standard, not every labeled cell contains the same number of grains. This is to be expected due to the variance in the amount of messenger RNA expressed in a population of neurons and the variation that arises from the ISHH method itself. The calibration routine provides a means of determining that variance. (3) It is important to stress the nonlinear relationship between grains per cell and measured transmission. This is to be expected as a consequence of the nature of the light reflectance that is generated from grains that are concentrated over individual neurons. As the number of grains per cell increases, reflectance from groups of grains begin to cancel each other such that the relationship between measured transmission and grain number is nonlinear. This finding also suggests that other means of producing standards for ISHH that rely on the relationship between known amounts of radioactivity applied to sections and grains may produce an error in analysis. Such a procedure may be well suited to studies using autoradiography to analyze receptor binding in brain sections in which the receptor-binding sites are more homogeneously distributed in tissue. Even with receptor-binding techniques, the problem of saturation (in which light transmission is produced by densely packed silver grains), may be a problem. However, for the case of ISHH in which the label is generated over discrete cells, which are analogous to discrete objects, the problem of saturation may be enhanced. For instance, cells that are very densely labeled show a rim of

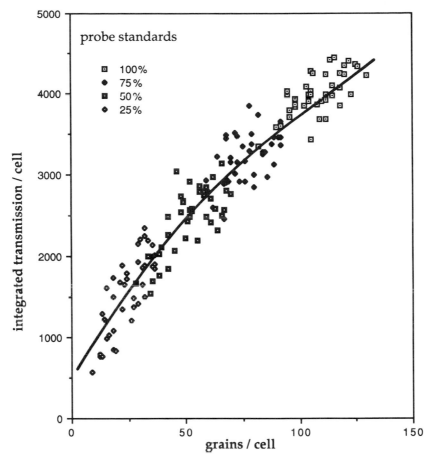

FIG. 3   Graph showing the relationship between the number of ISHH-generated grains per cell (counted manually at high magnification) and integrated transmission per cell (measured at low magnification as shown in Fig. 2) for 40 cells each from striatal sections to which had been applied probe standards containing ratios of radioactive : nonradioactive probes of 100 : 0 (100%), 75 : 25 (75%), 50 : 50 (50%), and 25 : 75 (25%). The curve fit for this distribution is a second-order polynomial with the equation: integrated transmission = 549 + 43.6 − 0.11 (grain number)^2 ($R = 0.96$).

bright labeling surrounding a dark center, in which the reflectance of grains in the center is canceled. In the examples used for this chapter, the exposure times for autoradiography were such that the labeling produced with the 100% standard was less than that which is often encountered. Thus, the nonlinearity of the curve shown in Fig. 3 is actually less than that which may be encountered if cells are heavily labeled. The method for generation of standards and the analysis of labeling produced by those standards described here provides a means of measuring the relationship between relative amounts of detectable mRNA expression and the histochemical label generated. Additionally, it allows the experimenter to determine, and thus avoid, ISHH conditions that would lead to saturation of label in sections.

Counting Labeled Cells with Image Modification

The second part of procedures to quantify ISHH for analysis of average changes in mRNA levels per cell can be done in one of two ways. The most straightforward means is to count the number of grains per cell and to establish a background level, under which cells are determined to be unlabeled. However, this procedure is cumbersome and limits the utility of the method for analysis. A second method is to utilize image analysis procedures of relatively low-magnification images. Again, the magnification that has been chosen, ×100, provides the ability to analyze a field of some 200 neurons (in the striatum). It is not within the scope of this chapter to provide an overly detailed description of the analysis routines that may be applied. Detailed descriptions of image analysis processes may be found elsewhere (7). Such routines are dependent on the specific image analysis system that one has available. Rather, a short description of the strategy that may be used is provided.

Image analysis provides a means of quantifying histochemically stained sections because each point of the digitized image (each pixel) is encoded with a value of light transmission (or a related function such as optical density, which is an inverse logarithmic function of transmission). The functions of an image analysis program provide procedures for manipulating the transmission values of each pixel in such a way as to allow groups of pixels to be counted as definable objects and also to measure the relative transmission of definable objects. A string of sequential image modification operations, termed a macro, may be designed to transform the original digitized images into a form that may then be analyzed by the computer to extract the desired data. There are two basic types of modification routines.

One type applies modification algorithms directly to the image. Among these are routines that increase edge detection (increase contrast) and smooth an image (reduce contrast). These routines operate by a process called kernal convolution. Kernals are a matrix of either 3×3 or 5×5 (or more) pixels in which each pixel is weighted and averaged with the other kernal pixels. Kernal convolution operates by applying such matrices to each of the pixels in the image and reassigning the value generated by the kernal to each pixel. For example, using a smooth kernal, each pixel is reassigned by an equal averaging of its surrounding pixels, which serves to reduce the difference between adjacent pixels of differing value.

Another type of modification routine includes processes that are applied to a histogram of the transmission levels of an image. Such histograms display the numbers of pixels for each transmission level. Typically, transmission levels between 0 and 255 are displayed on the x-axis of the histogram and the number of pixels at each level displayed on the y-axis. Procedures may then be applied directly to the histogram, which then alter the image accordingly. A simple procedure is to multiply the histogram by a number. For example, if the histogram is multiplied by 2, then the value of each pixel in the image acquires a new value that is twice as large as the original, which is reflected in the histogram as a spreading out of the bins for each transmission value (the bin containing the number of pixels with a transmission value of 10 is moved to a transmission level of 20). Another use of this type of procedure is the generation of binary images in which all pixels falling within set boundaries of transmission levels (a process called thresholding) are assigned a value of one and all pixels falling outside these boundaries are assigned a zero value. Such binary images may be manipulated in special ways. For example, two binary images may be added or subtracted together to generate a third binary image. Binary images may also be modified with routines that allow objects of certain sizes to be saved and others to be eliminated.

Stringing together sequences of modification functions allows the original images to be transformed according to the type of information that is required. This is dependent on the manner in which the image analysis system is able to extract data. For example, in the system that we use, the system is able to count objects if the objects are of a certain minimal size and separated from adjoining objects. The construction of specific image modification macro routines is dependent on the original image, and the type of data that is to be extracted. For the purposes of developing a proper routine, it is necessary to check the process against data obtained by visually analyzing the original tissue. An important note is that a strategy has been chosen that applies image modification macros to images without the necessity of experimenter mediation, once the routine has been set. This is necessary for quantitative analysis from many images, in that if a procedure required the modification to be altered, even slightly, for each image it would negate the possibility of such analysis. The specific capabilities of each image analysis system dictate the type of strategy that is used for image modification.

Bright-Field Modification

A macro modification procedure is used to transform an original bright-field image of a field of Nissl-stained cells into an image from which the computer can count the number of neurons in that field. The strategy of this procedure is based on the characteristics of Nissl staining of brain sections. Glia are small (less than 10–15 μm diameter) intensely stained (dark) cells. Neurons are generally larger and less intensely stained (lighter) owing to the larger volume of the cells. The strategy for counting neurons with image analysis takes advantage of both the size disparity between neurons and glia and the relative intensity of staining. Modification routines are established that allow an image of Nissl-stained cells to be transformed into one that eliminates glia based on their size and density of label but retains neurons, and separates them into countable objects. Useful modification procedures used in these routines include contrast enhancement, to separate cells, and the generation of binary images, which are used to eliminate small cells (glia) and used as a template for later dark-field modification.

Dark-Field Modification

Modification of the dark-field image, which displays the grains as light dots (high transmission levels), is straightforward. The modification of this image for quantification of intensity of label is accomplished with a thresholding procedure (described above for the calibration procedure). The dark-field image is also modified to generate an image in which labeled versus unlabeled neurons are displayed. Modification procedures used for this procedure first smooth the grains over a local area, and then use the binary image created for the generation of neuron objects as a mask. The rationale for this strategy is that grains will be localized over neurons that are identified with the bright-field modification and, due to scatter produced by the emission of the radioactive nuclide, over a small domain outside the neuron object field. Smoothing the image averages grains both directly over and outside the domain of labeled neurons, and using the bright-field mask not only regenerates the actual shape of the labeled neurons but identifies labeled cells. These routines must be checked visually to determine if the modified images identify the appropriate histochemical features.

Quantify Procedures

Modification macros are applied to sets of ISHH images from an experiment. In this case, the sections are from normal adult rat striatum, to which had been applied the probe standards. It is important to stress that the macro routines are applied to each set of ISHH images in the same way so that the parameters of modification are identical for each set. This generates a new set of images which include the modified bright-field image, "neurons" and the modified dark-field image, "labeled neurons." Figure 4 shows bright-field and dark-field images that have been modified to produce images of discrete objects that may be counted by the computer as cells. In the quantify part of the procedure four images are displayed (see Fig. 6). The first image is a template on which areas are selected for measurement. The

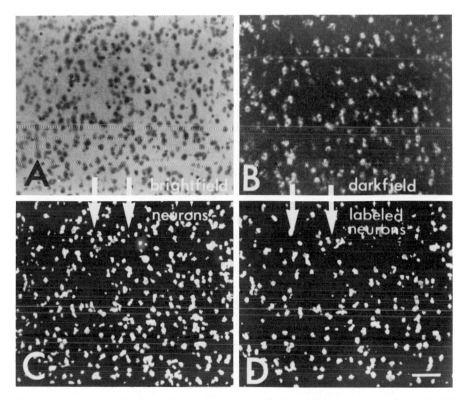

FIG. 4 Computer display showing an area of the striatum counterstained with thionin (Nissl stain) and containing ISHH labeling for enkephalin mRNA digitized at low magnification (×100) under bright-field (A) and dark-field (B) illumination. These images were then subject to the image modification routines described in the text to generate modified images displaying all Nissl-stained neurons (C, neurons) and ISHH-labeled neurons (D, labeled neurons). These images are of the type that are used in the quantify routines. It can be noted that small dark objects in A, which are stained glia, are eliminated from the modified neuron image in C. Bar, 100 μm.

second image is the modified bright-field image "neurons" from which are counted the total numbers of neurons that are in the area selected. The third image is the modified dark-field image "labeled neurons" from which are counted the number of neurons that contain ISHH-generated label. The fourth image is the original dark-field image of the ISHH grains, which after thresholding to select only that portion of the image that contains grains, is used to generate the relative intensity of label in labeled cells. The values that are used in this function may be determined by the experimenter, but typically are integrated transmission values, which sum the transmission values for all the pixels in the selection area.

There are several notes concerning the method of quantification by the image analysis system. First, the method of quantification is termed redirection, in that the same area selected in the template is selected in each of the second, third, and fourth images. Second, the portion of each displayed image that is subject to quantification may be selected using a threshold function, similar to that described above for generating binary images. For the modified "neurons" and "labeled cells" images the entire image is selected. For the fourth image containing grains, a threshold is set that selects only those transmission levels for the dark-field display of grains. This threshold, once set, is then used for all images in a given experiment. Third, the image analysis system has an algorithm that counts objects based on their size; small objects of a selected size may be ignored. Additionally, merged objects may in some cases be counted as discrete objects if the parameters of the counting algorithm are able to detect distinct inflection points as it traces around the perimeter of an object. However, in some instances, this algorithm is not able to break down complex objects sufficiently. This must be recognized as a potential source of error; however, with careful comparison with the original image, it may be estimated how large this error is. In the case of the images that we have prepared this error is less than 5%.

The modification procedures described above are used to convert the digitized images from which are counted the total number of neurons in each area, the number of neruons that contain detectable amounts of label, and the relative amount of transmission (density of label) per labeled cell. Using these procedures, the percentage of labeled cells per field is determined, as is the average transmission level per cell. This latter number may be correlated with the numbers of grains per cell according to the above described routine. Figure 5 shows a graphing of the average percentage of labeled cells obtained for each probe standard, the average number of grains per cell, and the average transmission level per cell. Using the standards for analyzing enkephalin mRNA expression in the striatum it is determined that the image analysis system is able to detect cells over a 4-fold range as

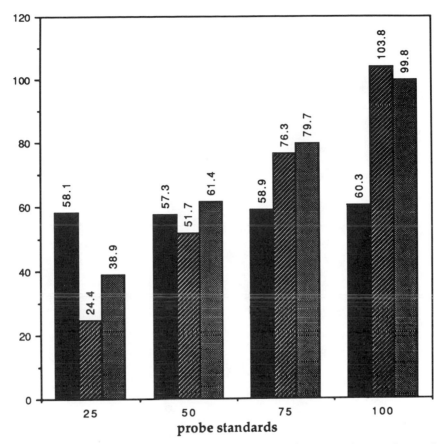

FIG. 5   Graph comparing averages of the percentage of neurons that are detected to contain ISHH-generated label [percentage labeled cells (■)], the number of manually counted grains per labeled cell [average grains per cell (▨)], and the integrated transmission per labeled cell (▦) measured at low magnification from adjacent sections to which had been applied probe standards containing 25, 50, 75, and 100% radioactive probe standards. These data are derived from 10 sample areas for each probe standard. The percentage of detectable labeled neurons does not vary significantly across the four probe standards, the average number of grains per cell varies in a linear manner over the range of probe standards, whereas the integrated transmission per cell varies in a nonlinear manner.

containing label. Importantly, as discussed above, while the average number of grains per cell is related linearly to the amount of radioactivity in the probe standards, the measure of average integrated transmission per cell is nonlinear.

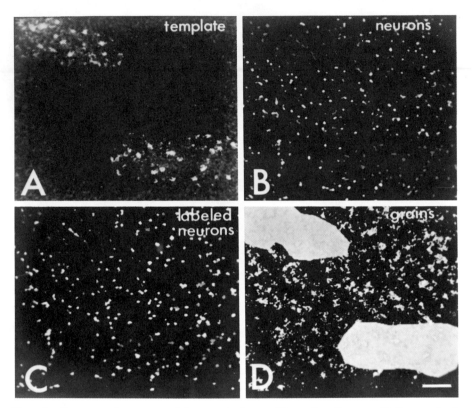

FIG. 6   Computer images used for a typical quantify routine for quantitative analysis of ISHH. In this example, the template image displays μ-opiate receptor binding in the striatum (A, template), which is from the matched area in a section adjacent to one in which enkephalin mRNA has been localized. The ISHH-labeled section was first digitized in bright-field, whose image was modified to display Nissl-stained neurons (B, neurons), and then digitized in dark-field, whose image was modified to display enkephalin mRNA labeled neurons (C, labeled neurons), and thresholded, whose image was modified to display ISHH-generated grains (D, grains). In this example, two μ-opiate receptor-rich patch areas had been selected in the template image, and the quantify routines counted the total number of neurons from B, the number of labeled neurons in C, and determined the sum of the integrated transmission levels for the labeled cells in the selected regions in D. Objects marked in two patches in A are redirected neurons, labeled neurons, and grains from the selected regions of B, C, and D, respectively. Bar, 100 μm.

For the purposes of providing an example of calibrating the image analysis system for measurements of average relative label per cell, the quantify redirected sampling routine selected the entire image as a template for sampling. Other sampling methods may be applied. Figure 6 shows a matched set of images in which the template (Fig. 6A) is a matched image displaying μ-opiate receptor binding in patches in the striatum. In this set of images, the modified image containing neurons is displayed in Fig. 6B, the modified image containing ISHH-labeled enkephalin neurons is displayed in Fig. 6C, and the thresholded dark-field image containing ISHH-generated grains is displayed in Fig. 6D. In Fig. 6, the two opiate receptor patches have been selected and the number of neurons, the number of labeled neurons, and the integrated transmission of grains have been counted.

Acknowledgments

Dr. Mike Brownstein generously supplied the oligonucleotide probes used in our ISHH studies and Dr. Scott Young provided valuable discussions of the strategies to be used for quantifying ISHH.

References

1. C. E. Gee, C. -L. C. Chen, J. L. Roberts, R. Thompson, and S. J. Watson, *Nature (London)* **306,** 374 (1983).
2. W. S. Young III, E. Mezey, and R. E. Siegel, *Neurosci. Lett.* **70,** 198 (1986).
3. C. R. Gerfen and W. S. Young, *Brain Res.* **460,** 161 (1988).
4. W. S. Young III, T. I. Bonner, and M. R. Brann, *Proc. Natl. Acad. Sci. U.S.A.* **83,** 9827 (1986).
5. K. L. Valentino, J. H. Eberwine, and J. D. Barchas (eds.), *In Situ* Hybridization: Applications to Neurobiology." Oxford Univ. Press, London and New York, 1987.
6. G. R. Uhl (ed.), "*In Situ* Hybridization in Brain." Plenum, New York, 1986.
7. H. L. Loats, D. G. Lloyd, M. Pittenger, R. W. Tucker, and J. R. Unnerstall, *in* "Imaging Techniques in Biology and Medicine" (C. E. Swenberg and J. J. Conklin, eds.), p. 1. Academic Press, San Diego, California, 1988.

[6]   *In Situ* Hybridization: A Methodological Guide

Joseph T. McCabe and Donald W. Pfaff

Introduction: Basic Principles

This chapter summarizes the most important procedural steps of the *in situ* hybridization histochemical technique for localization of specific mRNA molecules at the single-cell level. It derives from work with double-stranded, complementary DNA (cDNA) probes radiolabeled by nick translation, work with polymerase-labeled single-stranded RNA probes, and work with oligonucleotides, i.e., short, single-stranded DNA molecules. The specific methodological steps which are outlined here will generate a strong label over the appropriate cell types and preserve tissue integrity. A collection of recent publications will convince the investigator that the individual methodological steps for *in situ* hybridization (1, 2) have been continually changed and, at times, rediscovered. To the neuroscientist not familiar with this technique, therefore, this detailed protocol is provided to describe specifics of the procedure that are often left out of other publications and to provide some rationale for the specific steps.

The first section will outline the complete procedures for work with cDNA probes, RNA probes (riboprobes), and oligonucleotides. Later sections discuss control procedures for validation, and briefly, the use of the hybridization technique in combination with other histochemical methods. Finally, the *Appendix* describes in detail how various solutions and buffers are prepared and lists needed reagents and equipment.

Laboratory Environment

For *in situ* hybridization, clean, safe, and consistent laboratory practices are essential for minimizing exposure to hazardous materials (radioisotopes, organic and flammable solvents, tissue fixatives) as well as for maximizing the chances of producing clean autoradiograms. In particular, one must be wary of conditions that will destroy the unique target of *in situ* hybridization: cellular RNA. The most common source of tissue mRNA degradation, and consequent diminution of identifiable signal, is the ribonucleases (RNases). RNase contamination from equipment, solutions, or from the investigator

Methods in Neurosciences, Volume 1

must be scrupulously avoided by the following precautions. All solutions are prepared with *autoclaved, nanopure-distilled* water. All glassware, microfuge tubes, and pipette tips are autoclaved, and consumable supplies and reagents are kept exclusively for *in situ* hybridization. Disposable gloves should be worn during all procedures since the mRNA in tissue samples may be degraded by RNase on your skin. For further discussion, see Blumberg's review (3).

Tissue Preparation

For cryostat-cut material, stronger labeling more frequently appears to result from the use of fresh-frozen tissue, compared with preparation of tissue by perfusion (4–6). If *in situ* hybridization will not be used for other histochemical procedures, such as immunocytochemistry which requires perfusion fixation, the use of fresh tissue is recommended in the initial trials.

Proper tissue freezing is an important first step. The block must be quickly frozen without cracking the block or distorting its shape. Two procedures can be used for tissue freezing and for tissue storage. First, we customarily freeze single blocks of tissue for storage in 100-ml glass beakers in liquid nitrogen by wrapping each block in aluminum foil. A water-resistant marker (Sanford Sharpie permanent fine-point marker # 30001; Sanford Corp., Bellwood, IL) is used to label the aluminum foil. After the marker ink has dried, it will remain on the foil even after freezing and thawing (the black marker is the most permanent), and this enables the investigator to store many different samples in a single beaker. The marking is placed twice on the foil to ensure at least one legible record. When the animal becomes unresponsive to paw pinch after administration of anesthesia (sodium pentobarbital, 60 mg/kg body weight), the animal is decapitated and the brain is quickly removed from the skull on a chilled petri dish (place the dish on top of water ice). The brain is blocked with a new, clean, razor blade. New razor blades are coated with oil, and hence should be washed with soap, and then thoroughly rinsed. When possible, it is useful to work with small blocks of tissue. Not only are they easier to section on a cryostat, but they should increase the speed at which you freeze the entire tissue block.

If the blocks are to be stored for a long time period, the blocks are gently placed on top of the piece of aluminum foil in which it will be wrapped. The foil is placed level, atop crushed dry ice. While holding the tissue sample between clean forceps, place the tissue block onto the foil while taking care not to distort the anatomical configuration of the block. As the block freezes, evident by the whiteness of the tissue, loose crushed dry ice is placed around the block to fully freeze the tissue. After 5 min, the dry ice is gently brushed away from the tissue block and foil, and the block is carefully wrapped in the foil. It is convenient to have the foil so labeled that one can easily identify the tissue block. At no time should the tissue be allowed to warm: surround and immerse the wrapped block in crushed dry ice until it is placed in liquid nitrogen.

If one is to immediately use a tissue sample, it is often easier to mount the block directly onto a cryostat chuck. Before killing the animal, the chuck should be prepared: a layer of water-soaked Gelfoam (Upjohn Company, Kalamazoo, MI) is frozen to the chuck, and a thin layer of water is frozen over the Gelfoam to form a flat platform of ice by placing the chuck on a flat bed of powdered (finely crushed) dry ice. The tissue can be attached to the chuck/Gelfoam/water platform (which is already frozen) by placing a few additional drops of water on the platform, putting the base of the brain into the water, and allowing the water to freeze. As soon as the base of the brain has frozen to the platform (that is, the base of the brain is anchored in ice—do not freeze the entire brain), immediately begin to steadily surround the tissue with finely powdered dry ice. Allow the brain to freeze for about 30 min with dry ice and place in the cryostat.

An *alternative* to the "dry ice method" just outlined is to use Freon (chlorodifluoromethane) (7). While this method is more complicated, it avoids the potential for freeze–thawing of the perimeter of the tissue. The purpose of this procedure is to preserve tissue morphology by rapidly cooling the tissue. The cooling rate of Freon (in °C/sec) is orders of magnitude greater than that of liquid nitrogen. Therefore, freezing the brain directly in liquid nitrogen is not advisable. The rapid cooling rate by Freon greatly reduces the formation of large ice crystals (7), and thus avoids disruption of an intracellular matrix that helps to hold mRNA in place.

After removing the brain from the skull, one can either place it directly into foil or freeze it onto a Gelfoam/water platform and then on a chuck. Before placing the brain on a labeled piece of foil, shape the foil to form a "pocket" in which to seat the tissue block, and pierce the bottom of the pocket so that Freon can enter the foil through the bottom. Slowly submerge the unfrozen brain (with or without a chuck) into a beaker containing rapidly stirring liquid Freon that is chilled by liquid nitrogen. That is, place the beaker of Freon into a vacuum flask or other insulated container that is partially filled with liquid nitrogen. The purpose of placing the Freon beaker into a bath of liquid nitrogen is to lower the temperature of the Freon further (but not to the point that the Freon begins to freeze). The beaker containing the Freon also contains a stir-bar (VWR Type 58948-251) and the Freon is stirred (on a Magnetstir, Ace Scientific 22-2475) so that the Freon is swirling about in the beaker. The purpose of stirring the Freon is to increase substantially the cooling rate of the tissue by rapidly removing warmer

Freon away from the brain surface and allowing unwarmed Freon to constantly contact the brain surface (7). Note that the brain and chuck are not plunged into the Freon. That is, use long metal thongs to hold the chuck and slowly lower the chuck into the Freon. Closely watch that the tissue is freezing just ahead of when it is actually submerged in the Freon by observing the "whiteness" of the tissue migrate up the tissue. After the tissue has been carefully lowered into the Freon, suspend it there for approximately 1 min. Then, remove the chuck from the Freon and briefly blot it on tissue paper. Slowly submerge the chuck into a second beaker filled with liquid nitrogen.

Perfused and Embedded Tissue

Animals are anesthetized by intraperitoneal injection of 60 mg/kg sodium pentobarbital (e.g., Nembutal, Abbott Laboratories, North Chicago, IL). The chest cavity is opened to expose the heart, 0.5 cm^3 of heparin is delivered transcardially, and the animal is then perfused with 100 mM phosphate-buffered saline (PBS; see preparation in *Appendix*) until blood clears from the perfusate, and then with 4% paraformaldehyde in 100 mM PBS (see *Appendix*). The brain is removed from the skull, blocked, and placed in 15 or 30% sucrose (w/v) 100 mM PBS overnight. The tissue block is then frozen as described earlier. An extensive perfusion, which often was found essential for other histochemical procedures (or when combining *in situ* hybridization with immunocytochemistry or tract-tracing), can result in "overfixation" that reduces probe access to tissue RNA. This may then require the use of deproteinization or acid-treatment steps, which partially compromises membrane integrity but allows tissue mRNA to hybridize with the probe. Finally, it may be that perfusion and fixation with higher salt molarities (>100 mM) in PBS solutions are beneficial for RNA retention. Several recent publications outline protocols for the use of paraffin- and plastic-embedded tissue (8–10).

Tissue Sectioning

Sections (6–10 μm) are cut on a cryostat at −20 to −24°C (Bright cryostat, Hacker Instruments, Fairfield, NJ) and mounted directly from the knife onto chrome–alum-subbed microscope slides. Slides are not autoclaved, but you may want to include 0.02% diethyl pyrocarbonate in the chrome–alum solution (see *Appendix*). Some investigators report lower background and/or better tissue adherence with poly(L-lysine)-coated slides (11), but due to the positive charge of lysine, one will have to include an acetylation step (see below). At lower temperatures (<50°C) chrome–alum-coated slides may be adequate since the slides appear cleaner compared with poly(L-lysine)-coated slides. However, gel-coated slides will be problematic at higher temperatures that melt the gel and detach the tissue. If you are not using fresh-frozen tissue, and the tissue was perfused with a high-salt solution and/or is sucrose cryoprotected, tissue will cut better at lower temperatures (−25 to −30°C). However, you will have to experiment to actually find what cryostat temperature produces the best sections. As the tissue is mounted, the slides are stored on a slide warmer (39–48°C) for up to 3 hr before fixation. Rapid drying is important. During a routine cutting procedure, adjacent sections are alternately mounted (three sections/slide) on two slides. One of the pair of the slides is fixed and then immediately used for hybridization while the other slide is fixed and stored (see below). It is difficult to handle more than 60 slides in a single hybridization experiment.

Fixation of Sectioned Tissue

Freshly sectioned tissue should now be fixed with paraformaldehyde. The following protocol has been found to work very well for *in situ* hybridization with single-stranded probes (12) as well as for oligomers (13, 14). However, we have not determined if this is indeed the *optimal* tissue fixation procedure with fresh-frozen tissue for *in situ* hybridization with single-stranded probes, or whether optimal conditions vary with particular probes.

Sections are treated as outlined below with solutions which are 800–1000 ml volumes in separate 1-liter autoclaved, glass beakers with autoclaved aluminum foil covers. Be sure that your sections have completely dried on the slides before proceeding. While wearing gloves, place the slides in autoclaved metal slide racks. Slide racks (# 113, Lipshaw, Detroit, MI) have a capacity for 30 slides and conveniently fit into 1000-ml beakers.

1. Five minutes in 4% paraformaldehyde, 100 mM PBS with 0.02% diethyl pyrocarbonate (160 μl/800 ml).
2. Five minutes in 100 mM PBS.
3. Five minutes in 100 mM PBS.
4. Five minutes in 5 mM dithiothreitol in water.
5. Two minutes in 70% ethanol.
6. Two minutes in 95% ethanol.
7. Two minutes in 100% ethanol.
8. Two minutes in 100% ethanol.

    When dried, freeze sections (−70°C: see below) or for short-term (few days) storage, place in a vacuum desiccator.

    An *alternative* fixation procedure is the "ethanol–acetic acid" procedure (15). Utilizing both cDNA and oligomer probes, we have found that this procedure can produce quite striking, high-quality autoradiograms when the gene product (e.g., rRNAs or mRNAs to neuropeptides) is abundant (16–19).

1. Place sections in 100% ethanol : acetic acid [3 : 1 (v/v), pH 1.5] for 15 min.
2. Next, place the sections in 160 μl of diethyl pyrocarbonate (DEP), freshly prepared in 800 ml of 2× SSC : acetic acid (pH 3.5), for 30 min at 70°C. That is, a 2× SSC solution is prepared and titrated with acetic acid to adjust the pH to 3.50. SSC is sodium chloride/sodium acetate (see *Appendix*).
3. Then place in 1 μg/ml pepsin in 2× SSC : acetic acid (pH 3.5) for 15 min at 37°C.
4. Rinse for 1 min in 0.2× SSC at room temperature.
5. Rinse for 1 min in autoclaved nanopure water containing 5 mM dithiothreitol (DTT 0.771 g/liter) at room temperature.
6. Air dry in a vacuum desiccator overnight.

Tissue Storage

    For access to additional tissue, particularly if the samples are important for experimental reasons, it is convenient to save some of the sectioned tissue samples. After tissue fixation, slides may be stored frozen (−70°C), at room temperature (under vacuum in a desiccator), or submerged in 70% ethanol at 40°C (20). For brain tissue, no investigation has thoroughly determined the most efficient means for storing tissue sections, but two factors can destroy message: moisture, which allows potential low-level, tissue RNase activity, and, when the sections are frozen, lyophilization. When the tissue is to be frozen, the slides should be stored in slide boxes with Humi-caps (see *Appendix*) and sealed with electrical tape.

Prehybridization and Hybridization

Probe and Hybridization Buffer Preparations

    Probe preparation has been described elsewhere (18, 21–23). The probe must be dissolved in the appropriate hybridization buffer. This will probably call for precipitating the probe from the solution it is stored in and then redissolving the probe in hybridization buffer. If the present diluent of the probe will comprise too large a proportion of the hybridization solution (>20% of total volume), then the probe must be concentrated or precipitated. Before precipitation, it is suggested that one to three 1-μl samples of the solution are taken for scintillation counting. One-microliter samples of the supernatant are also taken after the tube has been microfuged and the supernatant is poured from the tube containing the probe. From these counts, one can assess the efficiency of precipitation. You may find that the "pellet" of probe you have formed is invisible. Therefore, measures of radioactivity of the probe solution before and after precipitation are important to monitor the location of the radiolabeled material.

To precipitate the probe, the salt concentration of the probe solution is first adjusted to 0.3 mol sodium acetate. Next, 100% ethanol is added to the tube so that the volume ratio of (salt) water to ethanol in the tube is 1 : 2 (DNA probes) or 1 : 2.5 (RNA probes) (24). The nucleic acid is precipitated to the bottom of the tube by placing the tube in the freezer ($-70°C$) or in dry ice for 20–30 min, and then microfuging the tube for 15–30 min. (A microfuge that is kept in a 4°C cold room is highly recommended.) Next, the supernatant is carefully poured out of the tube so that the pellet is left undisturbed. The tube containing the probe pellet is dried to remove any remaining water and ethanol by placing the tube in a vacuum desiccator for 15–30 min.

At times it is difficult to precipitate smaller cDNAs or oligomers. To facilitate precipitation, one can add, as a carrier, approximately 50 μg yeast tRNA/300 μl probe solution and then cool the solution for 30 min and spin down. The tRNA (Sigma Chemical Company, Type X #R-9001) may allow one to see a faint pellet. Also, precipitation can be extended (overnight) to increase yield. The probe can also be centrifuged for a longer time period (30 min) or spun at higher speeds (for example, use a Sorvall centrifuge). Addition of magnesium chloride to form a 0.01 M $MgCl_2$ solution (before adding the ethanol) can improve yield. Consult Wallace (24) and Maniatis *et al.* (25) for further information regarding nucleic acid concentration.

When tritium-labeled probes are utilized, scintillation counts will probably be less than you would expect. This is due to the fact that the β-particle emissions from the radiolabeled nucleic acid in the hybridization buffer are "quenched" within micelles of buffer. Therefore, the samples that are to be counted should first be hydrolyzed to disrupt micelle formation (see *Appendix*). It should be noted that RNA probes are best left concentrated (and in the unfrozen state as little as possible) since diluted RNA in warm aqueous solutions can rapidly degrade.

Tissue Pretreatment

Several publications review the rationale for tissue pretreatment (1, 2). These steps are applied to improve the probe's accessibility to the message while minimizing nonspecific binding and the loss of message by diffusion (26). Two tissue pretreatment protocols are outlined for use with riboprobes, since we have found great success with both of these methods. With respect to cDNA and oligomer probes, no further tissue pretreatments are used and prehybridization–formamide buffer is directly applied to dried sections (see below).

Tissue Pretreatment Method 1

Gibbs and co-workers (27) have recently localized nerve growth factor receptor mRNA in brain by greatly simplifying tissue pretreatment. The tissue is acetylated using the procedure of Hayashi and co-workers (28). For localization of this relatively rare message (few mRNA copies/cell), additional pretreatment steps diminished the signal.

Gloves are worn during all procedures. The selected, fixed slides are placed in autoclaved metal slide racks (Lipshaw #113) for acetylation. If tissue has been stored frozen, boxes that contain slides should be removed from the freezer and permitted to equilibrate to room temperature before they are opened (at least 1 hr). Add 13.3 ml of triethanolamine (Sigma T 1377) to 1000 ml autoclaved water to make a 0.1 M solution. Adjust the pH of the solution to 8.0 with HCl. While stirring rapidly, add 2.5 ml acetic anhydride (Fisher A-10) for a 0.25% solution, and place the sections in this solution for 10 min at room temperature (RT) with gentle stirring. If the sections were not stored, this treatment directly follows tissue fixation (see above).

Tissue Pretreatment Method 2

The following pretreatment has been used with single-stranded riboprobes to localize the mRNAs encoding vasopressin (12) and somatostatin (29). See the *Appendix* for details of the solutions.

Solution[a]	Time (min)	Temperature[b]
800 ml 0.1 M PBS + 160 μl DEP	3	RT
800 ml 0.1 M glycine in 0.1 M PBS	3	RT
800 ml 0.1 M glycine in 0.1 M PBS	3	RT

(continued)

Solution[a]	Time (min)	Temperature[b]
800 ml 0.1 *M* PBS	3	RT
800 ml 0.1 *M* PBS	3	RT
800 ml 0.3% Triton in 0.1 *M* PBS	15	RT
800 ml 0.1 *M* PBS	3	RT
800 ml 0.1 *M* PBS	3	RT
800 ml *predigested* proteinase K	30	37°C
800 ml 4% paraformaldehyde 0.1 *M* PBS	5	RT
800 ml 0.1 *M* PBS	3	RT
800 ml 0.1 *M* PBS	3	RT

[a] See *Appendix*.
[b] RT, Room temperature.

Prehybridization

Before prehybridizing, completely dry the region of the slide that surrounds the tissue section. You may do this by carefully wiping the slide with a clean, relatively lint-free tissue paper (e.g., Kimwipes, Kimberly-Clark Corporation, Roswell, GA), or you can place the slides in two water washes (2 min each) and then desiccate the slides. Alternatively, we have recently added the following steps to dry the sections rapidly, but we have not assessed how this affects signal strength. Slides are placed in two water rinses (2 min each), then in 70, 85, 95, 100, 100% ethanol (2 min each), and desiccated for 1 hr.

With RNA probes, the hybridization reaction will be carried out at higher temperatures (>25°C and as high as 50°C). One must not allow the prehybridization and hybridization buffers to drain from the tissue. Using a Pasteur pipette, one can "paint" a circle of nail polish (Wet 'N Wild Clear Nail Polish Protector, Pavion, Ltd., Nyack-on-Hudson, NY) around the sections. This works much better than encirclement of tissue with a wax ("china marker") pencil. [This approach is of course obviated by reaction conditions that use free-floating sections (9, 29, 30)].

A microfuge tube containing the prehybridization buffer (see *Appendix*) is heated to 100°C for 10 min by placing it in a heat block (Thermolyne Dri Bath Type 17600) or by carefully suspending the tube in boiling distilled water. The tube is then quickly cooled by placing it in a dry ice : 100% ethanol bath for approximately 1 min, followed by placing the tube into crushed (water) ice. The buffer is then diluted (1 : 1) with 100% deionized formamide (see *Appendix*). To apply the buffer to the tissue, place the slides flat in Nalgene storage boxes (Nalgene Cat. #5700-0500) which are first lined with filter paper. The filter paper is soaked with 4× SSC : formamide [1 : 1 (v/v)]. A

20-μl solution of the prehybridization buffer–formamide solution is carefully micropipetted onto the sections. The prehybridization incubation is for 2 hr at room temperature or 37°C.

When applying both the prehybridization and hybridization solutions to the tissue, one must be careful to not touch the tip of the pipette to the section. This will produce large gouges in the tissue. If you wish to spread a solution evenly over the section, this can be done with a clean Pasteur pipette where the tip of the pipette is smoothed and bent by "flaming" with a Bunsen burner.

In Situ Hybridization

Prehybridization buffer is drained from the slide by gently tapping the edge of the slide against a paper towel that is lying flat on a countertop. With a Kimwipe, excess buffer is then further removed from the slide by carefully blotting the buffer from the region surrounding the tissue. Sections should not be permitted to dry out at this time, nor should you touch the tissue. The hybridization buffer (see *Appendix*) is added to the microfuge tube that contains the "dried-down" probe. A sufficient amount of hybridization buffer–formamide is added so that the final concentration of probe is 0.2–12 ng/20 μl. That is, add hybridization buffer to the probe so that the probe concentration in the buffer solution is 0.4–24 ng/20 μl. In a subsequent step you will dilute the buffer by 50% with formamide and the final concentration of probe will be 0.2–12 ng/20 μl. The tube containing the probe with buffer is heated for 10 min (100°C), and then quickly placed in an ethanol–dry ice bath. Formamide is added to the buffer for a final concentration of 1 : 1 buffer : formamide and the solution is then kept on water ice. RNasin (0.5 μg/ml) can be added to the hybridization solution at this time to retard mRNA degradation. Twenty microliters of the formamide–hybridization buffer solution is then applied to each section. The tissue is hybridized overnight (19–20 hr) or for up to 3 days, in the dark, at room temperature or at 37–50°C (RNA probes) in the filter-lined Nalgene boxes.

For oligomers and cDNA probes, hybridization at room temperature works quite well and there is usually no problem with high background due to the low-stringency conditions. However, we have conducted hybridization reactions at temperatures as high as 45°C, and you may need to do this for higher stringency. For RNA probes, it is prudent to perform the hybridizations at higher temperature. This is due to the greater affinity of RNA probes, particularly since they are also usually longer in length, to bind nonspecifically to other nucleic acids and cellular proteins. [See discussions by Tecott *et al.* (31) and Angerer *et al.* (32) concerning hybridization kinetics.] Probes radiolabeled with ^{35}S may exhibit increased background due to the oxidation of the thiol group. Include 2-mercaptoethanol (33) or dithiothreitol (DTT) (4, 20, 34) in the prehybridization and hybridization buffers. Very high temperatures (>50°C) may destroy tissue quality and result in sections floating off the slide. Hence, increase the proportion of formamide in the hybridization mix to raise the stringency of the reaction further.

Posthybridization Treatments

Posthybridization Washes: RNA Probes

The slides are placed in metal slide racks and are washed in the following solutions. Slide racks and glassware exposed to RNase-containing solutions are used exclusively for these wash steps. We store this glassware and slide racks separately, and label all of this material "RNase Glassware."

Solution	Time (min)	Temperature
4× SSC with 5 mM DTT	20	RT
4× SSC with 5 mM DTT	20	RT
4× SSC with 5 mM DTT	20	RT
RNase treatment (see *Appendix*) in water bath/agitation	30	37°C
RNase buffer wash in water bath/agitation	30	37°C
2× SSC	10	RT
2× SSC	10	RT
0.1× SSC (2 liters) and 5 mM DTT 1.54 g/2000 ml	Overnight	RT

Posthybridization: cDNA and Oligomer Probes

Tissue is briefly dipped in a 2× SSC solution and then washed twice for 10 min each in a 2× SSC solution at room temperature. Slides are then washed overnight (at room temperature) in 2 liters of 0.1× or 0.5× SSC containing 5 mM DTT (1.54 g/2000 ml).

Final Slide Washes and Drying

The next day, slides are rinsed for 1 min each in the following solutions of 300 mM ammonium acetate (pH 5.5) : absolute ethanol—1 : 1 (v/v) (i.e.,

400 ml ammonium acetate plus 400 ml ethanol), a 3 : 7 (v/v), a 1 : 9 (v/v), and in absolute ethanol. The sections are then air-dried in a desiccator under vacuum. For ^{35}S- and ^{32}P-labeled material, expose tissue to autoradiographic film overnight if desired. After the tissue has thoroughly dried, slides are handled with gloved hands and placed in slide dippers (Plastic Slide Grips: #BG-5, Lipshaw, Detroit, MI) for coating in autoradiography emulsion.

Preparation of Autoradiograms

The following procedures are all performed in the darkroom under safelight conditions. Autoradiography emulsion is extremely light sensitive. It should be handled in a darkroom that is absolutely light-tight. Kodak sells their liquid emulsions (types NTB-2 and NTB-3) in a wide-mouth, light-tight container that allows one to dip slides directly into this receptacle. Great caution must be taken as one reuses emulsion, since it can potentially be contaminated with chemicals or isotope that will induce grain formation. Hence, careful records must be kept to monitor potential increases in background ("fog"). Kodak (at least unofficially) reports emulsion can be reused as many as 10 times.

The bottle of emulsion, normally stored at 4°C, is allowed to come to room temperature over a 2-hr period, and then placed into a 43°C water bath. The safelight, a Kodak No. 2 safelight filter, should be at least 2 m from the emulsion and dipped slides. Do not open the light-tight container of emulsion during the 3 hr when warming-up the emulsion.

When the emulsion has been warmed to 43°C, the slides can be dipped. Before using slides with hybridized tissue, test for bubbles in the emulsion by first dipping a number of blank slides. If you find an excessive number of bubbles on your test slides, you can try and skim them off the top of the emulsion with another test slide. Allowing the emulsion to stand undisturbed for an additional 15–30 min also works well. After dipping, the emulsion coated slides are air-dried for 2 hr, in the darkroom (in absolute dark), and then placed in light-tight slide boxes that contain the desiccant, "Humicaps" (United Desiccants-Gates, Pennsauken, NJ). The slide boxes are then sealed with black vinyl electrical tape and stored at 4°C in lead-lined boxes filled with Drierite (anhydrous calcium sulfate: W.A. Hammond Drierite Co., Xenia, OH). An alternative storage method is to place the slide boxes in a freezer (−20°C). In this case, the taped slide boxes are first wrapped in aluminum foil and sealed again with black tape. The exposure step is crucial to providing quality autoradiograms. Autoradiogram storage should be in a dry, dark, and cold environment. Exposures range from a few days for ^{35}S- and ^{32}P-labeled probes, and days to 1–2 months for tritium. We use the poured emulsion "full-strength" and do not dilute it (some investigators dilute emulsion 1 : 1 with ammonium acetate or water).

It is strongly suggested that you not develop all of your autoradiograms at one time. Autoradiograms often require longer exposure times for a signal to be clearly greater than background. The rate of grain development is related to the amount of radioactivity which can be quite low in instances where there are few mRNA copies/cell. We commonly develop no more than 20% of our slides in one developing run, paying particular attention to include a fair sampling of slides from different treatment conditions. You will also want to process "control slides" that include, for example, sections that received no radioactive probe and control sections for negative and positive chemography [see Rogers (35) and the section *Controls* below].

Development of the Autoradiograms

On the day you will develop the autoradiograms, remove the slide boxes containing the *in situ* slides from storage and allow them to warm up to room temperature. The tape sealing the slide boxes should not be removed at this time since moisture may leak into the boxes and condense on the slides. This condensation may loosen the emulsion and tissue sections from the slides, or worse, rearrange the positions of the silver grains. We customarily allow the tissue to warm up to room temperature over at least 2 hr and keep the slide boxes away from strong light.

When all darkroom preparations are completed and the slides have reached room temperature, make the darkroom dark and begin developing. If developing more than one box of slides, first remove the black tape from around all the slide boxes before opening the boxes. This will prevent the autoradiograms from being exposed to sparks that are generated as the black electrical tape is peeled off.

Exposed slides are developed using Kodak D-19 developer that is freshly prepared 1 day prior to use, by following the vendor's directions. In the darkroom under safelight conditions, the slides are loaded into slide racks (Lipshaw #120) and gently submerged in the D-19 (16°C) for 2 min, without agitation. Slides are then carefully dipped (10 sec) into water (19°C), and then placed in two rinses of Kodak fixer (19°C) for 8 and 10 min, respectively, with slight agitation after the initial 4 min of fixation. Slides are then rinsed in distilled water twice for 10 min each. [Kodak recommends another method for autoradiogram development. Dilute the D-19 1 : 1 (v/v) with water and develop the emulsion for 4 min. Next, place slides in water for a few seconds, then place slides in Kodak Fixer for 4 min. All solutions should be 15°C.] Development reagents are used once and discarded and no more than 120 slides are processed per 300 ml of developer solution. The developing trays (stainless steel instrument trays) and stainless steel slide racks are reserved for autoradiography procedures. At this time, therefore, the slides are transferred to a second set of staining racks for staining, clearing, and coverslipping.

Sections can be lightly counterstained with cresyl violet, but care must be taken that the silver grains overlying the sections are not obscured by the stain. Slides (stained or unstained) are then dehydrated through alcohols (70, 90, 90, 100, 100% ethanols) and then placed in three xylene (or other clearing agent) rinses for 5 min each. Without allowing tissue to dry out, coverslip the sections with Permount (Fisher Scientific Co., Cat. #SO-P-15).

One should of course use a staining station with clean reagents to ensure the staining solutions do not damage the autoradiogram. Exposure to strong basic solutions can cause the loss of grains or cause grains to move in the gelatin. Acid solutions also can result in the loss of grains. If some stain is adhering to the gelatin in the emulsion, a brief exposure to weak acetic acid (a few drops in 300 ml of 95% ethanol) can remove the stain. The effect of dirty staining solutions upon the clearness of the autoradiograms is exacerbated with RNase-treated tissue. Following RNase treatment, the amount of stainable cytoplasmic nucleic acid is negligible. Hence, investigators attempt to stain their material heavily by greatly curtailing the clearing time in ethanol. This can result in the deposition of a brown reaction product. If this is observed, place the sections into clean water, then destain in clean 70, 95 (2×), and 100% (3×) absolute ethanol.

For most applications it is unnecessary to stain the tissue *before* coating the slides with emulsion. If sections are prestained, one must be careful the stain does not desensitize the emulsion and inhibit grain formation (a form of negative chemography), or induce the formation of grains (positive chemography). The latter problem can result, for example, from prestaining the sections with methylene blue or toluidine blue (36).

Some comments concerning the technique of emulsion autoradiography: emulsions are extremely sensitive not only to light but also to certain chemicals and metals (iron, copper, mercury). It is very important that the darkroom is clean and absolutely light-tight. An ideal condition would be where the darkroom is used exclusively for microscopic autoradiography: you may find that an "ordinary" darkroom which works well for film autoradiography is not adequate. If after 20 min of dark adaptation, any light is seen within or entering the darkroom, rest assured that it can affect the emulsion. Check also for any sources of light that are generated by small "on" indicator lights of laboratory equipment in the darkroom, and do not wear a watch that has luminescent elements.

A second source of "background" grain formation can arise from drying emulsion too rapidly. As the emulsion dries, a certain degree of movement of both silver grains and gelatin occurs. With rapid dehydration of the emulsion, the sheer forces caused by movement of the drying emulsion can create background. Several publications discuss in more detail the methods for handling autoradiograms (37–39) as well as their use in the more rigorous, quantitative investigation (40–43). Finally, it is important that the autoradiography emulsion is relatively thin and evenly distributed over the tissue and slide. This will reduce problems with staining, and is essential for quantitation since grain density from a source is proportional to emulsion thickness.

Controls

As noted by Uhl (1), there is no single control that ensures the labeling is specific in all respects. The "tests" listed here, however, each add credence to the specificity of the findings.

1. Include some tissue where no probe and hybridization buffer are applied. Grain density should be extremely low and approximate the levels seen over clean glass.

2. Preincubate some tissue with "cold" probe, followed by hybridization with labeled probe (a "competition" or "blocking" experiment).

3. Use a different probe to identify another mRNA and label a different population of cells.

4. Test the extent of hybridization to a heterologous probe such as a plasmid. This should result in no grain formation.

5. Determine that one consistently labels the same neuronal population of cells in different tissue samples as well as in independent hybridization trials.

6. Include samples of other tissues which are thought not to contain the message.

7. Examine other brain sites where no grain accumulation is expected.

8. When possible, examine a "positive control": use tissue which contains an abundant amount of the message of interest.

9. Pretreat some sections with RNase A (up to 100 μg/ml solution). This of course removes all RNA from tissue and is not a test specific only to the message of interest. There is also the potential that signal will be removed by residual amounts of applied RNase that degrades subsequently applied RNA probes. Williamson (34) recommends that micrococcal nuclease be employed for this specificity test of riboprobes.

10. Use several probes complementary to different regions of the message.

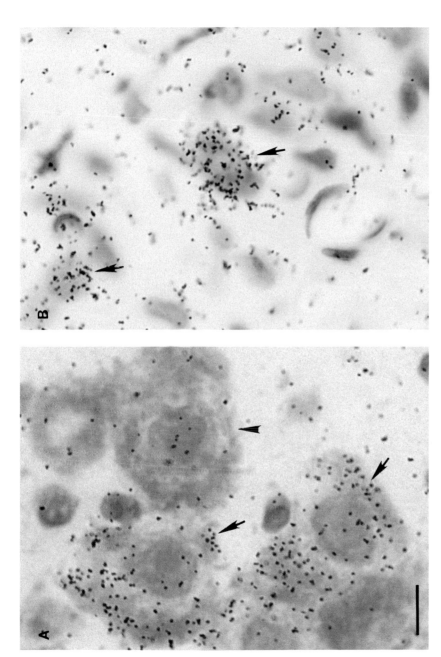

FIG. 1 *In situ* hybridization to identify oxytocin (A) and vasopressin (B) hypothalamic neurons. (A) Overlying grains are located primarily above the cytoplasm of oxytocinergic cells (arrows), while a neighboring, presumably vasopressinergic, cell is not labeled (arrowhead). (B) Depiction of label resulting from *in situ* hybridization to identify vasopressin mRNA. Grains extend beyond the visual limits of the underlying cell, since the probe was radiolabeled with the more energetic ^{35}S isotope. The two labeled cells (arrows) are also identified by diaminobenzidine reaction product from immunocytochemistry with a vasopressin antibody. Bar, ~10 μm. (A and B from Refs. 19 and 41, respectively.)

11. Test for "positive chemography" (the induction of grains by chemicals in the tissue) by incubating some sections in the hybridization–formamide buffer.

12. Test for "negative chemography" (loss of grains due to chemicals in the tissue) by exposing some autoradiograms of hybridized tissue to a light source, and then develop some of these slides at once and some of these slides at the time the experimental tissue is photodeveloped.

13. With cRNA probes, compare the extent of grain accumulation resulting from the probe (e.g., the "antisense" strand) to a control probe ("sense" strand) that is of the same length, same percentage of guanine monophosphate and cytosine monophosphate, and same specific activity.

14. Combine *in situ* hybridization with immunocytochemistry, or perform immunocytochemistry on adjacent sections to determine that cells which contain the protein also manufacture the message. This will not, of course, always be the case. Functionally significant proteins identified by the immunocytochemistry may be synthesized elsewhere and taken up by certain cells.

15. Use an experimental manipulation that is known to increase the cellular content of the particular message of interest to test if one can observe a quantitative increase in grain density over appropriate cell groups.

Analysis and Troubleshooting

Following development, staining, and coverslipping, autoradiograms are ready for light microscope analysis. The glass slide should appear clear and exhibit few overlying background grains (<4 grains/1000 μm^2). A higher concentration of grains in the emulsion over the tissue may be the result of background fog, plus nonspecific binding of probe to heterologous RNA. Several recent reports discuss the caution one must use in autoradiogram interpretation when the copy number/cell of the target RNA is low (44–46). With riboprobes and cDNA probes, one may observe a nonspecific "Nissl stain" pattern of label in certain brain areas, including the hippocampus and dentate gyrus, the granule layer of the cerebellum, the olfactory cortex and olfactory bulb, and over larger cells such as those of the oculomotor nuclei (27, 47, 48). These reports stress the importance of incorporating "sense control" tests. Tissue pretreatments and more stringent (low salt) posthybridization washes, with inclusion of formamide (49) or 2-mercaptoethanol (50) (^{35}S-labeled probes) in washing steps, can decrease nonspecific binding. Table I summarizes potential problems which can arise from *in situ* methods and what experimental procedures may alleviate the problem.

Signal will be evident by the accumulation of grains over the cytoplasm of labeled cells (Fig. 1). A cell is considered labeled when the number of grains

TABLE I Procedures for Optimizing *in Situ* Hybridization According to Problem Encountered[a]

Problem	Cause	Methodological change
No autoradiography grains	Latent image fading due to moisture while exposing	Improve autoradiogram storage conditions
	Negative chemography	Determine the chemical reagent(s) or treatment step(s) that prevent latent image formation
	Photodevelopment	Check expiration date of emulsion and photochemicals
	No hybridization	Verify the integrity of probe by gel electrophoresis
	Diffusion of tissue mRNA	Improve tissue fixation: brief paraformaldehyde or glutaraldehyde fixation will prevent the loss of mRNA from the tissue
	Loss of tissue mRNA	Decrease tissue deproteination from exposure to extremely acidic or basic solutions, or prolonged exposure to proteolytic enzymes (pepsin, proteinase K)
	Message degradation	Prevent RNase contamination: use autoclaved glassware and solutions; add dithiothreitol, diethyl pyrocarbonate to solutions. Wear gloves when handling tissue, and reserve glassware specifically for *in situ* hybridization
	Inaccessibility of tissue mRNA	Reduce tissue fixation: prolonged or high concentrations of paraformaldehyde or glutaraldehyde can produce excessive cross-linking, as can transcardial perfusion
	Inaccessibility of message	Increase protein denaturation and deproteination: use proteolytic enzyme treatments or *brief* exposures to 0.2 N HCl, 0.07 N NaOH, or 0.3% (v/v) Triton X-100
Low signal	Low copy number of tissue mRNA	Increase probe concentration in the hybridization buffer
		Use single-stranded probes
		Use a more energetic isotope, ^{32}P or ^{35}S, instead of ^{3}H
		Increase hybridization time

(*continued*)

114

TABLE I (*continued*)

Problem	Cause	Methodological change
		Use optimal hybridization temperature to increase rate of hybridization reaction and rate of diffusion of probe
		Include dextran sulfate in hybridization buffer
		Increase duration of autoradiogram exposure
		Use probes less than 500 base pairs in length. Probe sizes of 70–300 base pairs may be optimal
High "background"	Positive chemography	Determine the chemical reagent or treatment step that induces grain formation
	Problems with photodevelopment	Decrease autoradiogram exposure time; decrease development time and temperature
	Problems with emulsion over glass	Check emulsion has not been exposed to light, chemical(s), or isotope emission, any of which increases background fog. Consider the condition under which emulsion was dried (see *Preparation of Autoradiograms*)
	Nonspecific binding of probe to tissue protein or heterologous RNA	Pretreat tissue with acetic anhydride and/or glycine
		Decrease nonspecific hybridization: use prehybridization step, reagents in hybridization buffer that will bind nonspecifically to tissue [yeast total RNA, salmon sperm DNA, yeast tRNA, bovine serum albumin, poly(vinylpyrrolidone), Ficoll]
		For ^{35}S-labeled probes, include dithiothreitol, 2-mercapto-ethanol, or sodium thiosulfate in buffers
		Increase stringency of wash conditions, include formamide
Poor tissue morphology	Excessive deproteination	Decrease exposure to proteolytic enzymes
	Freezing artifact	Prevent improper tissue freezing techniques which produce large ice crystals

[a] Adapted from McCabe *et al.* (4).

over the cytoplasm is 3–5 times the grain density over neuropil (41, 42, 51). For probes radiolabeled with isotopes other than ^{3}H or ^{125}I, resolution will not be at the single-cell level. The track lengths of ^{35}S and ^{32}P, for example, result in the formation of grains in the emulsion surrounding labeled cells. As noted earlier, the ability to determine cytoplasmic localization with ribo-probes is greatly impaired by RNase treatment which removes stainable nucleic acids from the tissue.

Combination with Other Techniques, and Use of Nonisotopically Labeled Probes

In situ hybridization can be used in conjunction with other neuroanatomical methods. First, several reports describe the use of *in situ* hybridization combined with immunocytochemistry (5, 29, 41, 52). Several recent papers also describe the use of *in situ* hybridization at the electron microscope level (8, 53). *In situ* hybridization can also be combined with tract-tracing methods (54, 55). One can also combine *in situ* hybridization with the hemolytic phaque assay to assess gene expression and hormone secretion from individual cells (56). Several papers also describe the use of nonra-dioactive probes (9, 57–61).

Appendix

Directions are given for preparation of the hybridization (HB) and prehy-bridization (PHB) buffers, and how to prepare stock 20× SSC, formamide, and the reagents used for tissue fixation. A procedure for scintillation counting of tritiated probe material and the preparation of microscope slides are also summarized. A list of required materials and reagents (with catalog numbers) is also included (see Table II).

Prehybridization and Hybridization Buffers (2×)

The prehybridization and hybridization buffers (62) are almost identical and can be prepared at the same time. The main difference between these buffers is that the hybridization buffer contains dextran sulfate (E below) and polyadenylic acid [poly(A); L below] while prehybridization buffer does not. The buffers are prepared in two steps. First, make separate stock solutions of the reagents at the concentrations listed in the "stock solution"

TABLE II   List of Materials and Reagents (with Catalog Numbers)

Materials for slide preparation and storage
  Poly(L-lysine) (Sigma Cat. #P-2636)
  Permount (resin for coverslipping; Fisher Scientific Company)
  Humicaps (cylindrical desiccant capsules: anhydrous calcium sulfate, #245-2, Humi-Cap
      #386, 1.5 g; United Desiccants-Gates, United Catalysts, Inc. Group, Pennsauken, NJ)
  Metal slide rack #113, accommodates 30 slides (Lipshaw, Detroit, MI)
  Black slide boxes (slide storage) [Clay-Adams (Cat. #3843), Division of Becton,
      Dickinson, & Company, Parsippany, NJ]. Boxes should be checked for light-tightness
      by holding each half of box up to a strong light to determine if light can penetrate the
      plastic
  Vacuum desiccator Nalge #5310; desiccator plate #5312-0230
  Markers: Sanford Sharpie permanent fine point marker #30001 (Sanford Corp., Bellwood,
      IL)
  Gelfoam (for mounting tissue blocks to chucks; Upjohn Company, Kalamazoo, MI)
  Anesthesia: sodium pentobarbital (e.g., Nembutal; Abbott Laboratories)
Equipment
  Hybridization boxes (Nalgene Containers Cat. #5700-0500)
  Magnetstir (Ace Scientific 22-2475)
  Spin-bars (VWR 58948-251)
  Heat block (Thermolyne Dri Bath type 17600)
  Vortexer (Touch mixer, FisherBrand 12-810)
Reagents used in hybridization steps (Sigma reagent, unless noted)
  Acetic anhydride (Fisher Chemical Co. #A-10), 500 ml
  Ammonium acetate (#A-1542), 100 g
  Bovine serum albumin (Acetylated #B-2518), 25 mg
  Dextran sulfate (#D-8906), 10 g
  Diethyl pyrocarbonate (DEP; #D-5758), 5 ml
  dl-Dithiothreitol (DTT; #D-9779), 10 g
  EDTA (disodium salt #E-5134), 100 g
  Formamide (Fluka Chemical Corp., Ronkonkoma, NY; Formamide, Amide C_1, Catalog
      #47670, puriss)
  Ficoll type 400 (#F-2637), 5 g
  Glycine (essentially ammonia-free; #G-7126), 500 g
  Monobed resin stock #MB-1A (for deionizing formamide: Sigma's Amberlite "ion
      exchanger" Resin #MB-1A), 500 g
  Pepsin (#P-6887), 1 g
  Polyadenylic acid (#P-9403), 100 mg
  Poly(vinylpyrrolidone) (#P-5288), 100 g
  Proteinase K (protease, type XXVIII, #P-4914), 5 mg
  RNase A (type X-A; Cat. #R-5250), 100 mg
  Salmon testes DNA (type III, #D-1626), 1 g
  Sodium pyrophosphate (#P-8010), 500 g
  Triethanolamine (#T-1377), 500 ml
  Tris-HCl 7.6 (Trizma 7.6; #T-4253), 100 g
  Trizma 8.0 (#T-4753), 100 g
  Triton X-100 (Sigma), 100 ml
  Yeast tRNA (type X, #R-9001), 500 U (~25 mg)
  Yeast total RNA (type III, #R-7125), 500 mg

(continued)

TABLE II (*continued*)

Reagents of autoradiography
  Kodak NTB-3 autoradiography emulsion [4 fluid ounces (118 ml); Kodak Cat. 165-4441]
  Kodak NTB-2 autoradiography emulsion [4 fluid ounces (118 ml); Kodak Cat. 165-4433]
  Plastic slide grips (for dipping slides in emulsion) (#SG-5; Lipshaw, Detroit, MI)
  Kodak developer D-19 (to make 1 gallon) #146-4593
  Kodak fixer (to make 1 gallon) #197-1746
  Kodak darkroom lamp #152-1178
  Kodak safelight filter type 2 (5.5 in. diameter) #152-1525
  Slide rack and handle (accommodates 60 slides) (#120; Lipshaw, Detroit, MI)

column. Then to make a buffer, one combines each stock reagent in a sterile 50-ml tube by using the volume or amount given in the "volume added" column. That is, add to a 50-ml tube: 12 ml of 5.0 M NaCl solution, 1 ml of 1.0 M Tris (pH 7.6) solution, 167 μl of 6% BSA solution, etc. After adding all 13 reagents to the tube (or 11 reagents in the case of the prehybridization buffer), add enough distilled water to the tube to make a 50-ml volume. Note that all stock solutions are made with autoclaved, double-distilled water and are prepared in autoclaved glassware or microfuge tubes. All stock solutions are stored frozen ($-20°$C) and have never been thawed more than two times to make more buffer.

Reagents B through L are purchased from the Sigma Chemical Company (St. Louis, MO) and the catalog numbers are listed in the Reagent List (Table II). Sodium chloride, Tris-HCl 7.6, EDTA (ethylenediaminetetraacetic acid), and sodium pyrophosphate (NaPPI) are stored in their crystalline form, at room temperature, as purchased from the vendor. Sigma containers of bovine serum albumin (BSA), dextran sulfate, Ficoll, poly-(vinylpyrrolidone) (PVP), ammonium acetate, and salmon testes DNA are stored at 4°C. The RNA reagents and dithiothreitol are stored at $-20°$C.

Reagents	Volume added	Stock solution
A. Sodium chloride	12 ml of 5.0 M	5.85 g/50 ml
B. Tris-HCl 7.6	1 ml of 1.0 M	2.98 g/20 ml
C. BSA	600 μl of 1.6%	1.6% = 25 mg/1.5 ml
D. EDTA	400 μl of 250 mM	1.68 g/20 ml
E. Dextran sulfate	10 g[a]	Dry
F. Sodium pyrophosphate	500 μl of 5%	2 g/40 ml
G. Ficoll type 400	330 μl of 6%	60 mg/ml
H. Poly(vinylpyrrolidone)	330 μl of 6%	60 mg/ml

(*continued*)

Reagents	Volume added	Stock solution
I. Yeast total RNA	250 μl of 20 mg/ml 2.5 ml for PHB[a]	60 mg/3 ml
J. Yeast tRNA	100 μl of 50 mg/ml	25 mg/0.5 ml
K. Salmon testes DNA	1 ml of 10 mg/ml 5 ml for PHB[a]	60 mg/6 ml
L. Poly(dA)	330 μl of 15 mg/ml[a]	15 mg/ml
M. *dl*-Dithiothreitol	50 μl of 20 mg/ml	20 mg/ml
N. Add water to bring buffer to a 50 ml volume. Aliquot prepared buffers to 1.5-ml microfuge tubes and store at −20°C.		

[a] Delete dextran sulfate and poly(A) (polyadenylic acid) when preparing prehybridization buffer (PHB), but use 2.5 ml total RNA and 5.0 ml salmon testes DNA for PHB. Salmon testes DNA is diluted in sterile water, agitated for 2 hr, and sheared by passing through an 18-gauge sterile needle eight times. Place the tube with the DNA in a beaker of boiling water for 5 min and then allow to cool to room temperature.

Tables III and IV provide a convenient checklist for the preparation of buffers.

TABLE III   Preparation of 50 ml Prehybridization Buffer

Date:
Prepared by:
Tube label:

	1. Stock solution[a]	2. Amount stock to tube
A. _____	NaCl 5.0 *M*: 14.61 g/50 ml (RT)	_____ 12 ml to tube
B. _____	Tris 7.6: 2.98 g/20 ml (RT)	_____ 1 ml to tube
C. _____	BSA 1.6%: 25 mg/1.5 ml (CR)	_____ 600 μl to tube
D. _____	EDTA 250 m*M*: 1.86 g/20 ml (RT) (place in hot water to dissolve)	_____ 400 μl to tube
E. _____	NaPPI 5%: 2 g/40 ml (RT)	_____ 500 μl to tube
F. _____	Ficoll 6%: 60 mg/ml (CR)	_____ 330 μl to tube
G. _____	PVP 6%: 60 mg/ml (RT)	_____ 330 μl to tube
H. _____	Yeast tRNA: 50 mg/ml (F)	_____ 100 μl to tube
I. _____	Yeast total RNA: 20 mg/ml (F) (place in boiling water for 10 min before adding to tube)	_____ 2500 μl to tube
J. _____	Salmon testes DNA: 50 mg/ml (CR)	_____ 5000 μl to tube
K. _____	DTT: 20 mg/ml (F)	_____ 50 μl to tube
L. _____	Add autoclaved, double-distilled water to make 50 ml volume	
M. _____	Aliquot to labeled microfuge tubes and freeze	

[a] Storage site of reagents: CR, cold room or 4°C; RT, room temperature; F, freezer (−20°C).

TABLE IV   Preparation of 50 ml Hybridization Buffer

Date:
Prepared by:
Tube label:

1. Stock solution[a]	2. Amount stock to tube
A. _____ NaCl 5.0 M: 14.61 g/50 ml (RT)	_____ 12 ml to tube
B. _____ Tris 7.6: 2.98 g/20 ml (RT)	_____ 1 ml to tube
C. _____ BSA 1.6%: 25 mg/1.5 ml (CR)	_____ 600 μl to tube
D. _____ EDTA 250 mM: 1.86 g/20 ml (RT) (place stock in hot water to fully dissolve)	_____ 400 μl to tube
E. _____ Dextran sulfate 20% (CR)	_____ 10 g to tube
F. _____ NaPPI 5%: 2 g/40 ml (RT)	_____ 500 μl to tube
G. _____ Ficoll 6%: 60 mg/ml (CR)	_____ 330 μl to tube
H. _____ PVP 6%: 60 mg/ml (RT)	_____ 330 μl to tube
I. _____ Yeast tRNA: 50 mg/ml (F)	_____ 100 μl to tube
J. _____ Yeast total RNA: 20 mg/ml (F) (place in boiling water for 10 min before adding to tube)	_____ 250 μl to tube
K. _____ Salmon testes DNA: 10 mg/ml (CR)	_____ 1000 μl to tube
L. _____ DTT: 20 mg/ml (F)	_____ 50 μl to tube
M. _____ Poly(A): 15 mg/ml (F)	_____ 330 μl to tube
N. _____ Add autoclaved, double-distilled water to make 50 ml volume	
O. _____ Aliquot to labeled microfuge tubes and freeze	

[a] Storage site of reagents: CR, cold room or 4°C; RT, room temperature; F, freezer (−20°C).

20× SSC

20× SSC is a 20-fold stock solution of 0.15 M sodium chloride and 0.015 M sodium citrate in autoclaved, nanopure-distilled water. A 1-liter 20× SSC solution is freshly prepared for each hybridization experiment by adding 175.4 g sodium chloride and 88.2 g sodium citrate to an autoclaved flask and adding water to a 1-liter volume. To make a 0.5× SSC solution, add 50 ml of 20× SSC stock and enough water to make a 2000 ml volume (1 : 40 dilution of 20× SSC). Here is a list of the most common dilutions:

4× SSC (1 : 5 dilution)	160 ml 20× SSC, add water to 800 ml
2× SSC (1 : 10 dilution)	80 ml 20× SSC, add water to 800 ml
0.5× SSC (1 : 40)	20 ml 20× SSC, add water to 800 ml
0.1× SSC (1 : 200)	4 ml 20× SSC, add water to 800 ml

Deionized Formamide

Formamide (Fluka Chemical Corp., Ronkonkoma, NY) is purchased in 500 ml quantities. It is deionized by mixing approximately 5 mg monobed resin (Sigma Amberlite "ion exchanger" resin MB-1A) per 50 ml formamide and stirring the mixture on a Magnestir for 30 min until the pH is approximately 7. One or two repetitions of this procedure may be required to attain pH 7. The mixture is then filtered and stored (−20°C) in sterile microfuge tubes.

Solutions for Tissue Fixation and Pretreatment

0.1 M Phosphate-Buffered Saline (PBS)

Prepare the following solutions separately, and then add the amount designated below:

> Solution A: 13.8 g $NaH_2PO_4 \cdot H_2O$ (monobasic)/1000 ml H_2O
> Solution B: 14.2 g $NaHPO_4$ (dibasic)/1000 ml H_2O

Amount of reagent	Final volume 4000 ml	Final volume 8000 ml
Solution A	560 ml	1120 ml
Solution B	3440 ml	6880 ml
NaCl	36 g	72 g

4% Paraformaldehyde in PBS

Paraformaldehyde powder is dangerous to mucous membranes. When handling, avoid contact with eyes, wear gloves and a mask. To prepare paraformaldehyde fixative, warm PBS up to 65°C. Only then, with vigorous stirring, slowly add paraformaldehyde. Add 160 g paraformaldehyde/4 liters PBS, 40 g paraformaldehyde/1000 ml PBS, or 32 g/800 ml PBS. Gradually add a *few* drops of 6 M NaOH as a final clearing step, then filter with fluted filter paper. Do not allow the temperature of the paraformaldehyde solution to exceed 68°C and do not prepare paraformaldehyde too long before use (longer than 1 month) since it will polymerize. An alternative procedure is to prepare 2× paraformaldehyde in water. This paraformaldehyde will not polymerize as quickly, and can be used by diluting with 2× PBS.

3:1 Ethanol:Acetic Acid

Mix 3 vol of absolute ethanol (for example, 600 ml) to 1 vol acetic acid (200 ml). The pH will be about 1.50.

0.1 M Glycine

Add 7.5 g glycine/liter 0.1 *M* PBS, or 6.0 g glycine/800 ml 0.1 *M* PBS. Glycine (sodium salt: essentially ammonia-free) is from Sigma (Cat. #G-7126).

0.3% (v/v) Triton PBS

Add 2.4 ml Triton X-100 to 800 ml PBS.

Diethyl Pyrocarbonate (DEP) in 2× SSC:Acetic Acid

Prepare 2× SSC:acetic acid first by making an 800 ml solution of 2× SSC and then slowly adding acetic acid until the pH = 3.50. Then add 160 μl of DEP (Sigma D-5758). DEP should be purchased in small-quantity sizes (5-ml vials) and stored at 4°C. A 5-ml vial is usually used for 1 week since this reagent quickly decomposes. As per vendor's instructions, an opened vial of DEP should not be stored with the cap tight.

Pepsin in 2× SSC:Acetic Acid

Prepare 2× SSC:acetic acid by making an 800 ml solution of 2× SSC and then slowly adding acetic acid until the pH = 3.50. To that solution, add 20 μl of a 40 mg/1000 μl stock solution of pepsin (Sigma P-6887) made in 20× SSC. That is, the final pepsin concentration is approximately 1 μg/ml. Usually a larger volume of pepsin stock (40 mg/ml) is prepared, aliquoted to microfuge tubes, and frozen (−20°C). A tube of aliquoted stock solution is then thawed and used once. The pepsin should be added to the 2× SSC:acetic acid solution about 30 min before placing tissue in the solution to give the pepsin time to digest any contaminants that may exist in the solution.

Proteinase K Solution

The vial of proteinase K from Sigma [protease, proteinase K type XI, Cat. #P-0390] contains 10 mg of enzyme. Prepare a "stock" solution in the vial by adding 2 ml of a solution of 0.1 *M* Tris-HCl, pH 8.0, plus 50 m*M* EDTA directly to the vial. For tissue digestion, 0.4 mg of proteinase K (160 μl of stock) is added to a 800 ml (prewarmed 37°C) solution of 0.1 *M* Tris, pH 8.0 (11.2 g), 50 m*M* EDTA (14.9 g), and water, so that the final enzyme concentration is 0.5 μg/ml. The proteinase K should be predigested for >30 min (37°C) before use.

RNase Buffer

The RNase buffer contains 10 m*M* Tris-HCl, pH 8.0, 0.5 *M* NaCl, and 1 m*M* EDTA, pH 8.0, by adding 1.13 g Tris-HCl, 23.2 g NaCl, and 0.30 g EDTA into 800 ml prewarmed (37°C), autoclaved water.

RNase Solution

Add RNase A at a final concentration of 2.5–10 μg/ml RNase buffer. Therefore, add 140–560 μl of this stock to 800 ml of RNase buffer. This solution should be prewarmed to 37°C. Remember that the RNase treatment described is with agitation and at 37°C. To agitate the solution gently, the beaker containing the RNase buffer is set in a water bath which is placed on a rotating platform (Thomas Rotating Apparatus).

300 mM Ammonium Acetate

Ammonium acetate (300 m*M*) is 20.81 g/900 ml autoclaved water, pH to 5.5 with acetic acid.

Hydrolysis of Tritium Probes for Scintillation Counting

1. Aliquot 1 μl of probe into a scintillation vial.
2. Add 100 μl 3% (v/v water) perchloric acid to the 1-μl aliquot.
3. Hydrolyze at 80°C for 30 min, or at 100°C for 10 min.
4. Neutralize with 100 μl 0.3 *N* NaOH.
5. Add 5 ml Liquiscint (or equivalent fluor) and count. Note that the solution may be cloudy. Although this does not usually affect counts, we include "clouded" blanks.

Preparation of Chrome-Alum Subbed Slides

Place the glass slides in a slide rack and wash first with hot soapy water, and then in plenty of running water. Place 3.0 g gelatin in a beaker. Add enough boiling water to dissolve gelatin. Add water to total 600 ml. Add 0.3 g chromium potassium sulfate. Diethyl pyrocarbonate (0.02%) can be added to the solution as an added precaution against RNases. Dip slides in the chrome–alum solution for 10 min, then dry slides in an oven overnight at 40°C.

Preparation of Poly(L-Lysine)-Coated Slides

Prepare a solution of 50 μg polylysine/ml of 10 m*M* Tris 8.0. For 1000 ml solution, add 50 mg poly(L-lysine) (Sigma #P-2636) and 1.4 g of Tris 8.0

(Sigma #T-4753) in 1000 ml nanopure distilled water. Wash rack of slides in nanopure distilled water four times (5 min each). Immerse the slides in polylysine–Tris 8.0 for 10 min. Dry the slides in an oven (40°C) overnight. With gloved hands, place the slides back in their boxes for storage, wrap the boxes in foil, autoclave.

Acknowledgments

The authors thank Dr. Robert Gibbs for his valuable comments, and Ms. Carla Eng for her assistance in the preparation of this manuscript.

References

1. G. R. Uhl (ed.), "*In Situ* Hybridization in Brain." Plenum, New York, 1986.
2. K. L. Valentino, J. H. Eberwine, and J. D. Barchas (eds.), "*In Situ* Hybridization: Applications to Neurobiology." Oxford Univ. Press, London and New York, 1987.
3. D. D. Blumberg, *in* "Methods in Enzymology" (S. L. Berger and A. R. Kimmel, eds.), Vol. 152, p. 20. Academic Press, Orlando, Florida, 1987.
4. J. T. McCabe, J. I. Morrell, D. Richter, and D. W. Pfaff, *Front. Neuroendocrinol.* **9,** 145 (1986).
5. B. D. Shivers, R. Harlan, B. S. Schachter, and D. W. Pfaff, *J. Histochem. Cytochem.* **34,** 126 (1986).
6. W. S. Young III, *in* "Methods in Enzymology" (P. M. Conn, ed.), Vol. 168, p. 702. Academic Press, San Diego, California, 1989.
7. L. Terracio and K. G. Schwabe, *J. Histochem. Cytochem.* **29,** 1021 (1981).
8. M. Binder, S. Tourmente, J. Roth, M. Renaud, and W. J. Gehring, *J. Cell Biol.* **102,** 1646 (1986).
9. A.-F. Guitteny, P. Bohlen, and B. Block, *J. Histochem. Cytochem.* **36,** 1373 (1988).
10. M. Jamrich, M. A. Mahon, E. R. Gavis, and J. G. Gall, *EMBO J.* **3,** 1939 (1984).
11. R. H. Singer, J. B. Lawrence, and R. N. Rashtchian, *in* "*In Situ* Hybridization: Applications to Neurobiology" (K. L. Valentino, J. H. Eberwine, and J. D. Barchas, eds.), p. 71. Oxford Univ. Press, London and New York, 1987.
12. J. T. McCabe, K. Almasan, E. Lehmann, J. Hänze, R. E. Lang, D. W. Pfaff, and D. Ganten, *Neuroscience* **27,** 159 (1988).
13. S. K. Chung, J. T. McCabe, and D. W. Pfaff, unpublished observations, 1989.
14. B. D. Shivers, R. E. Harlan, J. F. Hejtmancik, P. M. Conn, and D. W. Pfaff, *Endocrinology* **118,** 883 (1986).
15. A. T. Haase, M. Brahic, L. Stowring, and H. Blum, *Methods Virol.* **7,** 189 (1984).

16. K. J. Jones, D. C. Chikaraishi, C. A. Harrington, B. B. McEwen, and D. W. Pfaff, *Mol. Brain Res.* **1,** 145 (1986).

17. M. Kawata, J. T. McCabe, C. Harrington, D. Chikaraishi, and D. W. Pfaff, *J. Comp. Neurol.* **270,** 528 (1988).

18. M. Kawata, J. T. McCabe, and D. W. Pfaff, *Brain Res. Bull.* **20,** 693 (1988).

19. J. T. McCabe, J. I. Morrell, R. Ivell, H. Schmale, D. Richter, and D. W. Pfaff, *Neuroendocrinology* **44,** 361 (1986).

20. J. B. Lawrence, R. H. Singer, C. A. Villnave, J. L. Stein, and G. S. Stein, *Proc. Natl. Acad. Sci. U.S.A.* **85,** 463 (1988).

21. M. E. Lewis, T. G. Sherman, and S. J. Watson, *Peptides* **6** (Suppl. 2), 75 (1985).

22. D. A. Melton, P. A. Krieg, M. R. Rebagliati, T. Maniatis, K. Zinn, and M. R. Green, *Nucleic Acids Res.* **12,** 7032 (1984).

23. P. W. J. Rigby, M. Dieckman, C. Rhodes, and P. Berg, *J. Mol. Biol.* **113,** 237 (1977).

24. D. M. Wallace, *in* "Methods in Enzymology" (S. L. Berger and A. R. Kimmel, eds.), Vol. 152, p. 41. Academic Press, Orlando, Florida, 1987.

25. T. Maniatis, E. F. Fritsch, and J. Sambrook, "Molecular Cloning: A Laboratory Manual," p. 461. Cold Spring Harbor Laboratory, Cold Spring Harbor, New York, 1982.

26. J. T. McCabe, J. I. Morrell, and D. W. Pfaff, *in* "Neuroendocrine Molecular Biology" (G. Fink, A. J. Harmer, and K. W. McKerns, eds.), p. 219. Plenum, New York, 1986.

27. R. B. Gibbs, J. T. McCabe, C. R. Buck, M. V. Chao, and D. W. Pfaff, *Mol. Brain Res.*, in press (1989).

28. S. Hayashi, I. C. Gillam, A. D. Delancy, and G. M. Tener, *J. Histochem. Cytochem.* **36,** 677 (1978).

29. H. Hoefler, H. Childers, M. R. Montimny, R. M. Lechan, R. H. Goodman, and H. J. Wolfe, *Histochem. J.* **18,** 597 (1986).

30. E. Ronchi, L. C. Krey, and D. W. Pfaff, manuscript in preparation (1989).

31. L. H. Tecott, J. H. Eberwine, J. D. Barchas, and K. L. Valentino, *in* "*In Situ* Hybridization: Applications to Neurobiology" (K. L. Valentino, J. H. Eberwine, and J. D. Barchas, eds.), p. 3. Oxford Univ. Press, London and New York, 1987.

32. L. M. Angerer, M. H. Stoler, and R. C. Angerer, *in* "*In Situ* Hybridization: Applications to Neurobiology" (K. L. Valentino, J. H. Eberwine, and J. D. Barchas, eds.), p. 42. Oxford Univ. Press, London and New York, 1987.

33. C. E. Bandtlow, R. Heumann, M. E. Schwab, and H. Thoenen, *EMBO J.* **6,** 891 (1987).

34. D. J. Williamson, *J. Histochem. Cytochem.* **36,** 811 (1988).

35. A. W. Rogers, "Techniques in Autoradiography," 3rd Ed. Elsevier, Amsterdam, 1979.

36. G. A. Boyd, "Autoradiography in Biology and Medicine." Academic Press, New York, 1955.

37. B. M. Kopriwa and C. P. Leblond, *J. Histochem. Cytochem.* **10,** 269 (1962).

38. H. Korr and H. Schmidt, *Histochemistry* **88,** 407 (1988).

39. A. W. Rogers, *in* "Methods in Brain Research" (P. B. Bradley, ed.), p. 79. Wiley, New York, 1975.

40. M. E. Lewis, W. T. Rogers, R. G. Krause II, and J. S. Schwaber, *in* "Methods in Enzymology" (P. M. Conn, ed.), Vol. 168, p. 808. Academic Press, San Diego, California, 1989.

41. J. T. McCabe, J. I. Morrell, and D. W. Pfaff, *in* "*In Situ* Hybridization in Brain" (G. R. Uhl, ed.), p. 73. Plenum, New York, 1986.

42. J. T. McCabe, R. A. Desharnais, and D. W. Pfaff, *in* "Methods in Enzymology" (P. M. Conn, ed.), Vol. 168, p. 822. Academic Press, San Diego, California, 1989.

43. G. R. Uhl, *in* "Methods in Enzymology" (P. M. Conn, ed.), Vol. 168, p. 741. Academic Press, San Diego, California, 1989.

44. H. G. Callan and R. W. Old, *J. Cell Sci.* **41**, 115 (1980).

45. M. A. McClure and J. Perrault, *J. Virol.* **57**, 917 (1986).

46. R. Patient, *Nature (London)* **308**, 15 (1984).

47. G. A. Higgins and M. C. Wilson, *in* "*In Situ* Hybridization: Applications to Neurobiology" (K. L. Valentino, J. H. Eberwine, and J. D. Barchas, eds.), p. 146. Oxford Univ. Press, London and New York, 1987.

48. M. Schalling, T. Hökfelt, B. Wallace, M. Goldstein, D. Filer, C. Yamin, and D. H. Schlesinger, *Proc. Natl. Acad. Sci. U.S.A.* **83**, 337 (1986).

49. M. E. Harper, L. M. Marselle, R. C. Gallo, and F. Wong-Staal, *Proc. Natl. Acad. Sci. U.S.A.* **83**, 772 (1986).

50. J.-M. Sequier, W. Hunziker, and G. Richards, *Neurosci. Lett.* **86**, 155 (1988).

51. J. I. Morrell, M. S. Krieger, and D. W. Pfaff, *Exp. Brain Res.* **621**, 343 (1986).

52. V. Chan-Palay, G. Yasargil, Q. Hamid, J. M. Polak, and S. L. Palay, *Proc. Natl. Acad. Sci. U.S.A.* **85**, 3213 (1988).

53. R. A. Wolber, T. F. Beals, and H. F. Massab, *J. Histochem. Cytochem.* **37**, 97 (1989).

54. J. S. Schwaber, B. M. Chronwall, and M. E. Lewis, *in* "Methods in Enzymology" (P. M. Conn, ed.), Vol. 168, p. 778. Academic Press, San Diego, California, 1989.

55. J. N. Wilcox, J. L. Roberts, B. M. Chronwall, J. F. Bishop, and T. O'Donohue, *J. Neurosci. Res.* **16**, 89 (1986).

56. J. T. McCabe, R. Holl, W. W. Chin, M. W. Thorner, and D. W. Pfaff, unpublished observations, 1989.

57. H. Arai, P. C. Emson, S. Agrawal, C. Christodoulou, and M. J. Gait, *Mol. Brain Res.* **4**, 63 (1988).

58. G. V. Childs, J. M. Lloyd, G. Unabia, S. D. Gharib, M. W. Wierman, and W. W. Chin, *Mol. Endocrinol.* **1**, 926 (1987).

59. R. W. Dirks, A. K. Raap, J. Van Minnen, E. Vreugdenhil, A. B. Smit, and M. Van Der Ploog, *J. Histochem. Cytochem.* **37**, 7 (1989).

60. A.-F. Guitteny, B. Fouque, C. Mougin, R. Teoule, and B. Bloch, *J. Histochem. Cytochem.* **36**, 563 (1988).

61. R. H. Singer, J. B. Lawrence, and C. Villnave, *BioTechniques* **4**, 230 (1986).

62. J. T. McCabe, J. I. Morrell, R. Ivell, H. Schmale, D. Richter, and D. W. Pfaff, *J. Histochem. Cytochem.* **34**, 45 (1986).

[7] Combination of *in Situ* Hybridization with Immunohistochemistry and Retrograde Tract-Tracing

Alan G. Watts and Larry W. Swanson

Introduction

The anatomical localization of specific gene expression is currently possible using either immunohistochemistry (IHC) to label the gene product, or *in situ* hybridization (ISH) to label the messenger RNA (mRNA) transcribed from the gene itself. When used within the central nervous system, IHC has proved to be an important and powerful tool for delineating chemically specific neural pathways, and within recent years the number of readily available antibodies has increased to cover most putative neurotransmitters and neuromodulators, as well as some of their associated metabolic enzymes and receptors. More recently, the increased sophistication of molecular cloning techniques and nucleic acid manipulation has led to the widespread use of ISH within all aspects of neuroscience, and it is now rapidly developing into a powerful tool for investigating the mechanisms of gene control in anatomically defined regions of the CNS. Currently, two types of probe are widely used to detect mRNAs by ISH: (1) synthetic complementary DNA oligonucleotides (cDNAs) can easily be constructed from a known sequence of the gene, or from that deduced from a known amino acid sequence (access to the cloned gene is not usually necessary); and (2) complementary RNA (cRNAs) probes are synthesized, using bacteriophage RNA polymerases (1), from the desired cloned gene fragment that has been inserted into a suitable transcription vector. When compared to cDNA probes, cRNA probes are usually longer and have the advantage of greater sensitivity, generally lower background, and the formation of higher stability hybrids (see Refs. 2–4 for a discussion on the comparisons between cDNA and cRNA probes).

Analysis of gene expression in the neural systems which underlie specific physiological processes requires the correlation of hybridization to specific cell types. This can be achieved initially by using a Nissl counterstain to reveal cell groups, but labeling of hybridized cells by IHC provides more precise biochemical identification.

Many groups have been successful in immunostaining cells for antigens that are sufficiently abundant to remain detectable after hybridizing with

Methods in Neurosciences, Volume 1

cRNA or cDNA probes (e.g., Refs. 5–7), or, alternatively, immunostaining cells before hybridizing with probes that detect relatively abundant mRNAs (e.g., Refs. 8–10). The greater rigor of cRNA ISH means that the immunostaining of sections after hybridization is generally difficult because of the resulting loss of the antigen and the reduction in quality of tissue morphology. Here we report modifications to the ISH and IHC protocols currently used in our laboratory (11–13) which allow hybridization with cRNA probes after the sections have been immunostained, thereby retaining the inherent qualities of IHC but without an appreciable loss to the sensitivity of cRNA ISH.

In addition to combining ISH with IHC, it is possible, in some situations, to hybridize sections from animals that have had intracerebral injections of retrogradely transported fluorescent dyes (14, 15). Technical modifications that allow this combination are also described.

Methodology

The method described in the present chapter relies on preserving the mRNA within the section during IHC by keeping RNase activity to a minimum, and by blocking any remaining activity with inhibitors. We use the VectorStain avidin–biotin peroxidase staining kit combined with a cobalt intensification procedure (16, 17) to maximize the immunostaining. By titrating the concentration of primary antibody, it is possible to attain a level of staining that does not mask the autoradiographic signal from the cRNA probe.

Our protocol for ISH (11, 13) has been modified in the present method to account for the different hybridization kinetics that result from previous immunostaining. The hybridization time is increased from 18–20 hr to at least 48 hr (preferably as long as 72 hr) and the temperature of the post-hybridization high stringency wash increased from 55°C to at least 70°C.

It should be stressed that the following protocol has been constructed to fit the combinations of probes and antibodies that are currently in use in this laboratory, and individual investigators are encouraged to obtain similar data for their own systems.

Procedure

1. Perfusion of animals with fixative. Rats are perfused transcardially with an ice-cold 4% (w/v) paraformaldehyde solution where the pH is changed from 6.5 (0.1 M acetate buffer) to 9.5 [0.1 M borate buffer containing 0.05% (v/v) glutaraldehyde]. Brains are removed and postfixed

overnight at 4°C in the pH 9.5 fixative + 10% sucrose, but without the glutaraldehyde. This fixation procedure has been successfully used in this laboratory for a wide range of applications (11–14) and is compatible with the ISH protocol described in this chapter. However, it is very likely that other fixatives are equally compatible with the methods described here.

2. Frozen sections cut and either stored in cryoprotectant, or incubated for 1 hr in cold blocking buffer containing BSA (2%) and the RNase inhibitors heparin (5 mg/ml) and RNasin (50 U/ml). *Note:* Precautions should be taken to avoid RNase contamination at every stage of the immunostaining procedure; consequently, gloves should be worn throughout the handling of sections and slides.

Frozen sections (12–20 μm thick) are cut and washed three times (at least 5 min per wash) in cold KPBS (0.02 *M* potassium phosphate, pH 7.2–7.4, 0.15 *M* sodium chloride). As an alternative to immunostaining at this stage, sections can be stored in cryoprotectant (modified from Ref. 18; the phosphate buffer is made from 0.1% diethyl pyrocarbonate-treated, filter-sterilized water, and both the glycerol and ethylene glycol are RNase free; Sigma Inc.) for at least 3 months without appreciable loss of immunoreactivity or detectable mRNA. Sections are transferred and incubated for 1 hr at 4°C in freshly prepared KPBS containing 0.3% Triton X-100, 5 mg/ml heparin (#H-9266 Sigma, from ovine intestinal mucosa), 50 U/ml RNase (Promega, Madison, WI), 2% bovine serum albumin (BSA; Cohn fraction V, Sigma Chemical Co., St. Louis, MO), and 0.5% dithiothreitol (DTT).

When sections were incubated in 2% normal goat serum (NGS; used to inhibit nonspecific antibody binding), subsequent hybridization was eliminated by the presence of RNase activity in the untreated serum. When the NGS was replaced with purified BSA, significant amounts of mRNA could be detected by hybridization. At the concentrations of primary antiserum regularly used in this laboratory, 2% BSA was capable of satisfactorily blocking nonspecific antibody binding. Further inhibition of remaining RNase activity was achieved by the addition of heparin and RNasin (19).

3. Incubation for 48 hr in cold primary antibody containing heparin (5 mg/ml). Sections are washed three times in cold KPBS and incubated for 48 hr at 4°C in the diluted primary antibody containing 5 mg/ml heparin. RNasin is omitted here because of the possible effects of DTT (the stabilizer of RNasin) on antibody structure. We have successfully used heparin to block serum RNase activity for antibody dilutions of 1:2000 or greater. More concentrated antibody solutions may require more RNase inhibition.

4. Development of immunoreactivity using the Vector ABC procedure, with heparin (5 mg/ml) in the biotinylated secondary antibody. After cobalt intensification and development with diaminobenzidine, sections are mounted on gelatin-subbed/poly(L-lysine)-coated slides.

The antigen–antibody complex is visualized with the avidin–biotin horse-radish peroxidase (ABC) method (20) used according to manufacturer's specifications (Vector Inc., Burlingame, CA). Haparin (5 mg/ml) is added to the biotinylated secondary antibody but not to the ABC reagent, as no serum products are present (see step 2 above).

To intensify the reaction product, the sections are washed three times in 0.1 M sodium acetate (pH 6.0) and then reacted with 1% cobalt acetate in 0.1 M sodium acetate for 10 min. The intensification step is usually necessary to counteract the reduction in the immunostaining caused by exposure of the section to the hybridization solution (see step 6). After further washes in sodium acetate, the sections are developed in 3',3'-diaminobenzidine-HCl (Polysciences, Warrington, PA) using 0.07 U/ml glucose oxidase (type VII, Sigma), 2 mg/ml glucose, and 0.4 mg/ml ammonium chloride. Finally, sections are washed at least three times in KPBS and then mounted on gelatin-subbed/poly(L-lysine)-coated slides, air dried, and stored overnight in a vacuum desiccator.

At this point, slides can either be stored for at least 3 months at $-20°C$ (or lower) in air-tight boxes containing desiccant without appreciable loss of hybridizable mRNA, or immediately prehybridized as described below.

The slides are now hybridized essentially as described by Simmons *et al.* (13) (the acetylation step described in Ref. 13 was omitted, as it was found not to be necessary for the present method). However, modifications are introduced to account for the presence of the immunostaining. These involve increasing the hybridization time to at least 48 hr and increasing the temperature of the final posthybridization high stringency wash (0.1× NaCl/ sodium citrate; SSC) to at least 70°C.

5. Prehybridization of sections using proteinase K. The slides are incu-bated at 37°C for 30 min in 0.001% proteinase K (Boehringer Mannheim, Indianapolis, IN) in 100 mM Tris, 50 mM EDTA, pH 8.0, washed in the same buffer without proteinase K, and then dehydrated in increasing concen-trations of clean ethanol. Slides are air dried and then placed in a vacuum containing desiccant for a minimum of 2 hr but no longer than overnight.

6. Hybridization at 55–60°C for between 48 and 72 hr. Hybridization solution containing the labeled cRNA probe is applied and the slides incubated at 55–60°C for at least 48 hr. The hybridization solution should be replaced at least every 24 hr because of the possibility of breakdown of the cRNA probe (S. Watson, personal communication), and the attendant increase in nonspecific hybridization. The hybridization solution is changed as follows. The slides are washed in 2× SSC for 20 min to remove coverslips, followed by a further two washes (10 min each) in 2× SSC. After dehydration through 50–100% alcohols (containing 0.001 M DTT and 0.08×

SSC up to the 95% ethanol), the slides are vacuum desiccated for 30 min. Fresh hybridization solution is applied and hybridization allowed to continue for a further 24 hr.

When vasopressin (VAS)-immunostained sections were hybridized with prepro-VAS cRNA, a minimum of 48 hr was required for significant hybridization, and as long as 68 hr was required for hybridization to reach 70% of control levels. This particular combination of antibody and probe was chosen because it represented the maximum immunostaining that the cRNA probe would have to penetrate; different intensities of staining probably present different kinetic profiles.

7. Removal of hybridization solution. The hybridization solution is removed from the slides and they are washed four times for 5 min each in 4× SSC. To remove nonspecifically bound single-stranded cRNA, the slides are incubated at 37°C for 30 min in 10 mg/ml of RNase A (#R550U, Sigma) in 0.5 M NaCl, 0.25 M Tris (pH 8.0), and 0.001 M EDTA (pH 8.0).

Slides are gradually desalted in decreasing concentrations of SSC (2× to 0.5×). All solutions contain 1 mM DTT.

8. Posthybridization, with a high-stringency wash (0.1× SSC) at 75°C. This temperature was chosen after hybridized immunostained sections had been washed at temperatures between 55 and 100°C. Figure 1 shows that the signal-to-noise ratio markedly improved between 70 and 80°C due to the reduction in background (see also Ref. 21). At temperatures approaching the theoretical melting point specific hybridization was significantly reduced.

Slides are dehydrated in increasing concentrations of ethanol (containing 0.001 M DTT and 0.08× SSC up to the 95% ethanol) and finally vacuum dried at room temperature for about 30 min.

9. Exposure of the sections to autoradiographic emulsion and (if required) X-ray film. The slides can be exposed to X-ray film to check the general quality of hybridization or for quantitative densitometric analysis, but to reveal the relationship between immunostaining and hybridization, the slides must be dipped in liquid autoradiographic emulsion, exposed, and developed. We routinely use Kodak nuclear track emulsion (NTB-2) diluted 1:1 with distilled water. Exposure times will obviously depend on the level of hybridization.

Results

We have successfully combined IHC, using a number of antibodies, and hybridization, using probes derived from the genes for VAS, corticotropin-

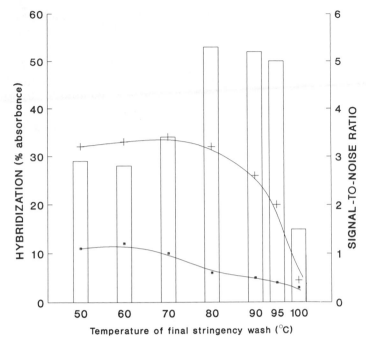

FIG. 1   The intensity of the hybridization and background signals (expressed in arbitary units as percentage absorbance) and the resulting signal-to-noise ratio in the rat thalamus as a function of the temperature of the posthybridization wash. All slides were immunostained with anti-CCK-8 serum [diluted 1 : 2000 (Immunonuclear Inc., MI)] and then were hybridized with a cRNA probe for ppCCK [see Simerly *et al.* (21) for preparation and characterization of this probe], according to the protocol described in this chapter. The figure shows the substantial increase in signal-to-noise ratio as the temperature of the posthybridization wash is increased from 50 to 95°C. (–■–) Background, (+) signal, (□) signal-to-noise ratio.

releasing hormone (CRH), tyrosine hydroxylase, cholecystokinin, preproenkephalin, and steroid hormone receptors. Figure 2 shows that excellent hybridization can be achieved with a number of these combinations without significant loss of either the immunohistochemical or ISH signals. When a heavy deposit of DAB polymer is present (e.g., when the combination of VAS immunohistochemistry and VAS *in situ* hybridization is used) this does not appear to present a barrier to probe penetration, provided sufficient time is allowed for hybridization.

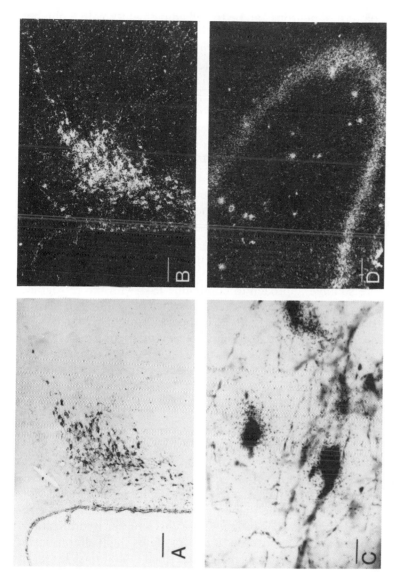

FIG. 2 (A and B) Photomicrographs from the same section showing CRH immunohistochemistry (A) and CRH ISH (B) in the paraventricular nucleus of a male rat adrenalectomized for 1 week before perfusion. Bar, 100 μm. (C) Photomicrograph of neurons in an accessory magnocellular group of a male rat hypothalamus stained using vasopressin immunohistochemistry and vasopressin ISH. Note the aggregation of silver grains in the vicinity of the immunostained cells. The presence of the heavy DAB deposit in some immunostained cells makes photography of the silver grains immediately over the cells difficult. Silver grains over less heavily stained cells (e.g., the cell on the right of the frame) are more easily visualized. Bar, 25 μm. (D) Photomicrograph of cholecystokinin (CCK) ISH in the CA3 region of the dorsal hippocampus on a section previously stained using an antibody against CCK-8. Note that the ISH signal remains strong in tissue that has been previously immunostained. Bar, 100 μm.

In Situ Hybridization Used in Combination with Retrogradely Transported Tracers

The projection pattern of neurons can be traced conveniently with a number of retrogradely transported fluorescent dyes (see Refs. 14, 15, and 22 for reviews concerning the choice and use of these dyes). By replacing the proteinase K step in the prehybridization step with a 30-min Triton X-100 incubation at room temperature (0.5% Triton X-100 in 100 mM Tris, 50 mM EDTA, pH 8.0), or no prehybridization treatment at all, fluorescently labeled cells can be detected after hybridization and autoradiography. When proteinase K was used, much of the fluorescent dye was lost.

In adrenalectomized animals injected with fluorogold (14) (Fluorochrome Inc., Englewood, CA) in the spinal cord and Fast blue injected intravenously to label cells that project to areas devoid of a blood–brain barrier (e.g., the median eminence), we have successfully detected fluorescently labeled cells in the paraventricular nucleus of the hypothalamus (PVH) after hybridization with ppVAS and ppCRH. However, it must be emphasized that this pretreatment does not work for all probes (especially for longer cRNA probes) in every application, and investigators should determine suitable parameters for different situations.

Perhaps a more suitable approach to combining ISH with the retrograde tracing of afferent connections is to use cholera toxin subunit B as the tracer and to detect the antigen with a monoclonal antibody and ABC staining (23). The immunostained sections can then be hybridized with the desired probe. Such an approach has been successfully used in this laboratory to label retrogradely the nigrostriatal pathway and then to hybridize the sections with ppTH to demonstrate the dopaminergic cells in this projection (H. Ericson, personal communication).

Summary

By carefully preserving mRNA within sections during immunohistochemistry, it is possible to immunostain tissue sections before hybridization with a variety of cRNA probes. If the immunohistochemistry is carefully controlled, there is no significant loss of immunoreactivity after hybridization. However, the presence of immunoreactivity necessitates slight alterations in the hybridization procedure, and under the described conditions, levels of hybridization of approximately 70% of control values can be obtained. Using immunostaining to delineate cell types biochemically will lead to a more accurate assessment of the physiological mechanisms controlling gene expression within the central nervous system.

Acknowledgments

We would like to thank Drs. J. Dixon, D. Ganten, and K. Mayo for the DNA constructs used to generate the probes employed in the methods described in this chapter.

References

1. D. A. Melton, P. A. Kreig, M. R. Rebagliati, T. Maniatis, K. Zinn, and M. R. Green, *Nucleic Acids Res.* **12,** 7035 (1984).
2. L. M. Angerer, M. H. Stoler, and R. C. Angerer, *in* "*In Situ* Hybridization: Applications to Neurobiology" (K. L. Valentino, J. H. Eberwine, and J. D. Barchas, eds.), p. 42. Oxford Univ. Press, London and New York, 1987.
3. K. H. Cox, D. V. DeLeon, L. M. Angerer, and R. C. Angerer, *Dev. Biol.* **101,** 485 (1984).
4. S. J. Watson, T. G. Sherman, J. E. Kelsey, S. Burke, and H. Akil, *in* "*In Situ* Hybridization: Applications to Neurobiology" (K. L. Valentino, J. H. Eberwine, and J. D. Barchas, eds.), p. 126. Oxford Univ. Press, London and New York, 1987.
5. V. Chan-Palay, G. Yasargil, Q. Hamid, J. M. Polak, and S. L. Palay, *Proc. Natl. Acad. Sci. U.S.A.* **85,** 3213 (1988).
6. J. F. Jirikowski, F. Ramalho-Ortigao, and H. Scliger, *Mol. Cell. Probes* **2,** 59 (1988).
7. M. Schalling, T. Hökfelt, B. Wallace, M. Goldstein, D. Filer, C. Yamin, and D. H. Schlesinger, *Proc. Natl. Acad. Sci. U.S.A.* **83,** 6208 (1986).
8. M. Brahic, A. T. Haase, and E. Cash, *Proc. Natl. Acad. Sci. U.S.A.* **81,** 5445 (1984).
9. B. D. Shivers, B. D. Harlan, D. W. Pfaff, and B. S. Schachter, *J. Histochem. Cytochem.* **34,** 39 (1986).
10. B. Wolfson, B. Manning, L. G. Davis, R. Arentzen, and F. Baldino, *Nature (London)* **315,** 59 (1985).
11. J. L. Arriza, R. B. Simerly, L. W. Swanson, and R. M. Evans, *Neuron* **1,** 887 (1988).
12. C. R. Gerfen and P. E. Sawchenko, *Brain Res.* **290,** 219 (1984).
13. D. M. Simmons, J. L. Arriza, and L. W. Swanson, *J. Histotechnol.* **14,** in press (1989).
14. P. E. Sawchenko and L. W. Swanson, *Brain Res.* **210,** 31 (1981).
15. L. C. Schmued and J. H. Fallon, *Brain Res.* **377,** 147 (1986).
16. K. Itoh, A. Konishi, S. Nomura, N. Mizura, Y. Nakamura, and T. Sugimoto, *Brain Res.* **175,** 341 (1979).
17. M. Sakanaka, T. Shibasaki, and K. Lederis, *J. Histochem. Cytochem.* **35,** 207 (1987).
18. J. S. De Olmos, H. Hardy, and L. Heimer, *J. Comp. Neurol.* **181,** 213 (1978).

19. S. H. Boyer, K. D. Smith, A. N. Noyes, and K. E. Young, *J. Biol. Chem.* **258,** 2068 (1983).
20. S. M. Hsu, L. Raine, and H. Fanger, *J. Histochem. Cytochem.* **29,** 577 (1981).
21. R. B. Simerly, B. J. Young, and L. W. Swanson, *Proc. Natl. Acad. Sci. U.S.A.* **86,** in press (1989).
22. L. W. Swanson, *in* "Methods in Enzymology" (P. M. Conn, ed.), Vol. 103, p. 663. Academic Press, New York, 1983.
23. H. Ericson and A. Blomqvist, *J. Neurosci. Methods* **24,** 225 (1988).

[8]   Localization of Neuronal mRNAs by Hybridization Histochemistry

Ruth E. Siegel

Introduction

In situ hybridization histochemistry is a technique that examines the expression of specific mRNAs in discrete cells and cell populations. The underlying principle of this procedure is straightforward. Tagged DNA or RNA probes complementary to the mRNA of interest are allowed to hybridize to a tissue section. A probe hybridizes specifically with its target RNA, and hybrid formation is subsequently detected with autoradiographic or histological procedures. Since the first use of *in situ* hybridization histochemistry several years ago to detect ribosomal DNA in squash preparations and cultured cells (1, 2), this technique has now been adapted to examine mRNAs expressed in the nervous system, including those encoding neuropeptides (3–8), enzymes of transmitter biosynthesis (9), and receptors (10–13).

Hybridization histochemistry adds a new dimension to the analysis of nervous system function. Because the brain is composed of heterogeneous cell types, techniques using tissue homogenates cannot adequately describe events in small populations. With a morphological approach such as *in situ* hybridization histochemistry, gene expression in discrete cells can now be examined. In addition, hybridization histochemistry identifies cell bodies in which neuron-specific molecules are synthesized. In contrast, immunohistochemistry localizes sites of product accumulation which may be in cell processes distant from the cell body. Thus, studies combining hybridization histochemistry and immunohistochemistry will provide a more complete understanding of the expression and regulation of neuron-specific molecules.

A variety of protocols have been used for *in situ* hybridization histochemistry. In our laboratory, highly reproducible procedures using ^{35}S-labeled single-stranded oligonucleotide and cRNA probles have been developed for examining the expression of a variety of neuroendocrine mRNAs. Procedures for tissue preparation and hybridization with these radiolabeled probes are described. In addition, a protocol is presented for combining *in situ* hybridization and immunhistochemistry for the simultaneous detection of both the mRNA and the encoded protein.

Solutions and Materials

To avoid RNase contamination, most solutions used for *in situ* hybridization are made from sterile components or are sterilized prior to use by filtration. Only the subbing solution, fixatives, and the reagents used following the completion of hybridization are used without sterilization.

> Gelatin-subbed slides: Slides that have been washed in mild detergent and extensively rinsed in deionized water are dipped in a solution containing 1.25 g gelatin and 0.125 g chromium potassium sulfate in 500 ml water. The slides are allowed to dry at room temperature for 45 min, dipped again in the gelatin solution, and air dried before use. Subbed slides can be stored up to 2 months before use
> 20× SSC: 3 *M* NaCl, 0.3 *M* sodium citrate, pH 7.0
> 5× tailing buffer: 500 m*M* potassium cacodylate, pH 7.2, 10 m*M* CoCl$_2$, 1.0 m*M* dithiothreitol
> Dithiothreitol (stock): 1.0 *M* in 0.01 *M* sodium acetate, pH 5.2
> TE buffer: 10 m*M* Tris, 1 m*M* EDTA, pH 7.5
> Yeast tRNA (stock): 25 mg/ml in water
> Acetic anhydride: 0.25% in 0.1 *M* triethanolamine HCl, pH 8.0 diluted just prior to use
> Hybridization buffer (oligonucleotide probes): 4× SSC, 50% formamide, 500 μg/ml sheared single-stranded DNA, 250 μg/ml yeast tRNA, 1× Denhardt's solution [0.02% Ficoll, 0.02% poly(vinylpyr-

rolidone), 0.02% bovine serum albumin], and 10% dextran sulfate (MW 500,000)

Hybridization buffer (cRNA probes): 2× SSC, 50% formamide, 1 mg/ml sheared single-stranded DNA, 1 mg/ml yeast tRNA, and 2 mg/ml bovine serum albumin. Both hybridization buffers are stable for several months at −20°C

RNase solution: 100 μg/ml RNase A and 1 μg/ml RNase T_1 in 2× SSC

PBS: Dulbecco's phosphate-buffered saline

Sodium phosphate buffer: 0.1 *M*, pH 7.3

Normal saline: 0.9% NaCl in water

Formaldehyde: 4% in PBS, made by dilution of 37% stock solution

Paraformaldehyde: 4% in sodium phosphate buffer

PBS/BSA: 1.0% bovine serum albumin, 0.3% Triton X-100 in PBS

Cresyl violet: 0.4% in water

Experimental Procedures

Tissue Preparation

To preserve mRNA, tissues are rapidly removed from the animal and frozen immediately. In most cases the tissue is placed on a layer of aluminum foil resting on powdered dry ice for several minutes. While this procedure is adequate for message preservation in small neuronal ganglia, larger tissues are generally cut, using sterile instruments, into small slices of approximately 3–4 mm for more rapid freezing. Alternatively, tissues can be removed from the animal and immediately immersed in isopentane cooled to −25–30°C. After a few seconds, the tissue is placed on dry ice for 10–15 min. For either procedure the frozen tissues are stored at −80°C wrapped in foil to prevent tissue desiccation, or sectioned immediately.

Prior to hybridization, 10- to 12-μm frozen sections are cut in a cryostat and thaw mounted onto twice-coated gelatin slides. The sections are allowed to dry at room temperature for approximately 1 min to ensure tissue attachment. The slides are then stored again at −80°C or processed immediately for *in situ* hybridization histochemistry.

Probe Preparation and Labeling

Highly reproducible hybridization signals are obtained using single-stranded DNA and cRNA probes. When radioactively labeled with ^{35}S, these probes allow detection of neuronal mRNA species with fairly good resolution.

Single-stranded DNA, or oligonucleotide probes, are widely used for examining the distribution of neuronal and endocrine mRNAs in tissue sections. These probes are chemically synthesized based on known sequences, thus avoiding the necessity of isolating a cloned cDNA. Many parameters are considered in the design of oligonucleotide probes. Most important, the stability of hybrid formation between the probe and the target mRNA is a function of both probe length and guanosine–cytosine (G–C) composition. In our laboratory, we have found oligonucleotides of 40–48 bases in length and 62–65% G–C produce strong hybridization signals. In addition to the parameters of hybrid formation, several aspects of probe specificity must be considered. For example, many neuronal proteins belong to gene families possessing significant sequence homology. In addition, some molecules are synthesized as part of larger precursors which undergo tissue-specific processing or alternative splicing to form bioactive products. Thus, a single mRNA may be differentially processed at different sites and the product mRNAs may contain both shared and unique regions. Despite these difficulties, highly specific oligonucleotide probes can be prepared with careful consideration of the sequences. A more detailed discussion of the strategies and parameters important in the probe design has appeared elsewhere (14).

Oligonucleotide probes are labeled on the 3′ end using terminal deoxynucleotidyltransferase (Tdt) and ^{35}S-labeled deoxyadenosine 5′-(α-thio)triphosphate (NEG 034H, New England Nuclear, Boston, MA). In a standard labeling reaction, oligonucleotide (final concentration = 0.1 μM), [^{35}S]dATP (70 μCi), 5× potassium cacodylate tailing buffer, and water to yield a final volume of 50 μl are combined in a sterile microcentrifuge tube. Terminal deoxynucleotidyltransferase (75–100 units) is added to initiate the reaction, which is carried out at 37°C for 10 min. The reaction is terminated with the addition of 400 μl of TE and 1 μl of tRNA, which acts as a carrier. The sample is extracted with 450 μl of phenol/chloroform/isoamyl alcohol (50 : 49 : 1, v/v). The aqueous phase containing the labeled probe is removed to a new tube and extracted with 450 μl of chloroform. The aqueous phase is again removed to another tube and the sample is precipitated by the addition of 0.05 vol of 4 M NaCl and 2.5 vol of ethanol and placed on dry ice for 30 min. After centrifugation for 30 min, the supernatant is discarded and the pellet is rinsed with ice-cold 80% ethanol. The pellet is dried briefly in air to remove the alcohol and then dissolved in 50 μl of TE and 1 μl of dithiothreitol. Labeled probes are stored at 4°C and can be used for 4–6 weeks.

Oligonucleotides prepared by this protocol have tail lengths of approximately 20–25 nucleotides. These probes hybridize readily to target mRNAs and generally allow moderately rapid signal detection. However, for reproducible labeling, the incubation time and amount of Tdt used for probe preparation should be adjusted for each new batch of enzyme. In addition, our protocol specifies tailing with dATP because, in our hands, probes labeled with either dCTP or dGTP produce high backgrounds when used for hybridization histochemistry.

Single-stranded cRNA probes have also been used successfully to localize neuronal mRNAs. The system for synthesizing cRNA probes consists of a bacteriophage polymerase and a plasmid cloning vector containing the appropriate promoter. To prepare the probe, the cDNA encoding the protein of interest is cloned into the vector downstream from the promoter. Large amounts of cRNA of uniform size and high specific activity can then be transcribed *in vitro* (15). In our laboratory, cRNA probes are transcribed in pGEM vectors (Promega Biotech, Madison, WI) from the *Salmonella* bacteriophage SP6 according to the manufacturer's protocol using ^{35}S-labeled uridine 5'-(α-thio)triphosphate (NEG 039H, New England Nuclear) with RNA polymerase. Probes ranging from 300 to 950 bases in length readily penetrate tissue sections and produce hybridization signals of high intensity (6, 16).

Tissue Processing

Prior to hybridization, several steps are performed to enhance both tissue preservation and the probability of hybrid formation. At all stages, care should be taken to avoid RNase contamination. For this reason, sterile solutions are used and all incubations are performed in plastic Coplin jars that have been treated with 0.1% diethyl pyrocarbonate (17) and subsequently autoclaved.

For *in situ* hybridization, the frozen tissue sections are allowed to warm to room temperature and are then fixed by immersion in 4% formaldehyde in 0.1 *M* sodium phosphate buffer (pH 7.3) for 5 min at room temperature. This short fixation both preserves tissue morphology and retains the mRNA in the tissue section. Hybridizations performed on postfixed sections yield more consistent results than those using tissues from paraformaldehyde-perfused animals. Following fixation, the tissue sections are washed in three changes of phosphate-buffered saline (PBS) to remove the formaldehyde. The sections are then incubated in 0.25% acetic anhydride in 0.1 *M* triethanolamine-HCl (pH 8.0) for 10 min at room temperature, a procedure which acetylates positively charged groups and decreases nonspecific binding of negatively charged probes (18). The sections are dipped once in 2× SSC and then dehydrated by incubation through a graded series of ethanol, a process that delipidates the tissue and increases access of the probe to its target mRNA. The tissues are incubated sequentially for 5 min each in 70,

80, 95, and 100% ethanol. The tissues are then immersed for 5 min in chloroform, incubated in 95% ethanol for 5 min, and then allowed to air dry.

To reduce nonspecific binding of the probe to the tissue, the processed sections are prehybridized in 45 μl of hybridization buffer for 1 hr at either room temperature (oligonucleotide probes) or 50°C (cRNA probes). Because the hybridization buffers are viscous when stored at -20°C, they are warmed to room temperature prior to use to improve accuracy of measurement. For this and all subsequent incubations in small volumes, the tissue sections are covered with small pieces of Parafilm to avoid tissue drying. In placing the coverslips over the sections, care is taken to avoid the formation of air bubbles. Following the incubation, the Parafilm coverslips are easily removed with a fine forceps or can be floated off the sections in 2× SSC.

Hybridization

Many protocols have been developed for *in situ* hybridization histochemistry. While these procedures have many similarities, the optimum procedure for a given experimental situation will depend on the tissue and the type of probe being used. In this section, procedures for hybridization histochemistry using single-stranded oligonucleotide and cRNA probes on postfixed mammalian tissues are described.

Oligonucleotide Probes

The following procedures have been developed for hybridizations with oligonucleotides 48 bases in length. While probes of this size are generally used, neuronal mRNAs can be successfully detected with much shorter probes (19, 20). Alterations in incubation conditions and the stringency of washes must be made to accommodate the shorter probes.

For hybridization, the tissue sections are covered with 45 μl of hybridization buffer containing probe (5 × 10^5 cpm) and 100 mM dithiothreitol. Each section is covered with a Parafilm coverslip and incubated overnight (20–22 hr) at room temperature in a humid chamber. Following hybridization, the Parafilm coverslips are removed and unhybridized probe is removed by washing in solutions of increasing stringency. The slides are washed four times for 15 min each in 2× SSC/50% formamide at 40°C followed by two washes for 1 hr each in 1× SSC at room temperature. Wash conditions of similar stringency can be obtained by lowering salt and formamide concentrations and by raising the temperature. However, these conditions may be detrimental for tissue preservation. After the final wash, the slides are dipped briefly in water to remove excess salts and are processed for autoradiography.

cRNA Probes

For hybridizations using cRNA probes, each tissue section is covered with hybridization buffer as above containing 5×10^5–10^6 cpm of probe and 10 mM dithiothreitol. The slides are incubated in the hybridization solution for 3 hr at 50°C on a slide warmer.

To remove the unhybridized probe, the coverslips are removed and the sections are rinsed in 2× SSC/50% formamide at 50°C for 5 min, followed by a second wash under the same conditions for 20 min. The slides are then placed on a slide warmer heated to 37°C and incubated under Parafilm coverslips with 40 μl of RNase solution for 30 min. The coverslips are removed in 2× SSC and sections rinsed twice for 12 min in 2× SSC/50% formamide at 50°C and twice for 5 min in 2× SSC at room temperature. After two quick rinses in water to remove remaining salts, the sections are allowed to dry.

Signal Detection

Hybrid formation is visualized by two methods: film autoradiography and liquid emulsion autoradiography. For autoradiographs of low resolution, the slides are placed against Kodak X-AR film and exposed at room temperature. This procedure provides rapid information concerning the regional distribution of mRNAs within a tissue (Fig. 1). Even with ^{35}S-labeled oligonucleotide probes, a signal can generally be detected within a few days. In addition, the intensity of the signal generated on film provides a guideline for exposure times necessary for liquid emulsion autoradiography. The time required for adequate grain densities is approximately four times longer than that producing the film image. While labeled cells in clusters are readily detected by film autoradiography, this technique lacks the sensitivity to detect single positive cells surrounded by unlabeled cells.

For higher resolution, the same tissue sections can be processed for liquid emulsion autoradiography following standard procedures (21) (Fig. 2). In most cases, the tissue sections are dipped in Kodak NTB3 emulsion diluted 1:1 with water and warmed to 43°C. The slides are hung in a vertical position and are allowed to dry at room temperature in the dark for 2–3 hr. The slides are then stored in a light-tight slide box containing desiccant, sealed with tape, and exposed at 4°C for varying lengths of time.

While the above protocol provides autoradiographs of good resolution, the coat of emulsion on dipped sections may be uneven and edge artifacts are sometimes observed. To obtain a more uniform coat of emulsion, a slight modification in the technique can be performed. Rather than dipping slides with tissue sections in the emulsion, thin coverslips are coated with

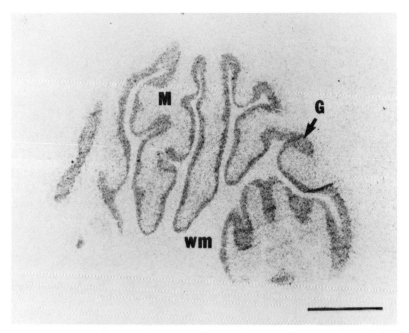

Fig. 1 Autoradiographic localization of the mRNA encoding the α1 subunit of the GABA$_A$ (γ-aminobutyric acid)/benzodiazepine receptor in the bovine cerebellum. Sections of bovine cerebellum were hydrized with an ^{35}S-labeled oligonucleotide probe complementary to bases 809–848 of the α subunit mRNA [P. R. Schofield, M. G. Darlison, N. Fujuta, D. R. Burt, F. A. Stephenson, H. Rodriguez, L. M. Rhee, J. Ramachandran, V. Reale, T. A. Glencorse, P. H. Seeburg, and E. A. Barnard, *Nature* (*London*) **328,** 221 (1987)]. Following hybridization, the section was placed against film and exposed for 5 days. The signal was greatest over the granule cell layer (G) but was also present over the molecular layer (M). No specific grains were observed over the white matter (wm). Bar, 5 mm.

emulsion and allowed to dry. The coverslips are then clamped against the tissue sections and processed as previously described (22). With either technique using liquid emulsion, the autoradiographs are developed in undiluted Kodak D19 for 2 min (at 17°C), rinsed briefly in water, and fixed in Kodak Fixer for 5 min. The slides are rinsed under a gentle stream of water for 20 min and then stained in 0.4% cresyl violet for the detection of cell bodies. Coverslips are placed over the dried tissues using DPX mounting medium (BDH, Poole, England) and observed.

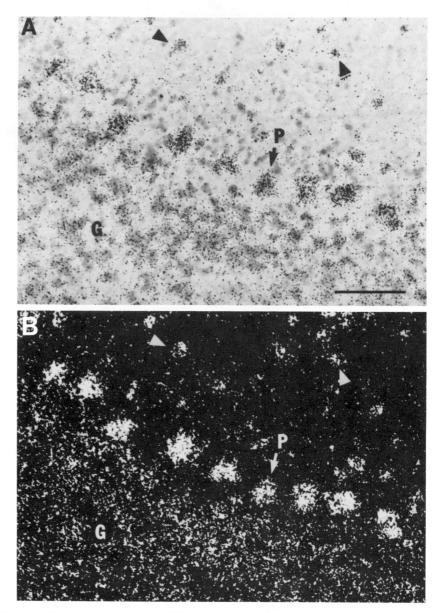

FIG. 2 Detection of the mRNA encoding the $\alpha 1$ subunit of the $GABA_A/$ benzodiazepine receptor in specific cell populations in the bovine cerebellar cortex following liquid emulsion autoradiography. Sections were hybridized as described in Fig. 1 and were exposed for 3 weeks for autoradiography. Bright-field (A) and dark-field (B) views of the same field reveal an intense signal over virtually all of the Purkinje cells (P). In addition, many cells in the granule cell layer (G) and some cells in the molecular layer (arrowheads) are labeled. Bar, 100 μm.

Colocalization of Neuronal mRNAs and Antigens

The colocalization of a mRNA and neuronal antigens in a tissue section can be accomplished by combining the techniques of *in situ* hybridization histochemistry and immunohistochemistry (Fig. 3). The best protocol in our hands is one in which the tissue is processed sequentially for *in situ* hybridization followed by immunohistochemistry (7). While there is some decrease in the intensity of the hybridization and fluorescence signals, this method still yields valuable qualitative information concerning the expression of a mRNA and antigen.

While procedures for hybridization histochemistry in the combined protocol are almost exactly as described above, there are a few differences. Most importantly, procedures providing the best preservation of the mRNA are not adequate for the preservation of many tissue antigens. For more consistent results, tissues are fixed by perfusion. Anesthetized rats are perfused via the ascending aorta at 25 ml/min with room temperature normal saline for 1 min. They are then perfused with 4% paraformaldehyde in sodium phosphate buffer for 5 min followed by perfusion with 10% sucrose in the buffered paraformaldehyde solution for 5 min. The tissue is then removed and soaked in the 10% sucrose solution in paraformaldehyde at 4°C for 30 min. For cryoprotection, the tissues are immersed for 30 min in 10% sucrose in PBS followed by a 60-min incubation in 20% sucrose in PBS at 4°C. The tissues are then frozen on dry ice.

Following fixation, cryostat sections are cut and processed for *in situ* hybridization. Because the tissue sections are already sufficiently fixed, the slides are dipped immediately in acetic anhydride following warming to room temperature. All subsequent steps for hybridizations and washes are exactly as described above.

After the last posthybridization wash in SSC, the slides are placed in PBS and processed for immunohistochemistry using the technique of indirect immunofluorescence (23). The tissues are incubated overnight at 4°C in primary antibody diluted in a solution of PBS containing 1% BSA and 0.3% Triton X-100 (PBS/BSA). They are then washed three times in PBS and incubated for 1 hr at room temperature in secondary antibody conjugated with tetramethylrhodamine and diluted in PBS/BSA. The slides are washed three times in PBS, dried, and processed immediately for autoradiography. After the appropriate period of exposure, the autoradiographs are developed and examined with phase and fluorescence optics. While rhodamine fluorescence is maintained throughout this process, less consistent results are obtained using secondary antibodies conjugated with fluorescein isothiocyanate.

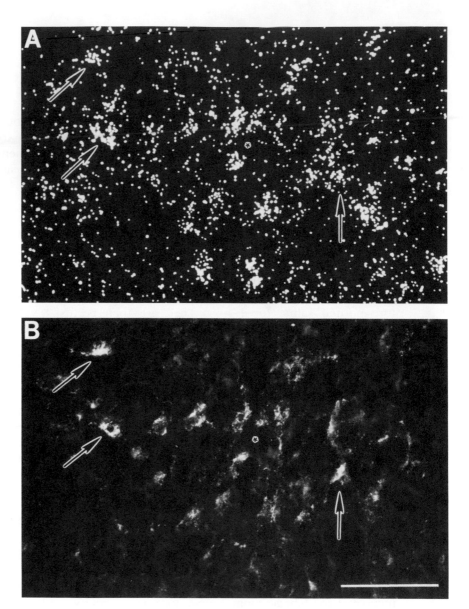

Fig. 3 Simultaneous detection of neurotensin mRNA and peptide in the paraventricular nucleus of the rat hypothalamus. Sections of rat brain were processed for *in situ* hybridization (A) using a ^{35}S-labeled oligonucleotide probe complementary to bases 477–524 of neurotensin mRNA [P. R. Dobner, D. L. Barber, L. Villa-Komaroff, and C. McKiernan, *Proc. Natl. Acad. Sci. U.S.A.* **84,** 3516 (1987)]. Following hybridization, the same tissue sections were stained for the neuropeptide by indirect immunofluorescence (B). Arrows indicate a few cells expressing both message and peptide. To aid in aligning the two photomicrographs, a star has been placed in the same position in both panels. Bar, 100 μm.

Quantitation of Results

Relative levels of mRNAs in tissue sections or individual cells can be obtained from film and liquid emulsion autoradiography. Two types of quantitative studies can be performed. In one approach, originally developed for the analysis of receptor autoradiography (24), the optical density of an image on film or a coverslip is measured by image analysis. Background densities obtained from adjacent tissue areas are subtracted from the values over positive areas to obtain a measurement of specificity. The optical density is then converted to an absolute amount of radioactivity by comparison to brain paste standards (6, 7) processed under identical conditions. Using this approach, it is possible to measure relative levels of a mRNA both within different tissue regions or in tissues maintained under different experimental conditions. A drawback of this procedure is that it disregards the fact that most brain regions are heterogeneous and that the level of mRNA expression may vary within the positive cell population.

Alternatively, the number of specific grains over positive cells following liquid emulsion autoradiography can be counted by visual observation or with an image analysis system. If all of the variables inherent in the technique of autoradiography are controlled, the number of grains over cells is proportional to the number of hybrids formed (25, 26). However, absolute quantitation is not possible for several reasons. For example, autoradiographic emulsion does not respond linearly to radioactivity at low signal levels (21). Thus, grain counts may underestimate the number of positive cells or the extent of labeling. Furthermore, reproducible quantitation is hindered by variation in emulsion thickness when using ^{35}S, an isotope of relatively high energy. This variable can be surmounted in part by using emulsion-coated coverslips rather than dipped slides. In spite of these limitations, relative numbers of positive cells and levels of message can be obtained if all samples in an experiment are processed identically.

While *in situ* hybridization has been used largely as a qualitative tool for mapping cell populations in the central nervous system and for comparing relative levels of mRNA, it ultimately may be used to quantitate the absolute number of mRNAs in specific neurons. However, many problems must be solved before this goal is achieved. First, it is possible that some message is lost during the hybridization procedure. Therefore, conditions must be perfected to allow the absolute preservation of the mRNA throughout tissue processing for hybridization and autoradiography. Second, conditions of hybridization must be established that result in the binding of the probe to all of the target mRNA. Finally, an image analysis system must be programmed to scan and store serial sections and provide a three-dimensional reconstruction of positive cells. This system must also be able to assign grains scattered beyond cell boundaries to a particular cell.

Controls for Specificity

Just as there is no single way to validate the specificity of immunohistochemistry, there is no perfect control for *in situ* hybridization histochemistry. Perhaps the best control is to use multiple probes synthesized to hybridize to nonoverlapping regions of the target mRNA. If more than a single probe complementary to a message reveals the same pattern of hybridization, it is probable that they recognize the same mRNA.

The specificity of the hybridization is further supported by the colocalization of the mRNA and the protein it encodes. However, situations may arise in which either the amount of mRNA or protein is below the level of detection by *in situ* hybridization histochemistry or immunohistochemistry. In the case of neuropeptide expression in the central nervous system, the peptide precursors are synthesized in the cell body but the peptide product is accumulated at distant sites in the nerve terminals. While the mRNA may be detected, the product may not be visible unless the animals have been pretreated with colchicine to prevent the transport of peptides out of the cell body.

In addition to these controls, other controls both support the specificity of hybridization and aid in establishing maximal hybridization conditions. For example, hybridization of the probe to tissues lacking the target mRNA or to tissues containing populations of both positive and negative cells, provides information concerning the background levels of the signal. Background levels can similarly be obtained by performing hybridizations using message sense probes homologous to the target mRNA.

Conclusions

In situ hybridization histochemistry is a powerful tool for examining many facets of nervous system function. While initial studies were limited to localizing a variety of neuronal mRNAs, other studies have now examined the regulation of specific mRNAs. Marked alterations in the expression of RNAs can be produced by drug treatments, surgical procedures, and experimental manipulations. By comparing changes in the levels of a mRNA and the product it encodes, new insights will be gained concerning cell function in the adult and developing nervous system. By examining the factors affecting the onset of expression of a particular mRNA, clues about the roles of trophic factors and other molecules in regulating growth and differentiation will be elucidated. Finally, examination of human postmortem tissues by hybridization histochemistry may reveal much about the pathophysiology of disease states.

Acknowledgments

I wish to thank Dr. Eva Mezey, Laboratory of Cell Biology, National Institute of Mental Health, Bethesda, Maryland, and First Department of Anatomy, Semmelweis University Medical School, Budapest, Hungary, for providing the photomicrographs used in Fig. 3. The work concerning the distribution of the GABA$_A$/benzodiazepine receptor mRNA was supported by grants from the Mathers Foundation and the National Institute of Mental Health 42173.

References

1. J. G. Gall and M. L. Pardue, *Proc. Natl. Acad. Sci. U.S.A.* **63,** 378 (1969).
2. H. A. John, M. L. Birnstiel, and K. W. Jones, *Nature (London)* **223,** 582 (1969).
3. C. E. Gee, C.-L. C. Chen, J. L. Roberts, R. Thompson, and S. J. Watson, *Nature (London)* **306,** 374 (1983).
4. R. E. Siegel and W. S. Young III, *Neuropeptides* **6,** 573 (1985).
5. B. Wolfson, R. W. Manning, L. G. Davis, R. Arentzen, and F. Baldino, Jr., *Nature (London)* **315,** 59 (1985).
6. W. S. Young III, E. Mezey, and R. E. Siegel, *Neurosci. Lett.* **70,** 198 (1986).
7. W. S. Young III, E. Mezey, and R. E. Siegel, *Mol. Brain Res.* **1,** 231 (1986).
8. R. T. Zoeller, P. H. Seeburg, and W. S. Young III, *Endocrinology (Baltimore)* **122,** 2570 (1988).
9. A. Berod, N. F. Biguet, S. Dumas, B. Bloch, and J. Mallet, *Proc. Natl. Acad. Sci. U.S.A.* **84,** 1699 (1987).
10. D. Goldman, E. Deneris, W. Luyten, A. Kochhar, J. Patrick, and S. Heinemann, *Cell* **48,** 965 (1987).
11. T. I. Bonner, N. J. Buckley, A. C. Young, and M. R. Brann, *Science* **237,** 527 (1987).
12. B. Fontaine, D. Sassoon, M. Buckingham, and J. P. Changeux, *EMBO J.* **7,** 603 (1988).
13. R. E. Siegel, *Neuron* **1,** 579 (1988).
14. M. E. Lewis, T. G. Sherman, and S. J. Watson, *Peptides* **6** (Suppl. 2), 75 (1985).
15. D. A. Melton, P. A. Krieg, M. R. Rebagliati, T. Maniatis, K. Zinn, and M. R. Green, *Nucleic Acids Res.* **12,** 7035 (1984).
16. R. E. Siegel, A. Iacangelo, J. Park, and L. E. Eiden, *Mol. Endocrinol.* **2,** 368 (1988).
17. T. Maniatis, E. F. Fritsch, and J. Sambrook, "Molecular Cloning: A Laboratory Manual." Cold Spring Harbor Laboratory, Cold Spring Harbor, New York, 1982.
18. S. Hayashi, I. C. Gillam, A. D. Delaney, and G. M. Tener, *J. Histochem. Cytochem.* **26,** 677 (1978).
19. G. R. Uhl, H. H. Zingg, and J. F. Habener, *Proc. Natl. Acad. Sci. U.S.A.* **82,** 5555 (1985).
20. M. L. Cohen, T. E. Golde, M. F. Usiak, L. H. Younkin, and S. G. Younkin, *Proc. Natl. Acad. Sci. U.S.A.* **85,** 1227 (1988).

21. A. W. Rogers, "Techniques of Autoradiography," 3rd Ed. Elsevier, Amsterdam, 1979.
22. W. S. Young III and M. J. Kuhar, *Brain Res.* **179,** 255 (1979).
23. A. H. Coons, in "General Cytochemical Methods" (J. F. Danielli, ed.), p. 399. Academic Press, New York, 1958.
24. J. R. Unnerstall, D. I. Niehoff, M. J. Kuhar, and J. M. Palacios, *J. Neurosci. Methods* **6,** 59 (1982).
25. M. Brahic and A. T. Haase, *Proc. Natl. Acad. Sci. U.S.A.* **75,** 6125 (1978).
26. L. M. Angerer and R. C. Angerer, *Nucleic Acids Res.* **9,** 2819 (1981).

[9]   *In Situ* Detection of Peptide Messenger RNA Using Complementary RNA Probes

A. Giaid, S. J. Gibson, J. H. Steel, and J. M. Polak

Complementary ribonucleotide probes have been transcribed from subcloned inserts of cDNA encoding amino acid sequences of various regulatory peptides. Using *in situ* hybridization, we have employed these probes to provide specific answers concerning mRNA production in several cell types. The peptides studied included calcitonin gene-related peptide (CGRP) in sensory and motor neurons, prolactin in the anterior pituitary, atrial natriuretic peptide (ANP) in cardiac myocytes, and neuropeptide Y (NPY) in cortical interneurons. These examples emphasize the value of *in situ* hybridization used in parallel with immunocytochemistry by elucidating sites of peptide production in the neuroendocrine system and their changes in different physiological states.

Methods in Neurosciences, Volume 1

Introduction

The general principle of the technique first described by Gall and Pardue in 1969 (1a) and used to demonstrate the spatial localization of ribosomal ribonucleic acid in *Xenopus* oocytes remains the basis of the *in situ* hybridization methods used today.

Every single strand of DNA (or RNA) has a predetermined complementary strand of nucleotides that will bind specifically to it. Thus, specific, labeled probes have been developed which can identify the presence of particular genes (DNA) or the transcription of those genes (mRNA) within tissue extracts, tissue sections, biopsies, or cell lines by binding to or hybridizing with their complementary nucleic acid *in situ*. The resulting hybrid can be detected according to the type of label used to tag the probe. These principles are analogous to the localization of a mature protein by specific labeled antibodies, as occurs in immunocytochemistry, a technique which has proven extremely useful in diagnosis and research (1). However, demonstration of the presence of an intracellular protein antigen does not necessarily indicate whether the corresponding gene is a product of that cell (2).

Different types of nucleic acid probes have been used for *in situ* hybridization to detect mRNAs. These include double-stranded DNA (3), single-stranded cDNA (4), complementary RNA (5), and oligonucleotides (6).

Single-stranded cDNA probes cannot self-hybridize, unlike the double-stranded probes in which self-reannealing and hybridization to the target sequences are in competition. On the other hand, it has been claimed that single-stranded cDNA probes give a high background due to entrapment of nonhomologous bacterial DNA sequences in the tissue (6).

The advantages of cRNA probes include high thermal stability and affinity of RNA–RNA hybrids (5), a constant probe size, no vector sequences, and the availability of RNase to remove unhybridized probes. Also, a probe with an identical sequence to the mRNA can be prepared as a sense probe for use as a negative control. Oligonucleotide probes have excellent properties of penetration into cells and tissues because of their small size, and have the advantages of single-stranded probes mentioned above. However, the use of single, short segments of DNA as probes limits sensitivity since only the complementary short segments of the target are available for hybridization (7).

Probes can be labeled with radioactive or nonradioactive tags; the most popular of the nonradioactive methods uses biotin-substituted nucleotides which are detected with labeled avidin. The sensitivity of this detection system is still not as good as that of the radioactive labeling method (8). We will outline the method we follow using radioactively labeled riboprobes and

give some examples of investigations of peptide mRNAs in the neuroendocrine system.

Methodology

Recombinant plasmids containing sequences corresponding to CGRP, prolactin, ANP, and NPY are isolated. A cDNA insert corresponding to a
known amino acid sequence from each peptide precursor is subcloned with
reverse orientation into the polylinker region of a vector using restriction
enzymes (e.g., *Hind*III and *Bam*HI). The plasmids are linearized with a
suitable restriction enzyme (*Bam*HI) and radiolabeled probes (cRNA
probes), complementary to the respective peptide coding sequences, are
transcribed from the linearized plasmid template (see *Synthesis of Single-
Stranded cRNA Probes for Transcription*).

All tissues used are fixed for 3–4 hr in 4% paraformaldehyde (pH 9.5) (see
Preparation of High-pH Paraformaldehyde), transferred to 0.1 *M*
phosphate-buffered saline containing 15% sucrose, and stored at 4°C for
24 hr. Cryostat sections (8–20 μm) are cut and mounted on clean, baked
(150°C overnight), poly(L-lysine)-coated slides and allowed to dry at 37°C
overnight before processing for hybridization. Tissue preparation, hybridization, posthybridization, autoradiography, enhancement of silver grains,
and control experiments are all described in the following sections (see *In
Situ Hybridization with cRNA Probes* through *Control Experiments*).

Synthesis of Single-Stranded cRNA Probes for Transcription

The following protocol is a modification of that given by Biotec for synthesis
of RNA probes. Note that all equipment and solutions are RNase free and
sterile.

1. To a sterile microfuge tube, at room temperature, add in the following
   order.
   4.0 μl 5× Transcription buffer (0.2 *M* Tris-HCl, pH 7.5; 30 m*M* MgCl$_2$,
     10 m*M* spermidine)
   2.0 μl 100 m*M* Dithiothreitol (DTT)
   0.8 μl RNasin (human placental ribonuclease inhibitor), 25 U/μl
     (Amersham Int., Bucks, UK)
   4.0 μl Nucleotide mixture [2.5 m*M* each of ATP, GTP, and UTP
     (Amersham)]

2.4 μl 100 m*M* Cytidine triphosphate (CTP) (Amersham)

1.0 μl Linearized plasmid template DNA (1 mg/ml) in water or Tris-EDTA buffer (1 μg)

5.0 μl Cytidine [^{32}P]triphosphate [10 mCi/ml (Amersham)]

0.5 μl SP6 RNA polymerase, T7 RNA polymerase, or T3 RNA polymerase, 10 U/μl (Amersham or Promega Biotec, Madison, WI)

2. Incubate for 1–1$\frac{1}{2}$ hr at 37–40°C.
3. To terminate transcription, add 1 μl RNase-free DNase (10 μg/μl) (Sigma, St. Louis, MO) and 1 μl RNasin. Incubate for 10–20 min at 37°C. All the solutions mentioned in steps 1–3 are stored at −20°C.
4. Add 1 μl total RNA: 10 μg/μl (Sigma), 175 μl DEPC-treated water, 5 μl 4 *M* NaCl. Extract with an equal volume (200 μl) of phenol-chloroform (1 : 1, v/v). Mix by vortexing. Separate the phases by centrifugation in microfuge (5 min).
5. Remove the upper aqueous phase (200 μl) and extract this with an equal volume (200 μl) of chloroform. Mix and spin as above.
6. To the upper aqueous layer add 100 μl 7 *M* ammonium acetate (2.5 *M* final concentration), 750 μl absolute ethanol (−20°C). Mix and leave at −20°C overnight.
7. Spin in microfuge for 30 min. Discard the supernatant. Dry the RNA pellet under vacuum. When dry, dissolve the pellet in 20 μl DEPC-treated water. Remove 1 μl for assessment of incorporation of radioactivity. Store ^{35}S probes at −70°C, ^{32}P probes at −20°C. The maximum storage time will depend on the radioisotope used.
8. Incorporation of radioactivity is estimated by determination of trichloroacetic acid (TCA)-precipitable counts. Take 1 μl labeled RNA probe and add 50 μl bovine serum albumin (10 μg/μl) and 1 μl 10% TCA.
9. Vacuum filter on GF/C (Glass microfiber paper, Whatman).
10. Wash the filter twice with 10% TCA and twice with absolute ethanol. Dry the filter.
11. Count the radioactivity on the filters and from this determine the percentage incorporation of radioactivity.

Preparation of High-pH Paraformaldehyde

Make 500 ml of 4% paraformaldehyde in 0.1 *M* borate buffer, pH 9.5.

1. Dissolve 19.1 g sodium borate and 2.0 g sodium hydroxide in 500 ml distilled water.

2. Heat to 60–65°C.
3. Add 20 g paraformaldehyde and stir.
4. Cool to room temperature or below.
5. Adjust pH to 9.5 with 1.0 M sodium hydroxide.
6. Cool to 10°C.

In Situ Hybridization with cRNA Probes

a. Tissue Preparation

1. Rehydrate in phosphate-buffered saline (PBS) (pH 7.2) for 5 min.
2. Immerse in 0.1 M glycine/PBS (5 min).
3. Permeabilize with 0.3% Triton X-100 in PBS (10–15 min).
4. Wash with PBS (2× 3 min).
5. Deproteinize by incubation with proteinase K solution [1 μg/ml protein-ase K (Sigma), 0.1 M Tris-HCl, pH 8.0, 500 mM EDTA, pH 8.0] for 20 min at 37°C.
6. Stop the enzyme reaction by immersion in 4% paraformaldehyde in PBS (freshly prepared).
7. To reduce nonspecific electrostatic binding of the probe, immerse sections in freshly prepared acetylation solution [0.25% (v/v) acetic an-hydride, 0.1 M triethanolamine, pH 8.0] for 10 min.
8. Prehybridize in 50% formamide in 2× standard sodium citrate (SSC) (37°C for 45 min) to decrease the melting temperature of hybrids, allowing a lower hybridization temperature to be used.

b. Hybridization

1. Drain slides briefly (do not dry).
2. Apply 20 μl of hybridization mixture preheated to 42°C containing 5 ng radiolabeled cRNA probe (5×10^5 cpm/section) diluted in hybridization buffer (8a).
3. Cover sections with suitably sized dimethyldichlorosilane-coated cover-slips.
4. Incubate sections in moist chambers at 42°C overnight.

c. Posthybridization Washing

1. Remove coverslips by immersion in 4× SSC.
2. Wash slides with 4× SSC (42°C, 3× 20 min) with gentle shaking.

3. Treat sections with RNase A solution (20 μg/ml, 0.5 M NaCl, 10 mM Tris-HCl, pH 8.0, 1 mM EDTA, pH 8.0) at 42°C for 30 min to remove unhybridized single-stranded cRNA probe.
4. Wash sections with 2× SSC (42°C, 30 min) with gentle shaking.
5. Wash sections with 0.1× SSC (42°C, 30 min) with gentle shaking.
6. Dehydrate with graded alcohol (70, 90, and 2× 100% ethanol) containing 0.3 M ammonium acetate (10 min each at room temperature).
7. Air dry for 1–2 hr.

Autoradiography and Quantification

a. Film Method

1. Expose labeled sections to radiation-sensitive film (e.g., Amersham): ^{32}P-labeled sections for 24 hr, ^{35}S-labeled sections for 48 hr, in darkness at 4°C. Labeled sections must be exposed with radioactive standard, either ^{32}P or ^{35}S.
2. Develop X-ray film in Kodak D19 developer prepared and used according to manufacturer's instructions (5 min at 18°C).
3. Rinse in distilled water containing 0.1% glacial acetic acid (30 sec).
4. Fix with AMFIX (photographic fixer) solution for 5 min, at 18°C.
5. Wash under running tap water for 15 min.
6. Dry and measure the optical density of each image using an image analysis system (IBAS, Magiscan, or Contex Vision).

b. Dipping Method

1. Dip section in an autoradiographic emulsion (Kodak NTB-2 or Ilford K-5) diluted 1 : 1 with double-distilled water at 42°C.
2. Air dry for 3 hr
3. Store slides in a lightproof box for 2–5 days depending on the radioisotope used (2–3 days for ^{32}P, 5 days for ^{35}S).
4. Develop with Kodak D19 for 3 min at 18°C.
5. Rinse in distilled water for 30 sec.
6. Fix with AMFIX solution for 4–5 min at 18°C.
7. Wash section under running tap water for 10–15 min.
8. Dehydrate, clear, and mount with DPX.
9. Count the number of labeled cells, number of grains, grain density per cell area, and background density for a similar size of unlabeled area using one of the previously mentioned image analysis systems.

Enhancement of Silver Grains

The level of positive labeling over the background ratio can be increased by the following manipulations.

1. The inclusion of dithiothreitol (50 mM) in one or all the following: prehybridization solution, hybridization mixture, or posthybridization washing. This reducing agent has a great effect on reducing background with the use of ^{35}S-labeled probes.
2. The addition of "cold" cytidine triphosphate to the prehybridization buffer.
3. Addition of an autoradiographic enhancer to the autoradiographic emulsion.
4. Decreasing autoradiographic exposure time or amount of probe used for hybridization.
5. Exposing sections to UV light prior to the hybridization step increases the density of positive labeling over the background level.

Control Experiments

Control experiments are very important in assessing the specificity of the hybridization and should include the following.

1. Sense probes: Probes identical to the coding strand of the mRNA under investigation are transcribed and hybridized as above. These are used as negative controls.
2. Ribonuclease treatment: Sections are treated with RNase A (20 μg/ml 37°C, 30 min) before the prehybridization step.
3. Inappropriate probe for the tissue in question.
4. Inappropriate tissue for the probe in question.
5. Northern blot analysis: The presence of the particular mRNA in the tissue may be confirmed by Northern blot hybridization.
6. Several probes, coding for different regions of the same gene.
7. Immunocytochemistry: The correlation of immunocytochemical results with those obtained by *in situ* hybridization can be a useful indication of the specificity of the signal.

Localization of Peptide mRNAs in the Neuroendocrine System

Calcitonin Gene-Related Peptide

Calcitonin gene-related peptide (CGRP) is a 37-amino acid peptide whose existence was predicted following analysis of the calcitonin precursor gene (9). Immunocytochemistry has shown CGRP to be one of the most abundant neuropeptides in primary sensory neurons and it was the first peptide immunoreactivity detected in motoneurons and motor end plates (10–13). Immunostained CGRP in motoneurons, however, has a granular appearance, making it difficult to assess whether the soma are themselves immunoreactive or whether the immunoproduct is formed by terminals of CGRP-immunoreactive fibers impinging on the soma. Therefore, *de novo* synthesis of CGRP in motoneurons remains to be confirmed. *In situ* hybridization was employed to determine whether motoneurons were authentic sites of CGRP RNA production, thereby adding strength to the recent hypothesis that CGRP derived from motoneurons can act as a long-term trophic factor at the neuromuscular junction (12, 13).

Following hybridization with human and rat CGRP probes, autoradiographs showed labeled cells in the dorsal root ganglia (Fig. 1A) and ventral spinal cord of man and rat (Fig. 1B). In the spinal cord these cells were identified as motoneurons by their size and location. In man, many more motoneurons expressed CGRP gene transcripts than were CGRP immunoreactive. In contrast, in rat, numbers of motoneurons labeled following hybridization were similar to the numbers of CGRP-immunoreactive motoneurons detected using immunocytochemistry (14).

In dorsal root ganglia (included as a positive control in the above experiment) of man and rat, 30–50% of the neuronal population expressed CGRP transcripts, with characteristically small- and medium-sized ganglion cells being labeled. The distribution and frequency of radiolabeled neurons paralleled those of immunoreactive neurons (14).

Prolactin

The aim of this study was to evaluate the use of *in situ* hybridization in investigation of endocrinological changes in a model system and to answer the question whether the technique allows a better understanding of the intracellular events which take place during hormonal gene transcription and translation.

Prolactin mRNA levels in the pituitaries of normal, pregnant, lactating,

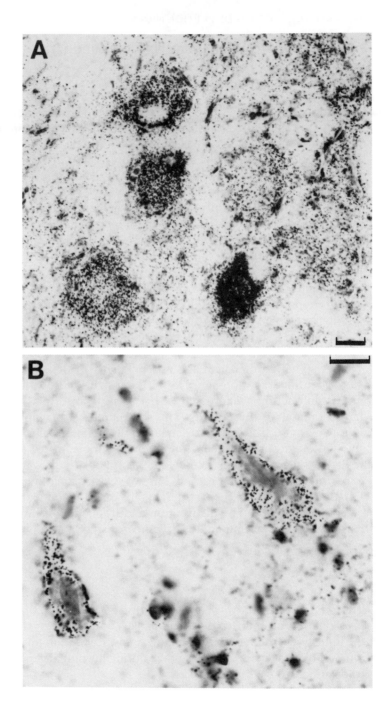

and ovariectomized female rats were investigated using *in situ* hybridization with a cRNA probe encoding prolactin mRNA (Fig. 2A–D). Large differences in labeling intensity and frequency of labeled cells were seen. In normal rats, prolactin cRNA labeled cells in the anterior pituitary were numerous and evenly distributed, with individual cells intensely labeled. Prolactin mRNA was greatly reduced in pregnant rats. A few silver grains were found over labeled cells in the anterior lobe, showing a generalized reduction in prolactin gene expression. In contrast, in ovariectomized rats there was an apparent reduction in labeled cells, while the intensity of hybridization in individual cells remained high. This suggests that ovariectomy turns off the prolactin gene in a subpopulation of cells (15). Anterior pituitaries of lactating rats showed such a strong hybridization signal that individual cells could not be distinguished beneath the silver grains, suggesting that the prolactin mRNA level in all the cells had increased. Quantification of the signal can be obtained from whole autoradiographs transposed onto film and measurements made using densitometry (Fig. 2E and F).

Atrial Natriuretic Peptides

Atrial natriuretic peptide (ANP) was originally identified in the atrium and consists of 151 and 152 amino acids in the human and rat heart, respectively (16–20). It has potent diuretic and natriuretic properties. ANP immunoreactivity has been localized to atrial myocytes of several mammals, including man (21). However, in nonmammalian species, ANP-like immunoreactivity occurs in the ventricles as well as the atria (22), and the results of mRNA blot analysis (23) and radioimmunoassay (24) together indicate at least some expression of the ANP gene in the ventricle of the rat.

To investigate whether ANP in the ventricle is synthesized by ventricular myocytes, tissue sections from rat and man and cultures of rat heart were processed for *in situ* hybridization using labeled cRNA probes for rat and human ANP.

Cultures of both rat atrium and ventricle showed positive labeling for ANP mRNA, with fewer labeled cells and reduced density of silver grains in ventricular cultures compared with myocytes in atrial cultures (Fig. 3A). In

---

FIG. 1 Autoradiographs following hybridization with ^{35}S-labeled antisense CGRP probes. (A) Primary sensory neurons in rat lumbar dorsal root ganglion and (B) motoneurons in human lumbar, ventral cord. Paraformaldehyde-fixed tissues; 20-μm cryostat sections. Hematoxylin counterstain. [From Gibson *et al.* (14) with permission.]

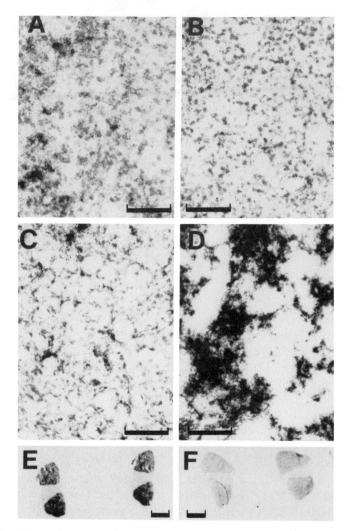

Fɪɢ. 2 Sections of rat anterior pituitary hybridized with a ³²P-labeled prolactin probe for detection of mRNA. (A) Control rat, (B) pregnant rat, (C) ovariectomized rat, (D) lactating rat, (E and F) film autoradiographs of sections of ³²P-labeled prolactin cRNA pituitary from (E) control and (F) pregnant rats. Paraformaldehyde-fixed tissues; 20-μm cryostat sections. Bars, A–D, 50 μm; E and F, 1 mm.

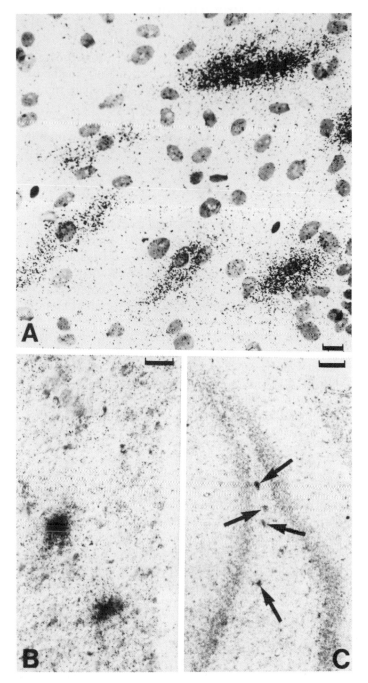

FIG. 3   (A) *In situ* hybridization of ANP mRNA in cultured myocytes of rat atrium using ^{35}S-labeled cRNA probes. (B) Several neurons labeled with NPY cRNA probe in cortex. (C) Labeled neurons (some indicated with arrows) in the dentate gyrus of the rat hippocampus after *in situ* hybridization with NPY cRNA probes labeled with [32]P. Cryostat sections (20 μm) fixed in paraformaldehyde and counterstained with hematoxylin. Bars, A and B, 10 μm; C, 50 μm.

sections from rat atria, numerous myocytes expressed ANP mRNA, whereas in the ventricles only scattered myocytes possessed ANP transcripts; these latter cells occurred mainly in the subendocardium of the interventricular septum. Sections of human right atrial appendage also displayed labeling of myocytes. The distribution of ANP transcripts in both cultures and tissue sections showed a close correspondence to the distribution of ANP immunoreactivity as revealed by immunocytochemistry (8a).

Neuropeptide Y

Neuropeptide Y (NPY) is a 36-amino acid peptide first isolated from the brain (25), its name being derived from its characteristic tyrosines at both N- and C-terminal ends. NPY is one of the most potent vasoconstrictors and it has a widespread distribution in the peripheral and central nervous systems (26). In particular, it is present in many cortical interneurons in a variety of mammals, including man (27). The function of these NPY-containing neurons is under investigation, as they exhibit numerical and morphological changes in certain neurological diseases (28).

In man, neurons expressing NPY mRNA were demonstrated in the deeper laminae (IV–VI) of the cerebral cortex in both surgical biopsy specimens and postmortem tissue. The distribution of these neurons was comparable to that of NPY-immunoreactive cells as shown in sections from the same region (29). In rat, NPY mRNA transcripts were localized to neurons of the cortex and hippocampus (Fig. 3B and C).

Conclusion

The recent development of *in situ* hybridization has provided further information on the function and gene expression of hormonal and neural peptides in tissues at the cellular level. In addition to defining the sites of peptide biosynthesis, it is possible to study the effects of physiological events on peptide mRNA expression. By performing *in situ* hybridization histochemistry in combination with other biochemical and histological procedures, much can be learned about gene expression within individual neurons in the adult and developing animal.

References

1. J. M. Polak and S. Van Noorden, "Immunocytochemistry: Modern Methods and Applications," 2nd Ed. Wright, Bristol, England, 1986.
1a. J. C. Gall and M. L. Pardue, *Proc. Natl. Acad. Sci. U.S.A.* **63,** 378 (1969).

2. G. Nilaver, "Brain *in Situ* Hybridization" (G. R. Uhl, ed.), p. 249. Plenum, New York, 1986.

3. M. L. Pardue, *in* "Nucleic Acid Hybridization" (B. D. Hames and S. J. Higgins, eds.), p. 179. IRL Press, Oxford, 1985.

4. J. G. Stevens, E. K. Wagner, G. B. Devi-Rao, M. L. Cook, and L. T. Feldman, *Science* **235**, 1056 (1978).

5. K. H. Cox, D. V. DeLeon, L. M. Angerer, and R. C. Angerer, *Dev. Biol.* **101**, 485 (1984).

6. J. P. Coghlan, P. Aldred, J. Haralambidis, H. D. Niall, J. D. Penschow, and G. W. Treger, *Anal. Biochem.* **149**, 1 (1985).

7. B. J. Morris, I. Haarman, B. Kempter, V. Hollt, and A. Herz, *Neurosci. Lett.* **69**, 104 (1986).

8. L. I. Larsson, T. Christensen, and H. Dalboge, *Histochemistry* **89**, 109 (1988).

8a. Q. Hamid, J. Wharton, G. Terenghi, C. Hassall, J. Aimi, K. Taylor, H. Nakazato, J. E. Dixon, G. Burnstock, and J. M. Polak, *Proc. Natl. Acad. Sci. U.S.A.* **84**, 6760 (1987).

9. S. G. Amara, V. Jonas, M. G. Rosenfeld, and E. S. Evans, *Nature (London)* **298**, 240 (1982).

10. S. J. Gibson, J. M. Polak, S. R. Bloom, I. M. Sabate, P. M. Mulderry, M. A. Ghatei, G. P. McGregor, J. F. B. Morrison, J. S. Kelly, R. M. Evans, and M. G. Rosenfeld, *J. Neurosci.* **4**, 3101 (1984).

11. M. G. Rosenfeld, J. J. Mermod, S. G. Amara, L. W. Swanson, P. E. Sawchenko, J. Rivier, W. W. Vale, and R. M. Evans, *Nature (London)* **304**, 129 (1983).

12. H. V. New and A. W. Mudge, *Nature (London)* **323**, 809 (1986).

13. B. Fontaine, A. Klarsfeld, T. Hökfelt, and J. P. Changeux, *Neurosci. Lett.* **71**, 59 (1986).

14. S. Gibson, J. M. Polak, A. Giaid, Q. A. Hamid, S. Kar, P. M. Jones, P. Denny, S. Legon, S. G. Amara, R. K. Craig, S. R. Bloom, R. J. A. Penketh, C. Rodek, N. B. N. Ibrahim, and A. Dawson, *Neurosci. Lett.* **91**, 283 (1988).

15. J. H. Steel, Q. Hamid, S. Van Noorden, P. Jones, P. Denny, J. Burrin, S. Legon, S. R. Bloom, and J. M. Polak, *Histochemistry* **89**, 75 (1988).

16. M. Yamanaka, B. Greenberg, L. Johnson, J. Seilhamer, M. Brewer, T. Friedmann, J. Miller, S. Atlas, J. Laragh, J. Lewicki, and J. Fiddes, *Nature (London)* **309**, 719 (1984).

17. S. Oikawa, M. Imai, A. Ueno, S. Tanaka, T. Noguchi, H. Nakazato, K. Kangawa, A. Fukuda, and H. Matsuo, *Nature (London)* **309**, 724 (1984).

18. S. A. Atlas, H. D. Kleinert, M. J. Camargo, A. Janaszewicz, J. E. Sealey, J. H. Laragh, J. W. Schilling, J. A. Lewicki, L. K. Johnson, and T. Maack, *Nature (London)* **309**, 717 (1984).

19. K. Kangawa, T. Tawaragi, S. Oikawa, A. Mizuno, Y. Sakuragawa, H. Nakazato, A. Fukuda, N. Minamino, and H. Matsuo, *Nature (London)* **312**, 152 (1984).

20. M. Maki, R. Takayanagi, K. S. Misono, K. N. Pandy, C. K. Tibbettes, and T. Inagami, *Nature (London)* **309**, 722 (1984).

21. K. Kikuchi, K. Nakao, K. Hayashi, N. Morii, A. Sugawara, M. Sakamoto, H. Imura, and H. Mikawa, *Acta. Endocrinol. (Copenhagen)* **115**, 211 (1987).

22. C. Chapeau, J. Gutowska, P. W. Schiller, R. W. Milne, G. Thibault, R. Garcia, J. Genest, and M. Cantin, *J. Histochem. Cytochem.* **33,** 541 (1985).
23. A. L. Lattion, J. B. Michel, E. Arnauld, P. Corrol, and F. Soubrier, *Am. J. Physiol.* **251,** H890 (1986).
24. D. G. Gardner, C. F. Deschepper, W. F. Ganong, S. Hane, J. Fiddes, J. D. Baxter, and J. D. Lewicki, *Proc. Natl. Acad. Sci. U.S.A.* **83,** 6697 (1986).
25. K. Tatemoto, *Proc. Natl. Acad. Sci. U.S.A.* **79,** 5485 (1982).
26. J. M. Allen and S. R. Bloom, *Neurochem. Int.* **8,** 1 (1986).
27. V. Chan-Palay, Y. S. Allen, W. Lang, U. Haesler, and J. M. Polak, *J. Comp. Neurol.* **238,** 382 (1985).
28. V. Chan-Palay, W. Lang, Y. S. Allen, U. Haesler, and J. M. Polak, *J. Comp. Neurol.* **238,** 390 (1985).
29. G. Terenghi, J. M. Polak, Q. Hamid, E. O'Brien, P. Denny, S. Legon, J. Dixon, C. D. Minth, S. L. Palay, G. Yasargil, and V. Chan-Palay, *Proc. Natl. Acad. Sci. U.S.A.* **84,** 7315 (1987).

[10]   Quantification of mRNA in Discrete Cell Groups of Brain by *in Situ* Hybridization Histochemistry

Margaret A. Miller, Janice H. Urban, and Daniel M. Dorsa

Introduction

In recent years, the rapid expansion of information concerning neurotransmitters in the central nervous system has necessitated the improvement of techniques which are useful in evaluating the function of these substances. The advent of molecular biology and its application to the neurosciences has introduced the possibility of examining genomic regulation of the biosynthesis of enzymes responsible for transmitter synthesis or, as is the case for neuropeptides, of protein precursors for the transmitter itself. In addition, the anatomical complexity of the brain makes it necessary to use techniques which allow a high degree of anatomical resolution as well as sensitivity and specificity. *In situ* hybridization histochemistry is a technique which affords the investigator the opportunity to visualize and quantify hybridization of labeled probes to mRNA contained within individual brain cells. The method is particularly useful when applied to situations in which the cells which express a particular gene are few in number compared to the adjacent neuropile. It is also useful in examining the regulation of populations of cells in a given nuclear region of the brain which may not respond uniformly to regulatory stimuli.

In this chapter, we will describe methods which we have found useful in evaluating the regulation of neuropeptide gene expression in discrete cell groups of the rat brain. While we have used these methods to study a wide variety of neuronally expressed genes, we will focus our attention on applications to the study of vasopressin-containing neuronal systems. This system provides an interesting model for several reasons, including the fact that the vasopressin gene is expressed both in well-defined nuclear groupings of cells in the supraoptic (SON) and paraventricular (PVN) nuclei of the hypothalamus and in scattered, low-density cells in extrahypothalamic brain regions including the bed nucleus of the stria terminalis (BNST) and medial amygdaloid nucleus (MA). Thus, hybridization can be quantified using both film and photographic emulsion-based methodologies. Several other laboratories have previously reported use of *in situ* hybridization methods to examine the effects of physiological stimuli on vasopressin mRNA levels in the SON and PVN of the hypothalamus (1–4).

In Situ Hybridization Protocol

Our laboratory has recently used *in situ* hybridization to localize and study the regulation of discrete vasopressin cell groups in the bed nucleus of the stria terminalis and the medial amygdala. The amount of signal present in these cells is relatively low and thus we needed to optimize our assay conditions in order to study these cells. We have tried different protocols and are currently using a method that is a combination of those previously described by Cox *et al.* (5) and Young *et al.* (6). It was fortuitous that our first attempt at *in situ* hybridization was performed on the vasopressin system. This system has been well-studied and the anatomical distribution of cell bodies containing this peptide has been identified using immunohistochemical methods. Furthermore, the amount of vasopressin mRNA present in the PVN and SON is easily detected on both film and emulsion-coated slides (see Fig. 1). It is our opinion that when first establishing this methodology the investigator should use a system that contains a large amount of target mRNA in a well-defined area. Once familiar with the method, it is easier to identify labeled cells and optimize assay conditions appropriate for visualizing mRNA in other less-studied systems. Although we will discuss methods for measurement of vasopressin mRNA, we have used this same protocol to study other gene products in the brain using both oligonucleotide and ribonucleic acid probes (with some modifications for riboprobes) and have found the method to be generally applicable.

Basic Methodology

When performing *in situ* hybridization, it is important to remember that RNA in the tissue is vulnerable to degradation by RNases. Therefore, to maintain a strong signal, precautions should be taken to decrease RNase activity. We use RNase-free procedures during all our prehybridization

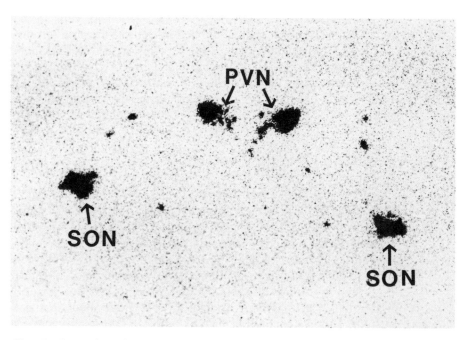

FIG. 1   Detection of vasopressin mRNA in the supraoptic (SON) and paraventricular (PVN) nuclei of the rat hypothalamus. The image shown is that which is obtained when the hybridized section is apposed to LKB-Ultrofilm. A ^{35}S-labeled 48-base oligonucleotide was used as probe.

steps. All our solutions are made with diethyl pyrocarbonate (DEPC)-treated water, and glassware (including slides, stir bars, spatulas) is baked overnight to destroy RNase activity. Chemicals are kept RNase-free, and gloves are worn throughout the procedure to prevent RNase contamination. Our assays are run using metal slide carriers (30 slides each) and glass staining dishes.

Tissue Preparation

Rats are decapitated and the brains rapidly removed and frozen on dry ice. Sections are cut on a cryostat maintained at $-20°C$. The tissue is blocked and mounted on the cryostat using mounting media. Coronal sections are cut (15 μm) and thaw mounted on gelatin-subbed RNase-free slides. The slides are placed in a black plastic box with a desiccant capsule and stored at $-70°C$. At this point it is important to keep the tissue cold and dry to reduce endogenous RNase activity and prevent breakdown of RNA in the tissue. Although we have not systematically studied the stability of mRNA over time, we have found no apparent reduction in hybridization signal in slides stored for several weeks at $-70°C$.

Prehybridization Treatment

Postfixing with 4% Paraformaldehyde

Slides are removed from the freezer, placed on foil, and sections are allowed to air dry for 10 min. Slides are then loaded into metal slide carriers and immersed for 5 min in a 4% buffered paraformaldehyde solution (pH 7.4) and subsequently rinsed in 0.1 M phosphate-buffered saline (pH 7.4). Both solutions are maintained in an ice-water bath.

Using an oligonucleotide complementary to mRNA encoding vasopressin, we have compared the hybridization signal over the SON and PVN in brain sections from rats perfused with 4% paraformaldehyde versus fresh-frozen brain sections postfixed as outlined. We have found essentially no variation in signal intensity in these cell groups. Furthermore, the cellular morphology in postfixed tissue is well preserved as identified by cresyl violet staining of emulsion-coated slides. The use of postfixed tissue alleviates the necessity of perfusing animals and allows serial tissue sections to be used for other studies, such as receptor localization. We no longer use proteinase K digestion or 0.1 N HCl treatment with our postfixation protocol. The choice of fixatives is dependent on the type of tissue and should be tested for different hybridization protocols (7). Refer to Angerer et al. (8) for a thorough review of fixation procedures used for in situ hybridization.

Acetic Anhydride

The tissue is briefly rinsed in 0.1 M triethanolamine (TEA, pH 8.0) at room temperature. Acetic anhydride (875 μl) is added to a dry, baked staining dish containing a magnetic stir bar. A tray of slides, which has been blotted to remove excess moisture, is put into the dish and immediately covered with 350 ml of 0.1 M TEA. The solution is stirred and slides are incubated at room temperature for 10 min. Slides are removed from the acetic anhydride solution and rinsed in 2× standard saline citrate (SSC).

The purpose of this step is to decrease nonspecific binding of the probe to the tissue. Treatment with acetic anhydride acetylates amino groups in the tissue and thus reduces electrostatic binding of the probe (9). Since acetic anhydride is hydrophobic, visual inspection should be made to ensure proper mixing of the solutions.

Dehydration and Delipidation

After the 2× SSC wash, the slides are dehydrated through a graded series of alcohol rinses (70, 95, and 100% ethanol), immersed in chloroform for 5 min to delipidate the tissue, and then brought back through 100 and 95% ethanol before being air-dried.

In our experience, we have found that chloroform delipidation significantly reduces background on the tissue. We have examined the effect of this procedure on background (nonspecific binding of probe) using semi-serial rat brain sections through the hypothalamus at the level of the SON and suprachiasmatic nucleus (SCN) that have either been delipidated with chloroform or not delipidated. We found that background was reduced by this procedure, and signal intensity was not altered. Apparently, for some probes, lipids in the tissue tend to hydrophobically bind probe (or label), thus increasing the background. Eliminating or reducing nonspecific binding elevates the signal-to-noise ratio which contributes to increased assay sensitivity. We typically apply probe to the brain sections immediately following the alcohol rinses. However, we have found that the tissue remains stable at this point and can be stored for at least 1 week (at room temperature, RNase-free) prior to application of probe.

Hybridization

Probe Considerations

When establishing an *in situ* hybridization assay there are a number of methodological considerations. Perhaps the most critical of these decisions is selection of a probe. Currently, there are three different classes of probes used: (1) oligonucleotide probes, (2) ribonucleic acid probes (riboprobes), and (3) complementary DNA (cDNA). We have chosen to utilize oligonucleotide probes in most cases. These are single-stranded DNA probes that are synthesized on automated DNA synthesizers.

With oligomers, it is not necessary to have extensive knowledge of molecular biological procedures. These probes can be labeled to high specific activities and form very stable hybrids with the target mRNA. The major advantages of using an oligonucleotide are that these probes are easily obtained and can be tailored to a specific size, generally 20–50 bases in length, and G–C content can be optimized.

Sequences of particular genes can be checked by computer for homology with other known sequences. Regions exhibiting low homology and high G–C content can be identified and probes synthesized. For arginine-vasopressin (AVP), we have synthesized a probe which is complementary to the region of mRNA encoding the last 16 amino acids of the glycopeptide tail. By directing the probe toward this region, we achieve a probe specific for AVP mRNA. Although there is a high degree of homology between AVP and oxytocin, the oxytocin gene does not code for a glycopeptide tail.

Before synthesizing an oligonucleotide probe, the gene sequence should be cross-checked since published sequences occasionally contain typographical errors. It is also important to remember that, according to convention, the published gene sequence is the same as the mRNA, not complementary to it. A thorough discussion on the use of oligonucleotide probes has been presented by Lewis *et al.* (10).

Labeling of Oligonucleotide Probes

Once the probe is obtained, it must be labeled to allow its detection after hybridization. Although other types of detection methods have been developed, radioactive labels are used most frequently. Probes can be radiolabeled at the 5'-hydroxyl terminus with T4 polynucleotide kinase. However, for studies that require high-resolution autoradiography using low-energy emitters such as ^{35}S and ^{3}H, terminal deoxyribonucleotidyltransferase (TdT) is the preferred method for labeling probe since it produces probes with a higher specific activity. TdT catalyzes the addition of radiolabeled deoxynucleotide triphosphates to the 3'-hydroxyl terminus of the DNA probe. Addition of multiple radiolabeled bases increases the specific activity of the probe and enhances the detection of mRNA *in situ* by low-energy emitters.

The labeling procedure is carried out in a microcentrifuge tube. [^{35}S]dATP (75 pmol) is added to the tube along with 15 pmol of our 48-base oligonucleotide probe. The probe and dATP are added in a constant molar ratio of 1:5. Five microliters of 5× potassium cacodylate tailing buffer (Bethesda Research Laboratories, Gaithersburg, MD) is added along with sterile water to a final volume of 25 μl including addition of the enzyme. This mixture is preheated at 37°C for 5 min prior to the addition of 20–40 units of TdT (BRL). The reaction is incubated for 1.5 hr at 37°C and is terminated by immersing the tube in a 65°C water bath for 5 min. The probe is loaded onto a NENSORB column (New England Nuclear, Boston, MA) with 0.1 M Tris (pH 8.0) and eluted with 50% (v/v) propanol. Dithiothreitol (DTT; 10 mM) is added to the probe, which is then stored at −70°C. We have found that the probe remains more stable when stored in propanol DTT instead of TED and can be used for up to 2 weeks.

Hybridization Procedure

The concentration of the labeled probe used in our assays was determined by performing a saturation curve and using the concentration where the label starts to saturate the tissue (see *Quantification Methods* below). Using a higher saturating concentration of probe may increase nonspecific binding and, therefore, lower the signal-to-noise ratio. For our studies, we apply 0.6 μg/ml per kilobase complexity. This concentration is two times that used by Cox *et al.* (5) for studying sea urchin embryos. However, this concentration is in agreement with other groups studying the expression of neuropeptide mRNA in the brain (11).

On the hybridization day, the labeled probe is thawed and added to a mixture containing 0.5 mg/ml yeast tRNA and TED (10 mM Tris, 5 mM EDTA, and 10 mM DTT) buffer. This solution is heated at 70°C for 3 min and quickly cooled on slushy ice to prevent the probe forming hybrids with other strands. The mixture is then added to the hybridization buffer containing 50% deionized formamide, 10% dextran sulfate, 0.3 M sodium chloride, 10 mM Tris, 1 mM EDTA, 1× Denhardt's [0.2% Ficoll, bovine serum albumin, and poly(vinylpyrrolidone)] and 10 mM DTT. This solution is applied to the tissue in a volume of 45 μl and the tissue is covered with a silanized coverslip. The slides are placed in a moist chamber and incubated overnight at 37°C. The hybridization proceeds at a temperature that is approximately 20°C below the calculated T_m (temperature at which 50% of the hybrids dissociate).

The temperature for hybridization affects the specificity of the hybridization reaction and is calculated with reference to the T_m of the formed hybrids. The primary determinants of the T_m are the percentage of guanine/cytosine (GC) content, the length of the hybrids, and base pair mismatches. Generally, GC base pairs are more stable than AT pairs and can survive higher temperatures as a result of the increased stability. Other factors that influence the hybridization efficiency are salt concentration and percentage of formamide in the solution. Increased formamide concentrations are used to decrease the temperature at which the reaction is run. It is advisable to run temperature curves for each probe under the conditions of the individual laboratory to optimize hybridization conditions.

Posthybridization

After incubation, the coverslips are removed by rinsing individual slides in 1× SSC at room temperature. The slides are placed in a staining dish containing 1× SSC (preheated to 55°C) and washed for 15 min. The dish is placed in an oscillating water bath to maintain the saline citrate solution at 55°C. This procedure is repeated four times, changing the solutions between each wash period. Wash temperature varies for each probe and is approximately 15°C below the T_m of the hybrids. After the hot washes, the slides are washed twice in 1× SSC for 1 hr each. A magnetic stir bar is placed under the slide tray and the solution is stirred at room temperature. After the second hour-long wash, the tissue is dehydrated through a series of alcohols (70, 95, and 100%) containing 300 mM ammonium acetate (final dilution) and air dried. The ammonium acetate is added to prevent denaturation of the hybrids. At this point, the slides are either apposed to film or dipped in Kodak NTB2 track emulsion.

Autoradiography

All autoradiography procedures are carried out in a darkroom illuminated with a Wratten red light filter. Emulsion is very sensitive to light so it is important that the work area be as light-tight as possible.

Preparing Emulsion

Kodak NTB2 nuclear track emulsion is first melted by placing the container in a water bath set at 42°C. The emulsion is then diluted 1 : 1 with 600 mM ammonium acetate also at 42°C and gently mixed. Emulsion is decanted into 20-ml scintillation vials. The vials are wrapped with aluminum foil and placed in a box that is then wrapped in black plastic and stored at 4°C.

Dipping Slides

The vials of emulsion are melted at 42°C for 30 min. One vial contains enough emulsion to cover approximately 60 slides. Once melted, the emulsion is slowly poured into the dipping chamber (Electron Microscopy Supplies, Pt. Washington, PA) and maintained at 42°C. Blank slides are dipped to remove air bubbles and are used to assess the quality of the emulsion.

The slides are dipped by holding them at the frosted end and slowly immersing them, twice, into the emulsion. This should be a continuous and smooth motion to ensure an even coating of emulsion. The bottom edge of the slide is slid across the rim of the dipping chamber to remove excess emulsion. Slides are placed upright in a scintillation vial box to dry for approximately 2 hr. The emulsion-coated slides are transferred to a black plastic slide box containing a desiccant capsule. The seams of the box are sealed with electrical tape and the boxes are wrapped in foil and stored at 4°C.

Developing Slides

These steps are carried out at 16°C; the developer, rinse, and fixer should all be at the same temperature to prevent cracking of the emulsion. Emulsion-coated slides are placed in slide carriers and developed in Kodak D-19 (diluted 1 : 1 with distilled water) for 4 min. The slides are rinsed in water for 1 min and then fixed in Kodak fixer for 5 min. Fresh developer, rinse water, and fixer are used for each tray of slides.

Staining

After a gentle but thorough rinsing, the slides are counterstained with cresyl violet acetate (0.5% in sodium acetate, pH 3.5) for 5 min and rinsed briefly in distilled water. Slides are stained lightly, since we have found that overstaining with cresyl violet can interfere with dark-field microscopy. The slides are dehydrated through 70, 95, 100% alcohol, rinsed in xylene or a xylene substitute (Hemo-De; Fisher Scientific, Pittsburgh, PA) and coverslipped using Permount. The slides are cleaned with xylene to remove excess Permount, and the emulsion is removed from the back of the slides with Formula 409.

Controls

A major problem facing researchers is the identification of false positives. With *in situ* hybridization, grain clusters that constitute the signal must be determined to result from the specific hybridization of probe with target mRNA. Background binding or noise can be due to the formation of incomplete hybrids or to the nonspecific interaction (i.e., not due to base pairing) of probe or label with other tissue components. As discussed in the methods section, assay conditions must be optimized to minimize the formation of incomplete hybrids and reduce binding due to hydrophobic interactions.

For systems in which peptide-containing cells have been localized using immunocytochemical techniques, an anatomical criterion of signal specificity can be used. The location of grain clusters by *in situ* hybridization should make anatomical sense. Double-labeling techniques allowing the colocalization of peptide and mRNA in the same cell have been developed (12, 13). When discrepancies are observed between the findings of immunocytochemistry and *in situ* hybridization, or when the anatomical distribution is not known, other types of control procedures become particularly important. If message levels are sufficiently high, it may be important to replicate the results of *in situ* hybridization by Northern analysis using similar hybridization conditions and wash stringencies. Ideally, only one major band of the appropriate size should be visible.

As discussed previously, the stability of DNA–RNA hybrids is temperature dependent and the T_m can be used as an index of hybridization specificity. The T_m value determined theoretically can be compared to that derived empirically (10). Using the T_m value, the assay conditions (hybridization temperature and posthybridization wash stringency) can be adjusted to reduce the formation of incomplete hybrids. Signal due to incomplete hybrids will melt off at a lower temperature. While the T_m curve provides extremely valuable information concerning the specificity of signal, it may be technically difficult to generate for some systems, especially those in which the number of labeled cells is very low.

One of the strongest tests for specificity of hybridization is to show that multiple probes complementary to nonhomologous regions of the message hybridize to the same cells. This is typically done in serial sections; however, combinations of radioactive and biotinylated probes can be used to establish colocalization.

Competition studies involving the displacement of labeled probe by excess unlabeled probe have also been used to determine specificity of signal. We typically displace with 100-fold excess unlabeled probe. We have interpreted the loss of signal in these slides to indicate that the labeled probe is binding to a limited number of binding sites. Theoretically, nonspecific background binding should not be reduced by competition. While this control suggests that the labeled probe is binding to mRNA, it does not verify that the signal is due to the formation of complete hybrids, only a melting curve or a Northern analysis can determine this.

Control procedures involving the hybridization of labeled sense probes are also frequently run. Using the complementary sense strand ensures a match for G–C content and probe length. The absence of signal over cells in sections hybridized with sense probes suggests that antisense probes are binding to mRNA and not just interacting with tissue components in a nonspecific manner. This control suggests that the labeled probe is base pairing with mRNA, but again it does not address the completeness of hybrid formation.

Another control commonly used is to hybridize tissue sections that have been pretreated with RNase to destroy mRNA. The loss of signal over cells in these slides indicates that grain clusters present in adjacent sections are due to the interaction of probe with RNA. Again, this control indicates that the signal is due to probe hybridizing with RNA but it does not assess the degree of mismatches.

All of the controls listed above provide important information concerning the specificity of hybridization. No single control is adequate and a combination of these procedures must be run to validate an assay, reduce the possibility of false positives, and optimize the use of *in situ* hybridization as a quantitative technique.

Quantification Methods

One of the most attractive features of the *in situ* hybridization methodology is that it affords the investigator the ability not only to localize cells expressing a given gene product, but also to quantify the amount of mRNA present in a discrete anatomical region of the brain. Quantification, however, poses one of the most technically challenging aspects of this technique. We discuss here some of the approaches which we have used in quantification of film and emulsion autoradiography.

Since autoradiography had previously been used extensively to quantify mRNA on nitrocellulose blots from Northern analyses, it was natural that it be applied to detection of hybridization of radiolabeled probes to mRNA in tissue sections. Likewise, much of the early work was performed using ^{32}P-labeled probes which afforded high specific activity, and therefore sensitivity, but poor anatomical resolution due to the high-energy emission spectra of this isotope. Tritiated RNA probes translated from DNA templates using ^{3}H-labeled nucleotides have also been used to enhance resolution so that single cells containing message can be identified. In this section, we will focus our attention on the use of ^{35}S-labeled DNA probes. This isotope offers the advantage of intermediate β particle emission energy (e.g., very similar to that of ^{14}C), high specific activity and labeling efficiency, and autoradiographic resolution rivaling that achieved using tritium.

Film

Apposition of slide-mounted brain sections to photographic film results in images containing useful anatomical information at the level of nuclear brain structure. When cells showing positive hybridization for a given mRNA are grouped in close proximity to one another, images similar to those shown in

Fig. 1 result. Vasopressin-producing cells of the SON and PVN of the hypothalamus show a clear hybridization signal, and the intensity of that signal, e.g., the optical density (OD) of the film overlying those nuclei is directly proportional (although not necessarily linearly) to the quantity of vasopressin mRNA contained within their confines in a particular section. Therefore, it should be possible to relate the OD of the film to the amount of radioactivity required to expose the film to that OD. Using the specific activity of the labeled probe, one should be able to calculate mRNA hybridized per unit area.

The quantification scheme described above requires that a method of standardizing the relationship between radioisotope concentration and film OD must be devised. One method which has been used by investigators performing tissue-based receptor autoradiographic studies involves the use of "brain paste" standards containing different amounts of radioactivity. These standards are apposed to the film along with the hybridized sections of interest. The problem with this approach is that, when ^{35}S is used, its short half-life would require making standards for each experiment. We have used an alternative approach. In order to express signal density in terms of microcuries/gram tissue equivalents, we have cross-calibrated commercially available plastic standards containing ^{14}C with ^{35}S-labeled brain paste standards. Increasing concentrations of [^{35}S]ATP were mixed with brain paste, molded, and sectioned on a cryostat. Some sections were mounted on microscope slides while others were used for scintillation counting to determine the amount of radioactivity (microcuries/gram). Slide-mounted sections were air dried, apposed to LKB-Ultrofilm along with ^{14}C plastic standards, and exposed for 1-, 3-, and 5-day intervals. Figure 2 depicts the resulting curves for 3- and 5-day exposures. The relationship appeared nearly linear and a conversion factor based on optical density measurements was derived for each exposure that would relate microcuries/gram plastic to microcuries/gram tissue. Thus, the plastic standards can be used alone over time for inclusion in subsequent assays to relate OD to radioactivity.

Figure 3 depicts data obtained in an experiment in which we attempted to establish the probe concentration required to saturate the hybridization signal of vasopressin mRNA in the SON of the rat hypothalamus. Here, serial sections of brain containing the hypothalamus and SON were exposed to increasing amounts of ^{35}S-labeled oligonucleotide probe complementary to mRNA encoding a portion of the glycopeptide tail of the vasopressin precursor. The processed sections were apposed to LKB-Ultrofilm and the resulting images analyzed using a computerized image analysis system (DUMAS). The image was magnified using a lens and a video camera. A square cursor was used to sample the total hybridization signal (directly over the SON) and the background signal (moving the cursor to an adjacent

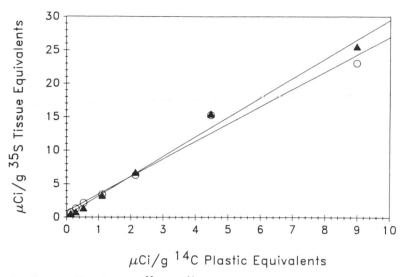

FIG. 2   Cross-calibration of ^{35}S to ^{14}C standards for use in quantitative film autoradiography. The curves shown were obtained by coexposing brain paste slices containing [35]S- and ^{14}C-impregnated plastic standards to LKB-Ultrofilm for (▲) 3 or (○) 5 days. The images were analyzed using a computerized image analysis system. See the text for further information.

region outside the SON). As Fig. 3 shows, the hybridization signal achieved in the SON was saturable. It is important to note that these readings were taken over the linear range of response of LKB Ultrofilm (e.g., less than 0.9 OD). If the investigator anticipates achieving greater OD values, other films may be more appropriate, such as Beta Max-Hyperfilm (Amersham Corp.). This film has a broader linear response range and offers the added advantage of a protective coating that prevents artifactual scratching which can easily occur when tritium-sensitive films are used.

Emulsion-Coated Sections

When the cells of interest are not densely packed or have low hybridization signal, little, if any, useful information can be obtained using films and emulsion coating of sections becomes preferable. Single-cell resolution can be achieved using either [35]S- or ^{3}H-labeled probes. Typically, what is observed is a radial pattern of grains above what can be verified as a cell soma using Nissl stains (see Fig. 4). The issue of quantification of hybridiza-

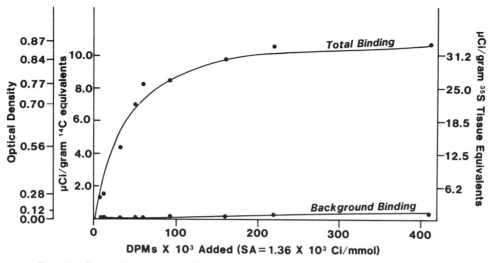

FIG. 3   Saturation of hybridization signal of AVP mRNA in the SON of the rat hypothalamus. Serial sections were exposed to increasing amounts of ^{35}S-labeled probe and then exposed to LKB-Ultrofilm. The resulting images were read for optical density. The curves in Fig. 2 were used to relate OD to ^{14}C and ^{35}S tissue equivalents.

tion signal becomes increasingly complex at this level. The problem requires relating silver grains in the emulsion overlying a cell to those associated with a known amount of radioactivity. One approach which has been used is to emulsion coat homogeneous radioactive sources such as the brain paste standards or plastic standards described above in order to construct standard curves. The potential flaw in this approach is that one can never be sure that the grain density associated with these continuous standards is similar to the pattern of grains due to radioactivity associated with probe in a single hybridized cell. The radioactivity in the latter case is more similar to a point source than to a homogeneous field of radioactivity. For this reason, we only quantify the number of cells showing hybridization signal and the number of grains per cell. Using this type of data, relative changes in mRNA levels in groups of cells can be assessed (e.g., -fold changes in signal or number of cells expressing a given gene product). Labeled cells are identified by the experimenter, and the grains are counted using an automated computer-based image analysis system. This system consists of a Data Cube IVS-12E video acquisition board (Data Cube, Inc., Peabody, MA) attached to an IBM AT computer. Video images are obtained by a Dage model 65 camera (Dage-MTI, Inc., Michigan City, IN) attached to an Olympus photomicroscope equipped with a dark-field condenser. Images are acquired in dark-field using the 40× objective.

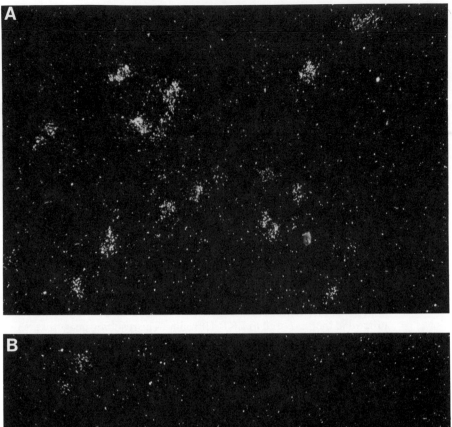

Fig. 4 Dark-field photomicrograph (100×) showing labeling of AVP mRNA in individual cells of the bed nucleus of the stria terminalis of male (A) and female (B) Wistar rats. The vasopressin system in this region of the brain is sexually dimorphic.

An automated grain detection program developed by Donald Clifton (Department of Obstetrics and Gynecology, University of Washington School of Medicine) is used to analyze the images. In this program, the center of the cluster of grains over a cell is found by determining the peak in the intensity profiles along the x and y axes of the image. Grains are assigned to pixels if its gray level value was greater than a predetermined threshold and that of the eight pixels surrounding it. Thus, background and signal grain density can be calculated, as well as the number of grains per cell (e.g., the number of grains over background present within a 32-μm radius of the center of the grain cluster). Many other equally effective grain counting systems are available.

Experimental Considerations

For some studies involving assessment of biosynthetic capacity, conventional filter or solution hybridization techniques may be adequate, and in fact the use of *in situ* hybridization in these studies could be considered technical overkill. For other studies, however, *in situ* hybridization is the technique of choice and allows the research to answer questions which cannot be addressed using other hybridization methods.

Since the quantitative information provided by *in situ* hybridization can be reduced to the cellular level, adequate and unbiased sampling becomes an important experimental consideration. This involves the selection of an appropriate sample and standardizing this sample between different treatment groups. First, tissue sections should be matched anatomically. This is facilitated by taking care to section the brains on the cryostat according to a standard atlas plane. We mount 3–4 serial brain sections per slide and leave a bank space on the slide if a section is lost during cutting. This enables us to account for all sections throughout our region of interest and facilitates the anatomical matching of slides. Once slides are matched, the subset of labeled cells or region to be sampled needs to be determined and standardized across groups. Limits on sample selection may be imposed by the particular software available to the researcher for quantification of the autoradiograms and emulsion-coated slides. In an attempt to reduce experimenter bias, our slides are then coded and read "blindly" by a single operator using the guidelines established for sample selection. Some recent studies have attempted to compare measurements of mRNA levels by *in situ* hybridization with those determined by Northern analysis and have found good agreement between the methods (14, 15). Clearly, the selection of which cells are sampled in any treatment group may dramatically influence the consistency of the findings and the degree of agreement between *in situ* and other methods of hybridization.

Hybridization studies generally fall into two major categories: (1) hybridization of a single probe in a particular subset of cells across two or more groups or (2) hybridization of multiple probes to the same cell or brain region. There are experimental considerations associated with each design. These considerations are particularly relevant when quantitative comparisons are to be made.

Most hybridization studies fall into the first category. When comparing across two or more groups using the same probe, group differences will be optimized by using a probe concentration which saturates mRNA levels in each group. This concentration of probe may need to be determined in a pilot assay. In addition, slides from each group need to be balanced within an assay and across assays to avoid introducing a systematic bias into the data. The assay itself must be standardized to minimize both inter- and intraassay variability. If possible, serial sections can be run in each tray as an internal control to assess intraassay variability. Since we currently run assays that include up to 600 slides, we balance our groups within the slide trays and change solutions after every four trays of slides in an attempt to reduce assay variability.

Quantitative studies involving hybridization of multiple probes within the same cells or brain regions present more complex experimental considerations than in simple localization studies. Assay conditions (including probe concentration, hybridization conditions, and wash stringencies) must be optimized for each probe. The use of oligonucleotide probes matched for length and GC content may facilitate running this type of study. Comparison of intensity of hybridization by multiple probes requires that differences in specific activity be controlled or taken into account. This might be easier to accomplish using oligonucleotide probes instead of riboprobes. Specific activity across probes could be matched by running end-labeled oligomers on a gel and only hybridizing with bands of a certain tail length.

Examples of Use

A major focus of our research has been to investigate the regulation of biosynthetic capacity of vasopressin (AVP) neurons in the bed nucleus of the stria terminalis (BNST) using *in situ* hybridization. Using a 48-base oligonucleotide probe complementary to the mRNA encoding the last 16 amino acids of the glycopeptide portion of the AVP precursor, we have verified the presence of AVP-synthesizing cells in the BNST. We have found that the sexual dimorphism of these cells recently shown by immunohistochemistry (16) results from a sex difference in the biosynthetic capacity of this cell group. Significantly more neurons are labeled in male rats ($p < 0.01$) than in female rats and labeled cells average more grains/cell in males ($p < 0.05$) than in females. Testosterone and/or its metabolites enhance the expression of the AVP gene in these cells, since we have found that long-term castration of adult male rats significantly reduces AVP mRNA levels in the BNST (cell number, $p < 0.01$; grains/cell, $p < 0.01$), while testosterone treatment reverses the effects of castration.

In addition to the BNST, we wanted to determine whether cells in the medial amygdala (MA) and locus coeruleus (LC) synthesize AVP. Other studies have shown the presence of AVP and neurophysin immunoreactivity in cells of the MA and LC (17), but direct evidence for AVP biosynthesis was lacking. Using methods described in this chapter, we were able to label AVP mRNA in cells in the MA but not in the LC. The lack of labeling in LC cells raises some important questions. Since our probe is directed at the glycopeptide region of the AVP gene it only labels the mRNA encoded by that particular gene sequence. Perhaps another gene, one that does not contain a glycopeptide region, is responsible for the synthesis of AVP in the LC. It is also possible that the amount of message produced in these cells is below the sensitivity limit of our assay. Alternatively, AVP may not be synthesized in these cells. The LC may take up and store AVP for release at a later time. Further studies will be required to thoroughly address this question. However, these results suggest that the combined use of *in situ* hybridization and immunocytochemistry together can provide valuable information on neuronal gene expression. *In situ* hybridization, when appropriately applied, can provide important information which cannot presently be obtained using other methods.

Acknowledgment

The authors wish to thank Maxine Cormier and Connie Evoy for typing this manuscript. We also wish to thank John Breininger for his skillful technical assistance. This work was supported by the Veterans Administration and NIH grant NS 20311.

References

1. H. H. Zingg, D. Lefebvre, and G. Almanzan, *Proc. Natl. Acad. Sci. U.S.A.* **261,** 12956 (1986).
2. T. G. Sherman, O. Cirelli, J. Douglass, E. Herbert, S. Burke, and J. J. Watson, *Fed. Proc., Fed. Am. Soc. Exp. Biol.* **45,** 2323 (1986).
3. P. J. Fuller, J. A. Clements, and J. W. Funder, *Endocrinology (Baltimore)* **116,** 2366 (1985).
4. G. R. Uhl, H. H. Zingg, and J. F. Habener, *Proc. Natl. Acad. Sci. U.S.A.* **82,** 5555 (1985).

5. K. H. Cox, D. V. DeLeon, L. M. Angerer, and R. C. Angerer, *Dev. Biol.* **101,** 485 (1984).

6. W. S. Young, T. I. Bonner, and M. R. Brann, *Proc. Natl. Acad. Sci. U.S.A.* **83,** 9827 (1986).

7. G. A. Higgins and M. C. Wilson, in *"In Situ* Hybridization: Applications to Neurobiology" (K. L. Valentino, J. H. Eberwine, and J. D. Barchas, eds.), p. 146. Oxford Univ. Press, London and New York, 1987.

8. L. M. Angerer, M. H. Stoler, and R. C. Angerer, in *"In Situ* Hybridization: Applications to Neurobiology" (K. L. Valentino, J. H. Eberwine, and J. D. Barchas, eds.), p. 42. Oxford Univ. Press, London and New York, 1987.

9. S. Hayashi, I. C. Gillam, A. D. Delaney, and G. M. Tener, *J. Histochem. Cytochem.* **26,** 677 (1978).

10. M. E. Lewis, T. G. Sherman, and S. J. Watson, *Peptides* **6** (Suppl. 2), 75 (1985).

11. K. V. Rogers, L. Vician, R. A. Steiner, and D. K. Clifton, *Endocrinology (Baltimore)* **122,** 586 (1988).

12. W. S. Young, M. Warden, and E. Mezey, *Neuroendocrinology* **46,** 439 (1987).

13. W. S. T. Griffen, in *"In Situ* Hybridization: Applications to Neurobiology" (K. L. Valentino, J. H. Eberwine, and J. D. Barchas, eds.), p. 97. Oxford Univ. Press, London and New York, 1987.

14. T. G. Sherman, H. Akil, and S. J. Watson, in "Vasopressin" (R. W. Schrier, ed.), p. 475. Raven, New York, 1985.

15. J. E. Kelsey, S. J. Watson, S. Burke, H. Akil, and J. L. Roberts, *J. Neurosci.* **6,** 38 (1986).

16. G. J. DeVries, R. M. Buijs, and A. A. Sluiter, *Brain Res.* **298,** 141 (1984).

17. A. R. Caffé and F. W. van Leeuwen, *Cell Tissue Res.* **233,** 23 (1983).

[11] *In Situ* Hybridization Approaches to Human Neurological Disease

Gerald A. Higgins and Vei H. Mah

In situ hybridization has emerged as a powerful tool for the examination of cell type-specific gene expression in the human central nervous system (CNS). The CNS is the most highly differentiated of all tissues, with the human brain containing several thousand different cell types. *In situ* hybridization can be used to identify and analyze specific mRNA transcripts within individual cells or populations of cells within this complex structure. The human CNS presents a more formidable challenge for such *in situ* hybridization studies than do similar approaches in other experimental species. However, recent increases in the sensitivity of *in situ* hybridization methods, coupled with rapid autopsy procedures and the increasing availability of postmortem tissue, have begun to make it possible to pose experimental questions about gene expression that can be addressed directly within the context of known features of human brain organization. For example, disease-related changes in gene expression can be determined by comparing differences in the distribution and/or abundance of specific mRNA species between normal and diseased tissue. This approach is especially important in neurological disorders such as Alzheimer's disease, in which the pathology targets specific neuronal subtypes, and appropriate animal models are not available for analysis.

In situ hybridization can be used to examine the expression of previously characterized gene products in human neurological disease, such as studies of differential amyloid β-protein mRNA expression in Alzheimer's disease, but it also represents a rapid and sensitive neuroanatomical screening method (1) when used in conjunction with anonymous DNA probes generated from genetic linkage studies of neurological disease. For example, recent anatomical studies suggest that medium spiny neurons of the caudate/putamen are one of the first neuronal subtypes to be affected in Huntington's disease (HD) (2). Thus, the neuropathological consequences of the disease may involve expression of an abundant gene product within a specific striatal cell type. Protein-coding DNA probes, generated from the region of human chromosome 4 that contains the genetic marker associated with HD (3), could be screened on tissue sections for their localization to vulnerable neuronal cell types. Initial screening could be used to identify striatal cell type-specific gene products. Alternatively, changes in the abundance of a particular mRNA may be identified by comparative studies of unaffected versus diseased human brain tissue.

The use of human brain tissue for *in situ* hybridization studies poses special problems that require protection of laboratory personnel from infectious agents, knowledge of patient history, and optimization of technical sensitivity. Brain mRNA may be vulnerable to degradation during the delay between death and subsequent fixation or freezing of tissue samples. Individual differences in premorbid state and postmortem delays can also produce tremendous variability between cases. Superimposed on normal variability are disease-related phenomena which may not be predictable. For some experiments, it may be important to quantify changes in the level of an affected mRNA, often by comparison to a control mRNA transcript whose prevalance is presumably not changed by the disease process. However, appropriate controls are not always apparent in comparisons between normal and diseased tissue. For example, under conditions which result in accelerated neuronal death and reactive gliosis, the levels of any given "control" mRNA transcript may also be changed by the disease process, even within surviving cells that appear unaffected. Finally, it is often difficult to acquire tissue from early stages of a disease. In neurological disorders such as Huntington's disease and Alzheimer's disease, the investigator is often faced with examination of "end-stage" phenomena, from patients who have died as a result of a lengthy degenerative process. Thus, dynamic changes in gene expression related to primary events in the disease process may not be directly available for examination, unless it is possible to obtain postmortem tissue samples from patients who have died at early stages of the disease process.

Maintenance of RNA Integrity in Human Postmortem Brain Tissue

The most common sources of human brain tissue for *in situ* hybridization studies come from autopsy and biopsy material. For tissue samples obtained at autopsy, lengthy delays may intervene between death and subsequent freezing or fixation. Lengthy postmortem intervals, the premorbid agonal state of the patient, neuropathological sequelae such as cell death, as well as dissection, storage, and histological procedures, may enhance ribonuclease-mediated degradation of RNA in tissue samples used for *in situ* hybridization. Sources of ribonuclease include endogenous stores and exogenous contamination introduced by experimental manipulation of the tissue. Brain tissue contains a lysosomal acidic ribonuclease, as well as an alkaline ribonuclease (active at pH 7.2 to 8), whose activity may normally be regulated by a bound inhibitor (4). The acidic form of ribonuclease can be released by a variety of factors which rupture lysosomes, including premorbid hypoxia, freeze–thawing, and tissue disruption during dissection and microtomy. Release of "free" alkaline ribonuclease may also be caused by disruption of the nuclease–inhibitor complex (5). Both forms of brain ribonuclease survive conditions which may inactivate many other enzymes, and retain their activity in previously frozen tissue (6).

Despite the presence of endogenous ribonuclease, a consensus of recent experimental data shows that brain mRNA remains stable in intact brain tissue over lengthy postmortem intervals. Results from studies using a variety of methods, including *in vitro* translation, Northern blotting, cDNA cloning, as well as *in situ* hybridization of mRNA, in both human and rodent, suggest that the integrity of brain RNA is not simply a function of the length of the postmortem interval (7–10). However, yields of total cellular and poly(A)$^+$ RNA seem to be consistently lower from human brain tissue as opposed to that of other species (7, 8, 11). It has also been suggested that dissection of human brain tissue greatly enhances RNA degradation through release of ribonuclease from cells on the disrupted, cut surface of the tissue block (8). Both the yield and integrity of RNA appear to be compromised in some neurological disorders (12). It was originally suggested that increased RNA degradation in Alzheimer's disease may be due to alterations of the alkaline ribonuclease–inhibitor complex (5), but these findings have not been reproduced by more recent studies (13). Instead, it appears that the cell death and accompanying lysis which occur in the disease probably lead to increased levels of nonsequestered ribonuclease which is active during the isolation and extraction procedure. Therefore, it is imperative for tissue dissection and manipulation be kept to a minimum, and be performed quickly and under conditions that minimize RNA degradation.

In contrast to brain proteins, which vary widely in their spectrum of activity and sensitivity to proteolysis following death (14, 15), postmortem degradation of mRNA occurs essentially at random in both normal and neurologically diseased brain tissue (7). All mRNA transcripts appear to be similarly affected by degradative processes, allowing meaningful quantitative comparisons to be made among different mRNA species, and between normal and pathological states (see below). Thus, it appears that postmortem interval may not be as important a factor in maintenance of RNA stability as are the premorbid agonal state of the patient, the cellular impact of neuropathological disease processes, and the manipulation of tissue specimens prior to the *in situ* hybridization procedure.

Tissue Preparation

Human brain tissue must always be handled with caution and appropriate protective measures undertaken, such as the wearing of gloves, to avoid transmission of viral or pathological agents from brain tissue to laboratory personnel. Ideally, it is possible for the basic scientist to interact closely with the neuropathologist in obtaining autopsy material. Neuropathological evaluation should be performed to confirm diagnosis and to identify potentially hazardous tissue samples. Also, cases of disease "mimicry," mixed disease entities, or confounding influences of disease in the cases of what appear to be neurologically "normal" individuals, can be identified by neuropathological examination.

Morphological sampling should be used to characterize tissue samples destined for biochemical analysis. Often, one brain hemisphere is frozen for neurochemical analysis, while tissue blocks or slabs from the other hemisphere are placed in fixative for subsequent morphological studies. Interhemispheric comparisons should be undertaken with caution, however, in light of possible hemispheric asymmetries which may exist in the normal human brain and in neurological disease. Thus, correlative measurements taken from the same tissue samples strengthen conclusions regarding disease-related changes in gene expression.

Fixation

We have used both fresh-frozen and immersion-fixed human brain tissue for *in situ* hybridization. Alternatively, brain tissue may be fixed by vascular perfusion after death (16). Tissue embedded in paraffin has been used successfully for *in situ* hybridization studies, even after storage in paraffin for several years (17). Fresh tissue must be quickly isolated, preferably under ultralow temperature conditions, be snap-frozen in isopentane or liquid nitrogen, and stored at liquid nitrogen temperatures until ready for use. Following cryotomy, slide-mounted unfixed tissue sections must be stored frozen, and immediately placed in fixative upon thawing to prevent endogenous ribonuclease activity. Better results are obtained with tissue slabs, no thicker than 1–2 cm, which are fixed by immersion in either 4% paraformaldehyde in phosphate buffer (PB: 0.15 M, pH 7.4) or 2% PLP (10 mM periodate/37.5 mM lysine/2% paraformaldehyde) at 4°C for at least 48 hr. These are then rinsed in a series of graded sucrose solutions [10, 16, 18, up to 40% (use RNase-free sucrose) in PB]. The tissue samples can then be frozen in powdered dry ice and stored at −80°C, or tissue sections stored in cryoprotectant solution [100 mM PB, pH 7.2, 30% sucrose (w/v), 30% ethylene glycol (v/v)] at −80°C. Long-term storage of sucrose-infiltrated brain tissue at 4° is *not* recommended. Tissue slabs or sections stored in cryoprotectant storage solution must be thoroughly rinsed in PBS prior to *in situ* hybridization, as this treatment seems to produce an elevation in background "noise." We have obtained better results with monoaldehyde fixatives such as 4% paraformaldehyde or PLP, than with Carnoy's fixative (ethanol/acetic acid), fixatives containing glutaraldehyde, or with picric acid-containing fixatives such as Bouin's or Zamboni's fixatives.

Cryostat Sectioning

Again, gloves should always be worn during handling of the tissue and slides. Frozen tissue slabs are frozen to a layer of OCT compound (Tissue Tek, Naperville, IL) on a cryostat chuck placed on a freezing stage or on crushed dry ice. Frozen 10- to 20-μm-thick sections are collected from the cold knife blade and thawed directly onto chromalum-subbed slides and air dried. Alternatively, large tissue sections may be more easily cut on a sliding microtome with a freezing stage. Our experience suggests that robust hybridization signals can be obtained from tissue section stored on slides which are kept desiccated for several weeks at 4°C or up to several months at −80°C.

Subbing of Slides

Unfortunately, one of the most trivial, but difficult, problems faced by the novice attempting *in situ* hybridization methods is maintaining adherence of tissue sections to slides during the procedure. Fixed tissue sections are mounted on freshly prepared (less than 1 week old) chromalum-subbed slides. To prepare the subbing solution, 1% gelatin (Sigma; calf skin gelatin, Type III) is dissolved by stirring in distilled water (dH$_2$O) at 37°C (do not exceed 40°C), and CrKSO$_4$ is added to a final concentration of 1 mg/ml. The slides are held in a stainless steel rack, dipped briefly in subbing solution, and allowed to air dry overnight, or at 37°C if destined for immediate use. Alternatively, slides can be subbed with high-molecular-weight polylysine (18). For fresh tissue sections, freshly prepared acetylated Denhardt's subbed slides are used. Precleaned slides are incubated in 3× SSC and 1× Denhardt's [0.02% bovine serum albumin/0.02% Ficoll/0.02% poly(vinylpyrrolidone)] for 3 hr at 67°C, rinsed briefly in dH$_2$O, acetylated in a 3:1 ratio of absolute ethanol to glacial acetic acid, and air dried. These slides remain viable for 3–5 days.

In Situ Hybridization Procedure

RNA Probe Transcription

Plasmid templates are incubated with the appropriate RNA polymerase (i.e., SP6, T7, or T3) for production of ^{35}S-labeled single-stranded antisense or sense strand RNA probes. It is essential that plasmid DNA templates for RNA polymerase be completely linearized with the appropriate restriction enzyme. Supercoiled DNA is a more efficient template for transcription than is linearized plasmid, and sequences within certain transcription vectors may hybridize to glial cells within white matter regions of the CNS (see below). Transcription is performed in a volume of 25 μl containing 40 mM Tris-HCl, pH 7.5, 6 mM MgCl$_2$, 2 mM dithiothreitol (DTT), 5 U of ribonuclease inhibitor (Promega Biotech, Madison, WI), 400 μM of rATP, rGTP, and rUTP, 25 μM of [^{35}S]rCTP (800 Ci/mmol, Amersham, Arlington Heights, IL), 1 μg of linearized DNA template, plus 5–10 U of the appropriate RNA polymerase. The transcription reaction is incubated at 37°C for 1.5 hr, and incorporation is measured by trichloroacetic acid precipitation. Typical yields from these reactions containing limiting concentrations of labeled rCTP average 100–400 ng. The probe is then extracted, twice precipitated, and resuspended in small volumes of diethyl pyrocarbonate (DEPC)-treated (1 : 10,000 dilution) dH$_2$O prior to use. In the case of relatively short probe lengths, it is not necessary to remove nondenatured DNA template, because it does not seem to affect probe sensitivity or signal-to-noise ratio. However, better results can be obtained by using alkaline hydrolysis to reduce the size of RNA probes over 500 bases in length (19), and in these cases, denatured DNA template is removed by DNase treatment followed by purification by Sephadex G-50 spin chromatography (Pharmacia "Nick" columns).

Synthetic Oligonucleotide Probes

Synthetic oligonucleotide probes offer certain advantages over RNA probes in that they are easy to generate, their small size allows for greater penetration into the tissue, and they do not show some of the problems associated with certain RNA probes. However, they have greatly reduced hybrid stability and are less readily labeled to a high specific activity. For *in situ* hybridization, we routinely label oligonucleotide probes by addition of [^{35}S]dCTP to the 3′ end of the oligonucleotide with terminal deoxynucleotidyltransferase. The length of the added tail is controlled by the length of the reaction and the concentration of the reaction components. The reaction consists of [^{35}S]dCTP (800 Ci/mmol, New England Nuclear, Wilmington, DE); 5× tailing buffer containing 2 mM CoCl$_2$, cacodylate buffer, 100 mM

Tris (pH 7.5), and 5 mM DTT; 1 μg of oligonucleotide; 10 μl dH$_2$O; and 2 μl (20 U) of terminal transferase. The reaction is incubated at 42°C for 1 hr, and the reaction is terminated by heating to 67°C for 5 min. The labeled probe can be purified by polyacrylamide gel electrophoresis (12% for short oligonucleotides and 20% for longer oligonucleotides) under denaturing conditions. This allows visualization and size determination, and the probe can then be eluted from the gel for use.

Biotinylated Probes

In theory, biotinylated probes offer many advantages over radioactively labeled probes, including higher cellular resolution when combined with peroxidase detection methods, enhanced compatibility with immunocyto-chemical methods, and rapid results. However, it has been our experience that biotinylated probes are more than 10-fold less sensitive when compared side-by-side with high-specific-activity radiolabeled probes. This may be due to inherent problems associated with adding biotin molecules to nucleic acids, and maintaining subsequent accessibility to avidin. Recent increases in the sensitivity of detection and biotinylation methods may allow produc-tion of higher-specific-activity probes (20).

Amplification Procedures

DNA amplification methods may be applied to increase the sensitivity of *in situ* hybridization. *In situ* transcription involves annealing of short oligonu-cleotides to target mRNA, which can be used as a primer for reverse transcriptase-mediated amplification of the hybridization signal (21). In our hands, this method greatly increases the sensitivity of *in situ* localization of mRNAs, but does not offer any improvement in the signal-to-noise ratios that can be achieved by high-specific-activity (greater than 2×10^9 cpm/μg) radiolabeled RNA probes. However, recent advances in polymerase chain reaction (PCR) methods (22) can be applied to amplify the *in situ* transcrip-tion signal.

Hybridization Probes

A more detailed description of probe selection and hybridization kinetics can be found elsewhere (23). In general, we have chosen hybridization conditions consistent with published recommendations for single-stranded RNA and synthetic oligonucleotide probe hybridization (23, 24).

Preparation of Glassware and Reagents

All precautions are taken to maintain a ribonuclease-free environment in the laboratory (25). All Pyrex glassware is baked at 250°C for several hours. Phosphate-buffered saline (PBS) is prepared with DEPC and then autoclaved. In our experience, autoclaving does not completely eliminate DEPC from solutions. Thus, glassware or reagents to be used for enzymes such as proteinase K or ribonuclease are never pretreated with DEPC. Glass staining dishes are acid-washed, rinsed with dH$_2$O, soaked in dH$_2$O containing DEPC (1 : 10,000), rinsed with dH$_2$O, and baked at 250°C for 3–4 hr. The oven is then turned off and the staining dishes are allowed to cool to room temperature before they are removed from the oven. Metal slide racks are soaked in DEPC-treated dH$_2$O, and extensively rinsed in dH$_2$O before use. A separate set of glassware and metal staining racks are used for posthybridization treatments which use RNase A.

Pretreatment

Our method provides a compromise between permeabilization treatments to allow access of probe to mRNA, retention of mRNA within tissue, and preservation of cellular morphology. The current procedure has been more generally described elsewhere (1, 26). Pretreatment is performed on slides placed in metal racks in glass staining dishes. The slides are rinsed twice in PBS (0.15 M, pH 7.4, 145 mM NaCl) for 2 min each after each pretreatment step prior to dehydration. The pretreatment steps consist of (1) fixation in 4% buffered formaldehyde at room temperature (RT) (1 min for fixed tissue; 5 min for fresh tissue); (2) digestion in proteinase K [50 μg/ml in 5× TE (50 mM Tris, 5 mM EDTA), pH 8.0] for 7.5 min at 37°C; (3) 0.05 N HCl treatment for 7.5 min at RT (this step may be optional, but it seems to help reduce white matter background, and thus it may act as a delipidating as well as a deproteinizing agent); (4) postfixation in 4% buffered paraformaldehyde for exactly 5 min at RT; (5) dehydration in graded alcohols containing 0.33 M ammonium acetate (25 g/liter); and (6) air drying. We have also used acetic anhydride (0.25% in 0.1 M triethanolamine-HCl, pH 8.0) treatment, which reduces electrostatic binding of the probe to amino groups in tissue sections (27).

Prehybridization and Hybridization

In general, the prehybridization buffer consists of 50% formamide, 0.5 M NaCl, 25 mM PIPES buffer (pH 6.8), 25 mM EDTA, 250 mM DTT, 5×

Denhardt's solution, 0.2% SDS, and 10% dextran sulfate. Denatured yeast tRNA and salmon sperm DNA are added to 500 μg/ml. For short synthetic oligonucleotide probes, inclusion of homochromatography mix (250 μg/ml), which contains hydrolyzed tRNA fragments, appears to help reduce nonspecific absorption of the probe to other nucleic acids (23). Prehybridization buffer (750 μl) is carefully applied to cover the tissue sections on the slides, which are lying within a humidified plexiglass box, and are prehybridized for 1–3 hr. For both prehybridization and subsequent probe hybridization, the box is placed in a forced-air oven at the appropriate temperature (usually 45–60°C for RNA probes; 30–42°C for oligonucleotide probes, depending on the T_m).

For both RNA and oligonucleotide probes, the hybridization buffer consists of the prehybridization components plus labeled probe. The prehybridization buffer is removed by blotting of the slides, and 80 μl of hybridization buffer is added to cover the sections, followed by coverslipping. We have not found it necessary to siliconize or otherwise pretreat coverslips. The edges of the coverslips are sealed with Royalbond Grip contact cement (Indal Products, Los Angeles, CA), and the slides are placed into the humidified box for hybridization at the appropriate temperature. For ^{35}S-labeled RNA probes, the coverslips are removed at RT in 4× SSC containing 10 mM DTT or 250 mM 2-mercaptoethanol. Inclusion of high concentrations of reducing agents in the hybridization and posthybridization rinses helps to eliminate the nonspecific background associated with use of ^{35}S-labeled probes. Subsequent washing steps consist of incubation of the slides in (1) 4× SSC for 15 min at RT; (2) pancreatic ribonuclease [RNase A; can also include RNase T_1 (75 μg/ml in RNase buffer: 500 mM NaCl and 50 mM Tris, pH 8.0)] for 30 min at 37°C; (3) RNase buffer without ribonuclease for 30 min at 37°C; (4) 2× SSC for 15 min at 37°C; and (5) a high-stringency rinse, which can include 50% formamide, usually 0.2× SSC for 30 min at 42°C. For oligonucleotide probes, the coverslips are removed in 2× SSC, and the wash stringency taken to a combination of salt concentration and temperature appropriate for the probe. DTT (10 mM) is included in all washing steps with ^{35}S-tailed oligonucleotide probes. The slides are then air dried and are placed into a metal X-ray cassette for rapid exposure to X-ray film (DuPont Cronex 4) for 12–72 hr, depending on the amount of counts per second (cps) measured on the dried slides using a hand-held Geiger counter (e.g., 2–5 cps − 48 hr, 20 cps = 12 hr). The slides are then processed for emulsion autoradiography.

Two alternative approaches can be used for autoradiography. In the past, we have dipped the slides into Kodak NTB-2 or NTB-3 emulsion (diluted 1:1 with dH$_2$O) melted at 42°C, placed them into slide boxes containing Drierite, and exposed the slides at 4°C for a length of time 3- to 5-fold longer than that required to obtain a signal on the X-ray film. However, it has been argued that use of dry emulsion-coated coverslips may help to eliminate variability in the thickness of the emulsion coating over the tissue sections, which may arise from direct dipping of the slides in emulsion (28). Grain density may reflect emulsion thickness with a high-energy isotope such as ^{35}S, leading to possible errors in quantification by grain counting or optical density analysis. Thus, emulsion-coated coverslips may provide more useful quantitative information. Acid-cleaned coverslips are dipped in NTB-2 (Kodak) emulsion, dried, and stored in a light-tight box at 4°C until use. Coverslips are attached at one edge to the slides with superglue, and then clamped in place with Teflon binder clips for exposure. Autoradiographic development consists of (1) Kodak D-19 developer (diluted 1:1 with dH$_2$O) for 2.5 min at 16°C; (2) 20-sec rinse in dH$_2$O; (3) Kodak fixer for 5 min, followed by a running water rinse for 20 min. Selected slides are counterstained with cresyl violet for cytoarchitectonic orientation. Although much of the RNA may be lost during RNase treatment, sufficient cytoplasmic and nuclear staining is usually still apparent after Nissl staining to permit cellular localization.

Artifacts and Controls

We have previously shown that certain CNS structures containing high cellular and ribosomal RNA density exhibit elevated background signals with *in situ* hybridization (1), including the dentate gyrus and CA pyramidal fields of the hippocampal formation, granule cell layer of the cerebellum, primary olfactory and piriform cortices, medial habenular nucleus, and other regions which are stained intensely for Nissl substance. This is especially problematic when using RNA probes, as they appear to contain small sequences which hybridize to ribosomal RNA, even though corresponding DNA probe sequences do not recognize ribosomal RNA (24). Thus, *in situ* hybridization results showed elevated hybridization signals present in these regions should be interpreted with caution and confirmed by other methods. Hybridization to size-fractionated mRNA on Northern blots will recognize 28 S (approximately 5 kb) and 18 S (approximately 2 kb) rRNA bands if the probe contains homology to these sequences, and target mRNA transcript(s) can be discriminated from these signals if they are of a different size. White matter regions sometimes show nonspecific background noise, which may be related either to vector sequence hybridization (see above) or to "lipid-trapping" by myelin or electrostatic effects (27).

We have routinely used sense-strand sequences as a heterologous probe control for RNA antisense hybridization specificity. However, recent studies suggest that symmetrical gene transcription may be more common than was previously thought (29), and therefore specific mRNA transcripts may be detected by sense-strand probes. Additionally, pretreatment of the tissue with RNase to eliminate mRNA from the tissue sections should completely abolish specific hybridization. Some investigators have used "blocking" controls similar to those used in receptor binding or immunocytochemical studies to control for probe specificity; however, we feel that these are unnecessary, considering the specificity of nucleic acid hybridization versus that of ligand–receptor or antibody–antigen interactions.

Application of Quantitative *In Situ* Hybridization Methods for Study of Gene Expression in Human Neurological Disease

Under hybridization conditions where the probe is in vast excess, and therefore the abundance of target mRNA does not influence the rate of hybridization, the intensity of the resultant signal is an accurate representation of the abundance of the target RNA, even if the kinetics of the reaction are not ideal pseudo-first-order in nature (19). When true saturation of the target is reached under high probe concentrations, it may be possible to calculate directly the number of mRNA copies per cell based on extrapolations from probe specific activity, probe length, and efficiency of autoradiographic grain development (19, 30, 31).

Measurement of relative mRNA abundance between different neuronal subpopulations can be made both by densitometric measurement (26) and by manual grain counting. Previously, we used a computer-based video image analysis system (32) for comparisons of relative amyloid β protein mRNA abundance between tissue sections from human brains of normal aged individuals and patients with Alzheimer's disease. In a given 200× magnification field, measurements of optical density per cell were made from individual grain clusters in dark-field microscopic images of emulsion autoradiographs. Individual measurements were pooled for a given neuroanatomical structure and displayed as a scattergram for graphic illustration of the computer-generated mean and standard deviation. In cases of numerically large population differences and small standard deviations, the data may be displayed as ratios of optical density. In most cases, significant differences in comparisons of optical density/cell measurements between cell populations can be determined by analysis of variance (ANOVA). For initial experiments, it is often wise to perform manual grain counting on the same neuronal populations to verify the optical density measurements and comparisons. This analysis is best performed by a naive observer. It should be appreciated that photographic emulsion such as NTB-2 may not provide a linear measure of radioisotopic emission (28). Thus, it is important to include radioactive standards that can be coexposed with the tissue sections, in order to obtain a standard curve reflecting the responses of the emulsion to known amounts of radioactivity. "Brain-paste" standards containing a range of known amounts of isotopes such as ^{35}S can be frozen and sectioned along with the tissue sections for coexposure. Also, saturation overexposure of the emulsion can lead to "ceiling" effects and should be avoided by limiting exposure to three times the amount of time it takes to produce an X-ray film image.

Often, it is necessary to compare the relative prevalence of a single gene product between neurologically normal and pathological states. Under ideal circumstances, the expression of a particular mRNA transcript will be induced or changed only within circumscribed cell populations, but not within all cells of the same tissue section. For example, total amyloid β-protein precursor mRNA levels are increased within parasubicular neurons, but not CA3 pyramidal neurons, in the hippocampal formation in Alzheimer's disease (26). Thus, it is possible to construct "within-section" ratios of hybridization intensity of the same mRNA target sequence between affected and unaffected cell populations within the same tissue sections for comparisons between normal and disease states. This limitation of relative quantitative determinations to comparisons of cell populations within a section is important because of observed variability between *in situ* hybridization experiments, and sometimes between slides within an experiment. When such within-section ratios of hybridization cannot be made, it is critical to hybridize adjacent tissue sections with probes whose abundance is presumably not changed by the disease process, for example, by using probes for so-called "house-keeping" transcripts. Densitometric values can then be normalized to control probe hybridizations on adjacent sections from the same brains.

Studies in which changes in the levels of different mRNAs are compared are made more difficult because different mRNA species may differ in their efficiency of hybridization. Under these circumstances, probe length, G–C content, and probe specific activity should be similar for accurate comparisons between different mRNAs. In all cases, it is important to observe robust, qualitative differences in mRNA levels before preceding to relative quantitative analyses. Our rule of thumb is not to undertake detailed quantitative studies if differences in mRNA levels appear less than 2-fold. The application of other molecular techniques, such as RNA blotting, RNA protection analysis, and PCR quantification (33), when used in conjunction with *in situ* hybridization, provide the most compelling support for measuring changes in mRNA abundance. Additionally, immunocytochemical localization performed on adjacent tissue sections serves as additional confirmation for changes which might be observed in corresponding mRNA levels, as well as providing additional information on the biosynthetic relationship between changes in mRNA and protein levels.

References

1. G. A. Higgins and M. C. Wilson, *in* "*In Situ* Hybridization: Applications to Neurobiology" (K. L. Valentino, J. H. Eberwine, and J. D. Barchas, eds.), p. 136. Oxford Univ. Press, London and New York, 1987.
2. C. E. Ribak, J. E. Vaughn, and E. Roberts, *J. Comp. Neurol.* **187,** 261 (1979).
3. J. F. Gusella, N. S. Wexler, P. M. Conneally, S. L. Naylor, M. A. Anderson, R. E. Tanzi, P. C. Watkins, K. Ottina, M. R. Wallace, A. Y. Sakaguchi, A. B. Young, I. Shoulson, E. Bonilla, and J. B. Martin, *Nature (London)* **306,** 234 (1983).
4. P. Blackburn, G. Wilson, and S. Moore, *J. Biol. Chem.* **252,** 5904 (1977).
5. E. M. Sajdel-Sulkowska and C. A. Marotta, *Science* **255,** 947 (1984).
6. R. C. Imrie and W. C. Hutchinson, *Biochim. Biophys. Acta* **108,** 106 (1965).
7. M. R. Morrison and W. S. T. Griffin, *Anal. Biochem.* **113,** 318 (1981).
8. S. A. Johnson, D. G. Morgan, and C. E. Finch, *J. Neurosci. Res.* **16,** 267 (1986).
9. T. L. Wood, G. D. Frantz, J. H. Menkes, and A. J. Tobin, *J. Neurosci. Res.* **16,** 311 (1986).
10. C. A. Marotta, R. E. Majocha, J. F. Coughlin, H. J. Manz, P. Davies, M. Ventosa-Michelman, W.-G. Chou, S. B. Zain, and E. M. Sajdel-Sulkowska, *Prog. Brain Res.* **70,** 303 (1986).
11. J. G. Guillemette, L. Wong, D. R. Crapper McLachlan, and P. N. Lewis, *J. Neurochem.* **47,** 987 (1986).
12. G. R. Taylor, G. I. Carter, T. J. Crow, J. A. Johnson, A. F. Fairbairn, E. K. Perry, and R. H. Perry, *Exp. Mol. Pathol.* **44,** 111 (1986).
13. M. R. Morrison, S. Pardue, K. Maschoff, W. S. T. Griffin, C. L. White III, J. Gilbert, and A. Roses, *Biochem. Soc. Trans.* **15,** 133 (1987).
14. G. Liguri, P. Nassi, N. Taddei, C. Nediani, and G. Ramponi, *Neurosci. Lett.* **85,** 244 (1988).
15. P. J. Whitehouse, D. Lynch, and M. J. Kuhar, *J. Neurochem.* **43,** 553 (1984).
16. G. Terenghi, J. M. Polak, Q. Hamid, E. O'Brien, P. Denny, S. Legon, J. Dixon, C. D. Minth, S. L. Palay, G. Yasargil, and V. Chan-Palay, *Proc. Natl. Acad. Sci. U.S.A.* **84,** 7315 (1987).
17. L. M. Angerer, K. H. Cox, and R. C. Angerer, *in* "Methods in Enzymology" (S. L. Berger and A. R. Kimmel, eds.), Vol. 152, p. 649. Academic Press, Orlando, Florida, 1987.
18. D. R. McClay, G. M. Wessel, and R. B. Marchase, *Proc. Natl. Acad. Sci. U.S.A.* **78,** 4975 (1981).
19. K. H. Cox, D. V. DeLeon, L. M. Angerer, and R. C. Angerer, *Dev. Biol.* **101,** 485 (1984).

20. D. E. Schmechel, P. J. Marangos, B. M. Martin, S. Winfield, D. S. Burkhart, A. D. Roses, and E. I. Ginns, *Neurosci. Lett.* **76,** 233 (1987).
21. L. H. Tecott, J. D. Barchas, and J. H. Eberwine, *Science* **240,** 1661 (1988).
22. R. K. Saiki, D. H. Gelfand, S. Stoffel, S. J. Scharf, R. Higuchi, G. T. Horn, K. B. Mullis, and H. A. Erlich, *Science* **239,** 487 (1988).
23. J. Meinkoth and G. Wahl, *Anal. Biochem.* **138,** 267 (1984).
24. G. M. Wahl, J. L. Meinkoth, and A. R. Kimmel, *in* "Methods in Enzymology" (S. L. Berger and A. R. Kimmel, eds.), Vol. 152, p. 572. Academic Press, Orlando, Florida, 1987.
25. D. D. Blumberg, *in* "Methods in Enzymology" (S. L. Berger and A. R. Kimmel, eds.), Vol. 152, p. 20. Academic Press, Orlando, Florida, 1987.
26. G. A. Higgins, D. A. Lewis, D. Goldgaber, D. C. Gajdusek, J. H. Morrison, and M. C. Wilson, *Proc. Natl. Acad. Sci. U.S.A.* **85,** 1297 (1988).
27. W. Hayashi, I. C. Gillam, A. D. Delaney, and G. M. Tener, *J. Histochem. Cytochem.* **36,** 677 (1978).
28. M. J. Kuhar and J. R. Unnerstall, *Trends Neurosci. (Pers. Ed.)* **8,** 49 (1985).
29. J. P. Adelman, C. T. Bond, J. Douglass, and E. Herbert, *Science* **235,** 1514 (1987).
30. M. Brahic and A. T. Haase, *Proc. Natl. Acad. Sci. U.S.A.* **75,** 6125 (1978).
31. A. W. Rogers, "Techniques of Autoradiography," 3rd Ed. Elsevier, Amsterdam, 1979.
32. W. G. Young, J. H. Morrison, and F. E. Bloom, *Soc. Neurosci. Abstr.* **11,** 679 (1985).
33. J. Chelly, J.-C. Kaplan, P. Maire, S. Gautron, and A. Kahn, *Nature (London)* **333,** 858 (1988).

[12] Localization of Peptide Gene Expression by *in Situ* Hybridization at Electron Microscopic Level

Georges Pelletier, Yiai Tong, Jacques Simard,
Hui-Fen Zhao, and Fernand Labrie

Introduction

The localization and quantification of mRNA by *in situ* hybridization performed at the light microscopic level is now routinely used in a large number of laboratories (1–6). This technique is very useful to identify the tissues or cell types which produce specific mRNAs. Moreover, even in homogeneous tissues, this approach is most useful to demonstrate cellular heterogeneity in mRNA levels following modification of physiological conditions or pharmalogical treatments (4). However, there are conditions where high resolution is needed to identify the cells or organelles which contain specific mRNAs. Recently, a few laboratories have tried to use *in situ* hybridization to detect various kinds of nucleotide sequences directly in ultrathin sections of embedded tissues (7–10). Among these attempts, only a very few dealt with the localization of mRNAs (9, 10). In view of the importance of optimal ultrastructural preservation for detecting gene expression in heterogeneous tissues, such as endocrine glands and nervous system, we developed a preembedding technique similar to that used for immunocytochemistry to localize mRNAs at the electron microscopic level using radiolabeled cDNA probes. In this chapter, we describe the technique that we have recently used to detect the gene expression of a pituitary hormone, prolactin (PRL), and two hypothalamic peptides, proopiomelanocortin (POMC) and somatostatin.

Preparations of cDNA Probes

The plasmid containing the rat PRL cDNA cloned into the *Eco*RI site of pSP64 (11) was generously provided by Dr. Richard A. Maurer (Department of Physiology and Biophysics, The University of Iowa, College of Medicine, Iowa City, IA). The full-length cDNA encoding the rat preprosomatostatin inserted into the *Bam*HI–*Xba*I site of pSP65 (12) was kindly provided by Dr.

Methods in Neurosciences, Volume 1

Richard H. Goodman (Division of Molecular Medicine, Department of Medicine, Tufts–New England Medical Center, Boston, MA). The plasmid containing the full-length fragment encoding the exon III (13) of the POMC gene, which encodes all the peptides with known biological activity and was cloned into pBR322 vector, was a generous gift from Dr. Jacques Drouin (Department of Molecular Biology of Eucaryotes, Clinical Research Institute of Montreal, Montreal, Quebec, Canada). The above-mentioned plasmids were transformed using high-efficiency DH5α competent cells (14) (Gibco/Brl, Burlington). Large-scale plasmid preparation was performed by the Triton–lysozyme method and thereafter purified twice by CsCl–ethidium bromide centrifugation (14, 15). The PRL cDNA fragment (717 bp) obtained following a *Eco*RI digestion was fractionated electrophoretically through an 5% polyacrylamide gel (15), while the *Eco*RI–*Sal*I restriction fragment (0.56 kb) encoding the preprosomatostatin and the *Hin*dIII–*Xho*I restriction fragment corresponding to the exon III of the POMC gene (1.6 kb) were electrophoresed on a 1% agarose gel (15). Thereafter, the isolated fragments were highly purified by electroelution with an electroeluter Bio-Rad model 422 using the recommended supplier procedure. The fragments were then labeled with [α-^{35}S]dCTPαS (1000 Ci/mmol) (Amersham, IL) by the random primer method (16) to a specific activity ranging between 0.8 and 1.2 × 10^9 dpm/μg and used the same day for hybridization.

Fixation and Tissue Preparation

The most important requirements of the procedure are to retain nondegraded mRNA and preserve morphological integrity. Adult female rats were then perfused with 4% paraformaldehyde in 0.1 *M* phosphate buffer (pH 7.4) (4–6) containing glutaraldehyde at different concentrations: 0.1, 0.5, and 2%. Brains and pituitaries were carefully removed and postfixed by immersion in the same fixative for 4 hr at 4°C. They were then rinsed for 12 hr in the same phosphate buffer containing 5% sucrose. Thereafter, the brains and pituitaries were cut with a vibratome into 50-μm sections which were collected in vials containing the phosphate buffer.

Hybridization Procedure and Embedding

The floating sections were then prehybridized at room temperature for 1 hr in a buffer containing 50% (v/v) formamide, 5× SSPE (1× SSPE being 0.18 *M* NaCl, 10 m*M* NaH$_2$PO$_4$, pH 7.4, 1 m*M* EDTA), 0.1% (w/v) sodium dodecyl sulfate (SDS), 0.1% (w/v) bovine serum albumin (Bethesda Research Laboratories, Gaithersburg, MD), 0.1% (w/v) Ficoll, 0.1% (w/v) poly(vinylpyrrolidone), 200 μg/ml denatured salmon testis DNA (Sigma Chemical Company, St. Louis, MO), 200 μg/ml yeast tRNA, 20 μg/ml poly(A) (Boehringer Mannheim, Montreal, Canada), and 0.1% Triton X-100. Hybridization was carried out for 18 hr at 42°C in the prehybridization buffer which did not contain Triton X-100 but contained, in addition, 4% (w/v) dextran sulfate and the appropriate ^{35}S-labeled cDNA probe at a concentration of 10^7 cpm/ml.

Following hybridization, the sections were rinsed at room temperature for 2 hr in 2× SSC (1× SSC being 0.15 M NaCl, 0.015 M sodium citrate, pH 7.0), followed by 2 hr in 1× SSC and 30 min in 0.5× SSC at 37°C. Some sections were treated with pancreatic RNase A (Boehringer Mannheim) (20 μg/ml) for 30 min at room temperature prior to hybridization procedures.

In order to verify the quality of hybridization, a few sections were mounted onto glass slides and placed in contact with Kodak X-Omat films at 4°C. With the PRL cDNA probe, a strong signal was obtained after 2 hr of exposure (Fig. 1), whereas, when POMC (exon III) and preprosomatostatin probes were used, a reaction of similar intensity could be obtained only after 12 hr of exposure (Fig. 5). The sections were then successively postfixed in 2.5% glutaraldehyde (15 min) and 2% osmium tetroxide (30 min) before being dehydrated in ethanol and flat-embedded in Araldite. Semithin (1 μm) and ultrathin (0.1 μm) sections were taken from the outer 3 μm of the blocks and processed for light and electron microscope autoradiography using Kodak NTB-2 and Ilford L-4 emulsion, respectively, as previously described (17).

Combination of Immunocytochemistry and *in Situ* Hybridization

At the light microscopic level, a combination of immunocytochemistry and *in situ* hybridization histochemistry in the same section has been described (18). Since this double-labeling approach is very useful to establish the specificity of hybridization signal, we have developed a similar approach for studies at the electron microscopic level. Ultrathin sections obtained from vibratome pituitary sections hybridized with [^{35}S]PRL cDNA probe was pretreated with 5% H_2O_2 for 5 min, incubated with antiprolactin antibodies (1/500) for 12 hr at 4°C, and rinsed twice in 20 nM Tris–saline buffer containing 1% BSA for 10 min each time prior to incubation in 1 : 20 protein A linked to 20-nm colloidal gold particles (Janssen Products, Belgium) for 2 hr at 20°C (19). The immunolabeled ultrathin sections were then processed for autoradiography (17).

Localization of PRL mRNA

It has been recently shown that, in rat pituitary, immunoreactive PRL is present not only in the typical PRL cell characterized by the presence of large irregular secretory granules but also in another cell type containing small round secretory granules (20). Since we could not rule out the possibility that antibodies to prolactin can recognize epitopes which belong to peptides other than authentic PRL, we felt that it was of interest to study the localization of PRL mRNA by the *in situ* hybridization technique and to compare the results with those obtained by immunolabeling. In vibratome sections of tissue fixed in 4% paraformaldehyde and 2% glutaraldehyde, the labeling obtained after *in situ* hybridization with [^{35}S]PRL cDNA probe was very strong in the anterior lobe (Fig. 1A). The neurointermediate lobe remained unlabeled. When sections were treated with RNase prior to hybridization, no signal could be detected (Fig. 1B).

In semithin sections, several cells appeared to be labeled with a few grains. These cells were located close to capillaries or arranged in clusters (Fig. 2). At the electron microscopic level, silver grains were seen overlying the classical PRL cells which contained round or ovoid mature secretory granules of a diameter ranging between 600 and 900 nm (Fig. 3). In this cell type, the Golgi apparatus is well developed and is generally associated with immature small granules. The cisternae of the rough endoplasmic reticulum are abundant. Silver grains were also associated with another cell type which is characterized by the presence of round or slightly ovoid granules of about 150–250 nm in diameter (Fig. 4). In sections immunostained for PRL localization, radiolabeling was only observed in the two cell types which contained secretory granules decorated with gold particles (Figs. 3 and 4).

In both labeled cell types, the silver grains were relatively few in number (4–8 grains per cell) and generally localized over the rough endoplasmic reticulum and the nucleus. The other cell types were consistently devoided of grains.

Localization of POMC and Preprosomatostatin mRNAs

A technique identical to that described above for PRL mRNA localization was used to detect POMC and preprosomatostatin mRNAs in the rat hypothalamus. In vibratome sections hybridized with the [^{35}S]preprosomatostatin cDNA probe, a strong signal could be detected in the periventricular nucleus (Fig. 5), as expected from immunocytochemical studies (21) and recent hybridization studies involving use of oligonucleotides (22). In semithin sections, silver grains were detected over the cytoplasm and

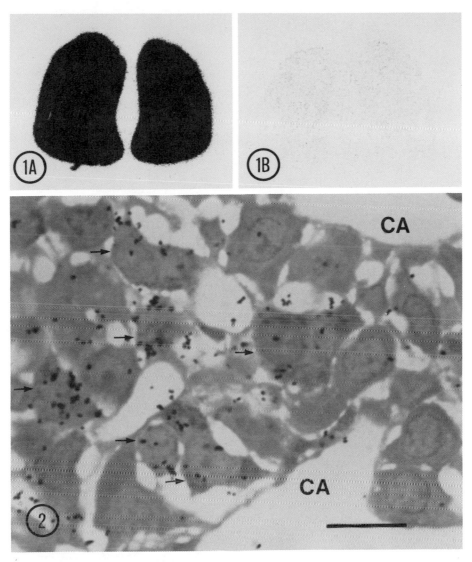

FIG. 1 (A) X-Ray autoradiogram illustrating the signal obtained after hybridization of [^{35}S]PRL cDNA probe to a vibratome section of the rat pituitary. Exposure time, 2 hr. (B) Vibratome section consecutive to that shown in Fig. 1A pretreated with RNase prior to hybridization. Only very weak labeling can be observed. Exposure time, 2 hr.

FIG. 2 Light microscope autoradiographic localization of PRL mRNA performed on a semithin section. Silver grains are overlying a few cells (arrows). CA, Capillaries. Exposure time, 36 hr. Bar, 10 μm.

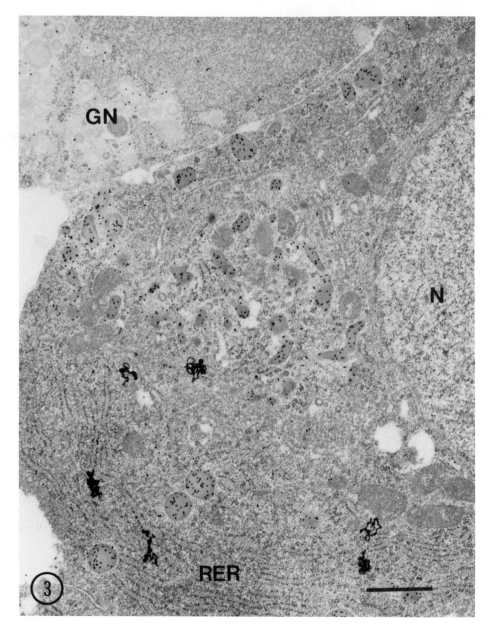

Fig. 3 Immunolocalization of PRL with the protein A–gold technique and PRL mRNA with autoradiography (see also Fig. 4). Exposure time, 14 days. Bar, 1 μm. Typical PRL cell. The large secretory granules are decorated with gold particles. Silver grains are found over the rough endoplasmic reticulum (RER). A gonadotroph (GN) is unlabeled. N, Nucleus.

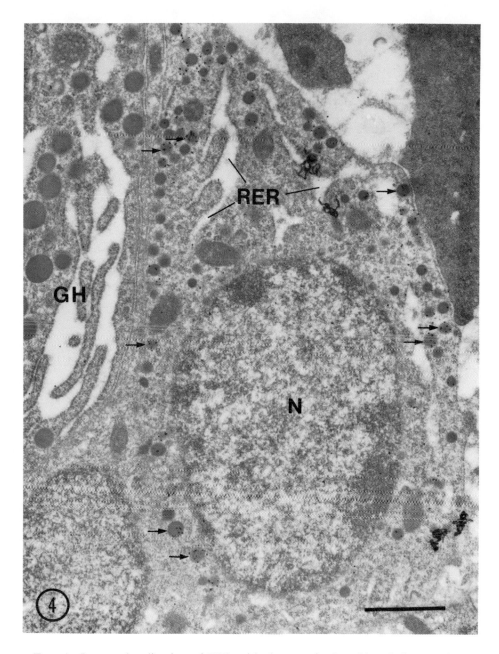

Fig. 4 Immunolocalization of PRL with the protein A–gold technique and PRL mRNA with autoradiography (see also Fig. 3). Exposure time, 14 days. Bar, 1 μm. In this cell type, the small secretory granules are labeled with gold particles (arrows) and silver grains are over the rough endoplasmic reticulum (RER). An adjacent growth hormone (GH)-secreting cell is unlabeled. N, Nucleus.

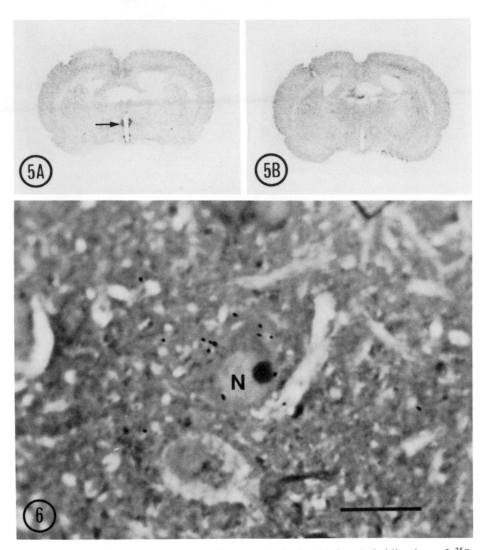

Fig. 5   (A) X-Ray autoradiographic signal obtained after hybridization of ^{35}S-labeled preprosomatostatin cDNA probe to a vibratome section of the rat brain. The reaction is located in the periventricular nucleus (arrow). Exposure time, 12 hr. (B) Pretreatment with RNase prior to hybridization has completely prevented the autoradiographic reaction. Exposure time, 12 hr.

Fig. 6   Localization of preprosomatostatin mRNA in a semithin section through the hypothalamic periventricular nucleus. Silver grains are overlying the nucleus (N) and cytoplasm of neurons. Exposure time, 14 days. Bar, 10 μm.

nucleus of a few neurons located along the third ventricle (Fig. 6). At the electron microscopic level, a few neurons displayed labeling over the rough endoplasmic reticulum as well as over the nucleus (Fig. 7). The ultrastructural characteristics of the positive neurons correspond very well to those previously observed using immunocytochemistry (21), especially the presence of the cytoplasm of large dense core vesicles of a diameter of 90–110 nm. The intensity of labeling showed variations from one cell to another one.

When the [^{35}S]POMC cDNA probe was applied to vibratome sections, hybridization signal could be detected only in the arcuate nucleus and the periarcuate region, as already reported by investigators who used immunocytochemistry (22) as well as *in situ* hybridization (3). In semithin sections, neuronal cell bodies were found to be labeled in the arcuate nucleus, the silver grains being located over both the nucleus and cytoplasm. At the ultrastructural level, labeling was observed over the rough endoplasmic reticulum and nucleus in neurons which had the characteristics of POMC neurons identified by immunoelectron microscopy (22). For both peptides, the best results were obtained in tissues fixed with the fixative containing 4% paraformaldehyde and 0.5% glutaraldehyde.

Discussion

The success of localizing specific mRNA sequences in tissue sections with high resolution depends on maintenance and adequate morphology during fixation and subsequent preparation of sections as well as maximal retention of cellular mRNA. In the present report, we have described in detail a preembedding technique performed in aldehyde-fixed tissue sections. The strong labeling obtained (Figs. 1 and 5) indicates that retention of mRNA is certainly adequate. On the other hand, since, after hybridization, the sections were postfixed in glutaraldehyde and osmium tetroxide before embedding in Araldite, an excellent ultrastructural preservation can be obtained (Figs. 3, 4, and 7), allowing identification of cells and organelles containing specific mRNAs. The nuclear labeling which has been routinely observed in pituitary and brain and was prevented when sections were pretreated with RNase probably indicates that nuclear mRNA can be detected with this approach.

We have also developed a technique for combining immunolabeling and *in situ* hybridization in the same ultrathin section. This approach appears to be a very powerful tool to establish beyond any doubt which cell type is involved in the biosynthesis of a specific peptide or protein. In fact, we have been able to demonstrate clearly not only that the typical prolactin cell

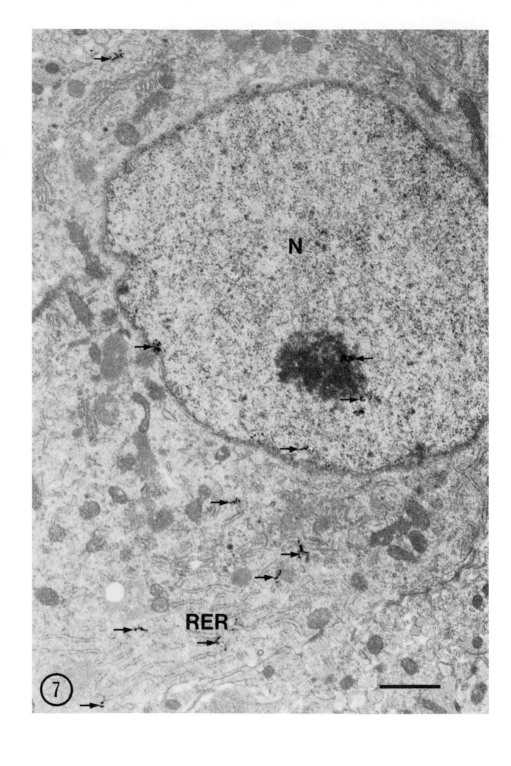

contains PRL mRNA but also that another cell type recently shown to be stained with PRL antibodies also showed a signal after hybridization with a [^{35}S]PRL cDNA probe. This double-labeling technique will be most useful to identify the different types of peptidergic and aminergic neurons using genetic probes to detect peptide and enzyme mRNAs.

References

1. B. Bloch, T. Popovici, D. Le Guellec, E. Normand, S. Couham, A. F. Guitteny, and P. Böhlen, *J. Neurosci. Res.* **16**, 183 (1986).
2. G. R. Uhl and C. A. Sasek, *J. Neurosci.* **6**, 3258 (1986).
3. C. E. Gee, C. L. C. Chen, J. L. Roberts, R. Thompson, and S. J. Watson, *Nature (London)* **306**, 374 (1983).
4. G. Pelletier, C. Labrie, J. Simard, M. Duval, M. G. Martinoli, H. F. Zhao, and F. Labrie, *J. Mol. Endocrinol.* **1**, 213 (1988).
5. G. Pelletier, N. Liao, N. Folléa, and M. V. Govindan, *Mol. Cell. Endocrinol.* **56**, 29 (1988).
6. G. Pelletier, N. Liao, N. Folléa, and M. V. Govindan, *Neurosci. Lett.* **94**, 23 (1988).
7. M. Binder, S. Tourmente, J. Roth, M. Renaud, and W. J. Gehring, *J. Cell Biol.* **102**, 1646 (1986).
8. J. Jacob, K. Gillies, D. MacLeod, and K. W. Jones, *J. Cell Sci.* **14**, 253 (1974).
9. M. Jamrich, K. A. Mahon, E. R. Govis, and J. C. Hall, *EMBO J.* **3**, 1939 (1984).
10. H. F. Webster, L. Lamperth, J. T. Favilla, G. Lemke, D. Tesin, and L. Manuelidis, *Histochemistry* **86**, 441 (1987).
11. E. J. Gubbins, R. A. Maurer, M. Lagrimini, C. R. Erwin, and J. E. Donelson, *J. Biol. Chem.* **255**, 8655 (1980).
12. R. H. Goodman, M. R. Montmigny, M. J. Low, and J. F. Habener, *in* "Molecular Cloning of Hormone Genes" (J. F. Habener, ed.), p. 93. Humana, Clifton, New Jersey, 1987.
13. J. Drouin, M. Chamberland, J. Charron, L. Jeanotte, and M. Nemer, *FEBS Lett.* **193**, 54 (1985).
14. H. Miller, *in* "Methods in Enzymology" (S. L. Berger and A. R. Kimmel, eds.), Vol. 152, p. 145. Academic Press, Orlando, Florida, 1987.
15. L. G. Davis, M. D. Dibner, and J. F. Battey, "Methods in Molecular Biology." Elsevier, Amsterdam, 1986.
16. A. P. Feinberg and B. Vogelstein, *Anal. Biochem.* **132**, 6 (1983).

FIG. 7 Localization of preprosomatostatin mRNA at the ultrastructural level. Silver grains (arrows) are located over the rough endoplasmic reticulum (RER) and nucleus (N) of a neuron located in the periventricular nucleus. Exposure time, 7 weeks. Bar, 1 μm.

17. G. Pelletier, *J. Cell Biol.* **62,** 185 (1974).
18. B. D. Shivers, R. E. Harlan, D. W. Pfaff, and B. S. Shachter, *J. Histochem. Cytochem.* **34,** 39 (1986).
19. J. Roth, M. Bendayan, and L. Orci, *J. Histochem. Cytochem.* **26,** 1074 (1978).
20. G. Pelletier, T. Antakly, and F. Labrie, *in* "Prolactin Secretion: A Multidisciplinary Approach" (F. Mena and P. C. Valerde, eds.), p. 75. Academic Press, London, 1984.
21. G. Pelletier, D. Dubé, and R. Puviani, *Science* **196,** 1464 (1977).
22. G. Pelletier, *Neurosci.Lett.* **16,** 85 (1980).

[13]   *In Situ* Hybridization for Detecting Gonadotropin-Releasing Hormone Messenger RNA and Measuring Physiologically Stimulated Changes

J. Fielding Hejtmancik, P. Michael Conn, and Donald W. Pfaff

Introduction

While the physiology of hypothalamic release factors has been studied in detail and control mechanisms at the protein level are well-established, questions about control of expression at the transcriptional level have remained largely unexplored until recently. Complementary DNA and genomic clones for gonadotropin-releasing hormone (GnRH) have now been isolated and contributed greatly to our understanding of the mechanisms of GnRH synthesis (1, 2). Availability of DNA probes for GnRH mRNA have begun to allow elucidation of the effects of steroid hormones on GnRH gene expression (3–7). GnRH is released from the median eminence into the portal circulation, where it stimulates synthesis and release of both luteinizing hormone (LH) and follicle-stimulating hormone (FSH) (8). At other brain

Methods in Neurosciences, Volume 1

sites GnRH may also facilitate mating behaviors (9). GnRH is found within circumscribed regions of the brain, including the preoptic–anterior hypothalamic and septal areas, with projections to the median eminence, the organum vasculosum of the lamina terminalis, and the olfactory system (10, 11). The preoptic area and the medial basal hypothalamus have been implicated in steroid hormone-mediated feedback on GnRH synthesis (12–14).

Although estrogen can regulate hypothalamic levels of GnRH, hypothalamic cells which bind estrogen contain no GnRH detectable by immunocytochemistry (15). A variety of studies have been consistent with an increased rate of GnRH synthesis following ovariectomy (15) or following estrogen replacement after ovariectomy (16). However, because of the difficulty of estimating GnRH synthesis and turnover in the face of changing rates of both synthesis and release, no clear answer to this question could be obtained.

While hormonal regulation of neuropeptides may include alterations in degradation rates, an estimate of the rate of GnRH synthesis would provide a strong suggestion of the effect of sex steroids on GnRH regulation, especially when one already has the ability to measure GnRH release. Steady-state levels of GnRH mRNA, and hence the rate of GnRH synthesis, can be assessed by *in situ* hybridization. Because hypothalamic neurons are heterogeneous in terms of neurendocrine activity, *in situ* hybridization is preferable to Northern or dot-blot analysis, which only detect message levels averaged over entire brain regions. For this technique to reflect mRNA levels accurately certain conditions must be met (17). First, the preparation of tissue samples must not allow significant degradation or masking of the RNA present. Second, the probe and hybridization conditions used must allow for annealing of complementary base pairs unique and sufficiently stringent to detect only the sequence of interest within the highly complex mixture of mRNAs in the brain (18). Third, since the levels of some neuropeptides may be low, especially under certain experimental conditions, the method must be sensitive. Finally, since subtle changes in GnRH mRNA levels might have major implications for GnRH action and release, the technique should be quantitatable.

With these factors in mind, we have used oligodeoxyribonucleotides and RNA complementary to coding regions of GnRH cDNA to identify cells in the rat and mouse hypothalamus that express GnRH and to quantitate the levels of this mRNA in these cells. These probes have been labeled with ^{3}H and ^{32}P and their specific hybridization detected by autoradiography using a film immersion technique. When carefully applied with appropriate controls, this technique allows a quantitative estimation of both the number of neurons expressing GnRH mRNA and the amount of GnRH mRNA within these cells relative to other samples analyzed in the same experiment. With this technique, one can demonstrate that, in contrast to what one would expect on the basis of a negative feedback model, long-term exposure to sex steroids actually increases GnRH mRNA levels and hence presumably the synthetic rate of GnRH.

Experimental Procedures

Tissue Preparation and Fixation

Sprague Dawley rats maintained on a 12-hr light/12-hr dark daily light cycle and give *ad libitum* food and water for at least 1 week were used in all experiments. Gonadectomy was performed under Metofane (Pitman Moore) anesthesia, with half of each sample group serving as controls. In some studies, female rats underwent replacement therapy by placement of an approximately 5-mm-long subcutaneous silastic tube filled with 17β-estradiol. Between 7 and 14 days later the mice were sacrificed by decapitation, and the brains were quickly (within 2 min) dissected and frozen with dry ice.

In order to avoid RNase contamination, gloves were worn, RNase-free materials were used, and equipment which came into contact with RNase was reserved for that use only. Throughout, many steps previously detailed by Shivers *et al.* (19) were used. Glassware and stainless steel microscope slides were treated for RNase by soaking with cleaning solution which can be purchased (e.g., Chromerge, CMS) or made by adding 150 ml of concentrated sulfuric acid to 850 ml H_2O in a 1000-ml graduated cylinder. After cooling, the solution is transferred to a Pyrex bottle containing 300 g of potassium dichromate and mixed. Soaking in cleaning solution should be followed by generous water rinses. In addition, glassware can be autoclaved for 30 min or baked at 180°C for 4 hr or longer. Some glassware such as Coplin jars cannot be heat treated. Plasticware was treated for RNase by soaking in 0.02% diethyl pyrocarbonate (DEPC; Sigma, St Louis, MO) followed by generous water rinses.

Brain tissue was sectioned and fixed as described (3) in 3% neutral-buffered paraformaldehyde containing 0.02% DEPC. Sections were then rinsed, dehydrated, and stored desiccated at −80°C. The microscope slides used were precleaned 3- by 1-inch slides with frosted ends. They were prepared by placing in a metal (RNase free) rack. Gloves were worn and the surface of the work area was covered. The slides were washed with acid–alcohol (0.2 *N* HCl in 95% ethanol) in glass staining dishes for 20 min. They were then subjected to three 2-min washes in distilled H_2O. The slides were then coated for 2 min with freshly prepared 0.02% DEPC-treated 0.5% gelatin/0.05% chrom-alum solution. This was prepared by dissolving 5 g of gelatin in 1 liter of boiling water, cooling, and adding 0.5 g of chromium potassium sulfate. The solution was filtered and 200 μl of DEPC was added before use. Finally, the slides were dried in a 60°C oven and stored in a dust-free box. This method of tissue preparation gives the greatest and most consistent hybridization signal with acceptable morphological appearance of cells.

Another technique which we have used is to subject the rats to Nembutal anesthesis and intracardiac perfusion with phosphate-buffered saline (PBS) for 5 min followed by 8 min with 3% neutral-buffered paraformaldehyde or buffered picric acid–paraformaldehyde solutions. Following the approach of Shivers *et al.* (3), the brain was removed, cryoprotected, sectioned, and stored desiccated at −80°C. The cell morphology of tissue treated in this fashion was superior to that of the frozen postfixed tissue. However, the hybridization signal intensity was less, and perhaps more important, the variation from sample to sample was greater so that this method was not routinely used. In addition, three other fixation conditions were tried and discarded (19). These involved freezing in a fashion similar to the technique initially described followed by fixation in glutaraldehyde, or Carnoy's solution, or ethanol–acetic acid (3 : 1, v/v).

Prehybridization Treatment

Tissue sections were removed from storage at −80°C and dried in a vacuum desiccator for 10 min. A ring of nail polish was applied around each section with a Pasteur pipette and allowed to dry (this can be successfully avoided by running reactions with free-floating sections). The sectons were prehybridized for 2 hr at room temperature in an equal mixture of 4× prehybridization buffer [1.2 M NaCl, 20 mM Tris-HCl, pH 7.5, 0.04% Ficoll (type 400), 0.04% poly(vinylpyrrolidine) (PVP-40, Sigma), 0.04% bovine serum albumin fraction V, 2 mM EDTA, pH 7.0, 0.1% yeast total RNA type III, 0.01% tRNA type IX, 0.1% herring sperm DNA, and 0.1% inorganic sodium pyrophosphate] freshly mixed with deionized formamide (19). The formamide was deionized by stirring together for 1 hr (not longer, in order to avoid degradation) at room temperature 22 g of Amberlite (MB-1A, Sigma) with one 442-ml bottle of formamide and filtering twice through Whatman 1MM paper. The deionization can be checked with a conductivity meter or by pH. Both the 2× prehybridization mixture and the formamide were stored in small aliquots at −20°C. After the two are combined and immediately before use, they are subjected to a heat denaturation step consisting of heating at 95°C for 10 min followed by snap cooling in an ice slush. After applying 20 μl of the combined prehybridization solution to each section, they were incubated with 4× SSC (NaCl/sodium citrate; 1× SSC is 150 mM NaCl + 15 mM sodium citrate) in 50% deionized formamide while humidified. Incubations were performed in the dark and, if necessary, could be extended overnight (19).

In order to increase penetration of the probe, a variety of agents including detergents and deproteinizing agents were tried, but under the conditions stated here they did not improve the signal strength and in some cases decreased it or damaged tissue morphology (19). However, other investigators have found deproteination methods to be helpful, and it may be beneficial in some cases (e.g., when using longer probes) to include a moderate deproteination step with a gentle postfixation step to stabilize the mRNA after protein removal.

Probes

Two types of probes have been used in studies of GnRH gene expression. The first was a 59-base oligonucleotide complementary to the sequence of human GnRH mRNA coding for amino acids −5 to 15 of the preprohormone, which code for the GnRH peptide (1). The amino acid sequence in this region is identical in the rat and human, while the nucleotide sequences differ by only 5 bases (1), all in the 3′-most 30 nucleotides. A 60-base oligonucleotide corresponding to amino acids 33–52 of the human GnRH precursor protein, including the region coding for GAP, was also used. This oligonucleotide probe, however, diverged in 17 of the 60 bases and gave no detectable signal when used in *in situ* hybridization in the rat. Oligonucleotide probes were labeled to specific activities of greater than 10^8 cpm/μg with ^{32}P or 1–2 × 10^6 cpm/μg with ^{3}H (when greater resolution of probe localization was required) as described below.

Oligonucleotides were synthesized with an Applied Biosystems DNA synthesizer (model 380) and deprotected with 2 ml of concentrated NH_4OH by incubating overnight at 55°C while well sealed. The sample was chilled to −20°C and opened carefully due to the potential for buildup of NH_3 gas. The sample was speed-vacuumed to dryness with the heater on (start while sample is still quite cold) and then resuspended to 1 ml with H_2O and taken to dryness again. The sample was resuspended in 0.5 ml of ethanol and speed-vacuumed to dryness with the ethanol step repeated twice. The oligonucleotide was then dissolved in 2 ml of 10 mM NH_4HCO_3 and applied to a disposable PD-10 column (Pharmacia) equilibrated with the same buffer. The vial was washed with 0.5 ml of the same buffer and this was also applied to the column. The column was eluted with 3.5 ml of the same buffer and the desalted oligonucleotide concentration measured by the OD_{260} of the eluted buffer measured against column buffer. In some samples, purification was stopped at this point, but occasionally a cloudy white precipitate appeared in the sample after storage at 4°C for days to weeks, For this reason, the oligonucleotides were further purified by preparative polyacrylamide gel electrophoresis. Electrophoresis was performed on a 30-cm-long preparative gel with 6-mm spacers and a 5-tooth comb with 2.5-cm-wide teeth. A 20% acrylamide sequencing-type gel was poured from a 25% acrylamide stock solution (181.25 g acrylamide + 6.25 g bisacrylamide + 394.14 g urea brought to 750 ml with H_2O and vacuum filtered through a 0.4-μm Millipore filter before storing at 4°C) by mixing 40 ml of the stock solution with 5 ml of 10 LGB (made by mixing 163.5 g Tris base, 27.8 g boric acid, 10.4 g EDTA, and H_2O to 1 liter), 4.65 ml H_2O, 0.35 ml of 10% ammonium persulfate (made fresh or stored at 4°C for less than 1 week), and 20 μl TEMED. Approximately 10 A_{260} units of oligonucleotide were speed-vacuumed to dryness, resuspended in 100 μl of 98% deionized formamide without loading dye, and loaded into each lane. A separate lane of tracking dye was run to assess electrophoresis without obscuring the oligonucleotides. The gel was run at about 600 V (so that the plates were hot but not painful to touch) until the bromphenol blue had migrated about 20 cm. The gel was placed on Saran wrap and the oligonucleotide identified by shadowing over a thin-layer chromatography plate using a hand-held long-wavelength ultraviolet lamp. The desired bands were excised and crushed with 1 ml of TE (10 mM Tris-HCl, pH 7.5, 1 mM EDTA) in an Eppendorf vial overnight with an average recovery of about 50% as estimated by assessing the A_{260}. If necessary, a larger volume can be used and concentrated by Speed-Vac or by isobutanol extraction. The oligonucleotide was then extracted with chloroform and desalted into TE as above. Some investigators prefer other methods of extracting the oligonucleotide from acrylamide gels, including crushing and phenol extraction or freeze–crushing. In addition, the oligonucleotides can be purified directly on an HPLC column if this is available. The oligonucleotide can be used directly or stored at 4°C without noticeable degradation for months to a year in most cases.

Oligonucleotides were phosphorylated using T4 polynucleotide kinase in a reaction containing 100 ng of oligonucleotide, 3 μl of [γ-^{32}P]ATP (straight from the bottle, crude 6000–8000 Ci/mmol from ICN), 66 mM Tris-HCl, pH 8.0, 10 mM magnesium acetate, 10 mM DTT, and 3 units of T4 polynucleotide kinase (Bethesda Research Laboratories, Gaithersburg, MD) in a total volume of 10 μl. The sample was incubated at 37°C for 30 min and 2 μl of urea dye [2 M urea, 0.1% bromphenol blue, 0.1% xylene cyanole, and 0.1% sodium dodecyl sulfate (SDS)] was added and the sample was loaded directly on a sequencing type 20% polyacrylamide gel as described above, but with a thickness of 0.2 mm (the same as used for sequencing). When the blue dye reached the bottom (usually an overnight run at about 750 V) the front glass plate was removed and the gel covered with Saran wrap. (Care must be taken because the lower well and the gel are both extremely radioactive. The gel should always be handled behind a shield blocking β emissions.) The labeled oligonucleotides were autoradiographed by overlaying with an 8 × 10 inch piece of Kodak XAR-5 film for 30 sec to 1 min. Orientation can be achieved with radioactive ink or by marking the edges of the film and Saran wrap with a Sharpie marking pen. After developing, the autoradiogram was placed under the glass plate and used as a guide to excise the labeled oligonucleotides. Care must be taken to view the bands from directly above as the glass plate is thick relative to the gel. If necessary, this difficulty can be avoided by transferring the gel to a used piece of X-ray film before autoradiography. The labeled fragments should be excised in as small a piece as possible, since any unlabeled oligonucleotide (which should be avoided in order to obtain as high a specific activity as possible) will migrate about 1 cm above the phosphorylated oligonucleotide. The gel fragment was placed in about 0.5 ml of TE and the fragment allowed to diffuse out overnight before use in hybridization. The Eppendorf tube was microfuged for several minutes and the probe in the supernatant concentrated by ethanol precipitation using yeast tRNA as a carrier. Crushing the gel was not found to increase probe diffusion out of the extremely thin gel and occasionally made obtaining uncontaminated supernatant fraction more difficult. This procedure was used to prepare probes which had essentially every molecule labeled. When this high specific activity was not required, the oligonucleotides were purified by loading on a 0.5-ml DEAE-52 column in 10 mM Tris, pH 8.0, 1 mM EDTA, 200 mM NaCl. After washing with at least 10 ml of the same buffer, the oligonucleotide was eluted with 10 mM Tris, pH 8.0, 1 mM EDTA, 500 mM NaCl. Alternatively, a NACS column (Bethesda Research Laboratories) was used for purification.

Tritiated oligonucleotide was obtained by tailing with [^{3}H]dCTP using terminal transferase. Tailing reactions were performed using 0.5 μg of oligonucleotide with 5 units of terminal transferase in 110 μl containing 2 mM [^{3}H]dCTP (50 Ci/mM, Amersham), 200 mM potassium acetate, 25 mM Tris-HCl, pH 6.9, 2 mM dithiothreitol, 0.5 mM cobalt chloride, and 0.25 mg/ml bovine serum albumin. The tritiated nucleotide comes stabilized in ethanol and must be lyophilized to dryness and resuspended in H$_2$O before use. The reaction mixture was incubated at 37°C until 10 residues had been added, in most cases about 15 min, although this should be determined in each individual reaction by running a time curve. Since the tailing reaction is very efficient, even at low dCTP concentrations, another way to limit the number of residues added is to limit the amount of dCTP present so that the nucleotide substrate is exhausted when 10 residues have been added to each oligonucleotide (that is, the molar ratio of tritiated nucleotide to oligonucleotide probe is 10 to 1). This has also worked well in our laboratories. The label incorporated into the probe is determined by either trichloroacetic acid precipitation in the presence of carrier DNA (200 μl of 5 mg/ml herring sperm DNA) or using a DEAE filter. Since tritium quenches significantly in aqueous buffers, the filters must be dried before scintillation counting. The reaction was then electrophoresed as above in order to separate the product from free nucleotide and unlabeled oligonucleotide. Regions of the gel corresponding to phosphorylated oligonucleotides 65–69 bases long (5–10 nucleotides longer than the original probe, as determined by the presence of standards end labeled with ^{32}P) were collected and allowed to diffuse from the gel as described above.

Hybridization and Washing

The prehybridization buffer was washed off briefly in 2× SSC and the sections were allowed to air dry. The probe was mixed in hybridization buffer (consisting of 2× prehybridization buffer with the addition of 20% dextran sulfate, 0.1 mg/ml polyadenosine, and 10 mM cold deoxyribonucleotides mixed with an equal volume of deionized formamide) and heat denatured as described above (3). Hybridization was carried out with solutions containing increasing amounts of labeled probe: approximately 6.5 × 10^4 cpm per section (3.2 × 10^6 cpm/ml in 20 μl), 9 × 10^4 cpm per section (4.5 × 10^6 cpm/ml in 20 μl), and 1.2 × 10^5 cpm per section (6 × 10^6 cpm/ml in 20 μl). The two highest probe concentrations in the series were demonstrated to be saturating, so that these values accurately reflected the amount of target mRNA present in the tissue. The background labeling was similar with all three probe concentrations. Tritiated probe was added at a concentration of 5 × 10^5 cpm/ml (12,000 cpm per section in 20 μl), an amount giving higher molar concentrations of probe than the highest concentration of ^{32}P-labeled probe. Sections were hybridized for 3 days at 37°C, which gave substantially greater signals than did shorter hybridization times such as 1 day or incubation for a similar time at room temperature. One disadvantage of a higher hybridization temperature is that the tissue section can detach from the microscope slide (19).

Use of single-stranded probes such as oligonucleotides or riboprobes has the advantage that the probe cannot reanneal to itself, as can double-stranded probes. This would decrease the sensitivity of the *in situ* hybridization procedure as well as compromise its quantitative nature, since, as described above, it is important to saturate the target mRNA. Single-stranded probes have been shown to have a lower background, since only the appropriate strand, which is capable of specific hybridization, is present (19). In addition, use of the complementary (antisense) probe serves as an excellent control for hybridization specificity.

Following hybridization, sections were rinsed twice for 10 min each in 2× SSC, 0.05% sodium pyrophosphate at room temperature. They were then rinsed in 0.5× SSC, 0.05% sodium pyrophosphate for 2 days with two changes of buffer. The nail polish was removed with a forceps and the sections were dehydrated in ethanol diluted with 300 mM ammonium acetate instead of water to maintain ionic strength and thus decrease the chance of probe loss (20).

Autoradiography

To detect radioactive probe the sections were dipped in Kodak NTB2 nuclear track emulsion at 43°C in a darkroom with a safelight. Because hybrids are stable after dehydration of the sections, it was not necessary to adjust the ionic strength of the emulsion. Dilution of the emulsion was found to decrease the sensitivity of the autoradiography, especially when using radioisotopes which emit high-energy particles (e.g., ^{32}P) (19).

After dipping the slides in emulsion, autoradiography was carried out. The slides were packed in black slide boxes with a desiccant (Drierite) and dried overnight in a large lightproof box also packed with the same desiccant and exposed at 4°C. When ^{32}P-labeled probes were used, the slides with sections were separated by blank microscope slides to decrease random exposure. An additional slide containing a section which was not hybridized but was dipped in emulsion was included in each box to estimate the background exposure.

Optimum exposure time depended on the radioisotope used, the amount and specific activity of probe added to the hybridization reactions, and the levels of GnRH mRNA in the sections. Thus, hybridization experiments were carried out in triplicate so that optimal exposure times could be determined empirically. When ^{32}P-labeled probes were used, sections were exposed for about 10 to 28 days. When ^{3}H-labeled probes were used, sections were exposed for about 60 days. The slides were brought to room temperature over 1.5 to 2 hr and sections were then developed under a safelight using Kodak D19 developer. After photo fixation, slides were rinsed in H$_2$O with one rinse for 2 min at 16°C and three more for 2 min each at room temperature. The sections were then stained with 0.5% cresyl violet and occasionally fast green, rinsed in H_2O, dehydrated in ethanol, cleared in xylene, and covered with a coverslip using Permount mounting medium. Sections were observed in a light microscope.

Analysis

All cells within each tissue section were analyzed for GnRH mRNA content in a "blinded" fashion. Initially, dark-field examination provided a general pattern of distribution of GnRH-containing cells to be established at low magnification. Then cells containing GnRH mRNA within each tissue section were determined quantitatively through light microscopic localization and counting of reduced silver grains using bright-field illumination. When tritiated probe was used, the relation of reduced silver grain content to cell structures were assessed. With ^{32}P-labeled probe precise localization is not possible, but accurate quantitation of mRNA content still can be carried out. When grain counts of individual labeled cell bodies and adjacent background areas (neuropil) were conducted with an eyepiece reticle, a neuron was considered positively labeled if the grain count overlaying the cell exceeded the background count 4-fold, a conservative estimate intended to exclude false-positive identifications. The product of the number of positive cells and the average grain count per cell was taken as an estimate of the total content of GnRH mRNA in a region. Often, this measure showed a significant difference between two conditions when either total labeled cell count or average grains per cell were different but by themselves achieved marginal or no statistical significance. For example, with the effect of estrogen on GnRH mRNA levels (5), there is a 40% increase in the grain count per labeled cell ($p < 0.05$) and a 36% increase in the mean number of cells per rat (suggestive but not significantly different), yielding a highly significant 90% increase in the produce of these two measures for estradiol-replaced rats. Statistical differences between test groups and control animals were estimated using Student's t-test and the Kolmogorov–Smirnov two-sample test (21).

Conclusion

Our positive results prove that this *in situ* hybridization approach is not only sensitive enough to detect a low-copy message (3), but also yielded quantitative results which are in good agreement with modern physiological approaches to feedback of steroid hormones on the brain. The *in situ* hybridization results showed that long-term exposure to estrogen in the ovariectomized female rat will actually increase mRNA levels for GnRH (5), and that long-term exposure to androgenic steroids in the male similarly will increase GnRH mRNA (4). Now, a variety of neuroendocrine physiological approaches show that negative feedback is not to be ascribed primarily to decreases in GnRH synthesis, but instead can be explained at the pituitary level. Increasingly, long-term sex steroid actions on the brain can be associated with increased synthetic activity of GnRH neurons.

The *in situ* hybridization results of Rothfeld *et al.* (5) in the human female have been replicated and extended with a protection assay (see below and Ref. 22). Assuming that this result is not due to direct sex steroid action on GnRH neurons (15), the GnRH message changes may be a consequence of increased release. Similarly, in the male, the demonstration of Rothfeld *et al.* (4) of a stimulatory effect has been replicated and extended (22, 23).

Physiological approaches to feedback mechanisms of hormones on the brain have undergone a revolution: portal blood sampling has given way to push–pull perfusion analysis and measurements taken through precisely engineered dialysis tube probes (24). It is now seen that effects of testosterone on LH release can be explained at the pituitary level by alterations in pituitary GnRH receptor content (25) in the male and, similarly, in the female, GnRH release as measured with push–pull cannulae indicates that negative feedback effects of ovarian steroids must be due to changes in the pituitary itself (26). GnRH release was not increased 4 or 8 days following ovariectomy (27). In contrast, hypophysectomized rats with pituitary grafts below the kidney capsule could demonstrate estrogen inhibition of luteinizing hormone release, suggesting strongly that pituitary mechanisms are sufficient for negative feedback (28). Predictions based on negative feedback at the level of the GnRH neuron itself have not been confirmed: e.g., following castration of male rats, mean GnRH pulse amplitude and mean GnRH levels were not different (29), with the best suggestion being that long-term castration can actually result in decreased biosynthesis of the GnRH prohormone (30). Likewise, in an experiment by Kream *et al.* (31), GnRH levels in the mediobasal hypothalamus were directly correlated with testosterone levels in the blood. Immunocytochemically, ovariectomy or castration resulted in decreases in the number of immunopositive GAP or GnRH neurons, directly opposite to the prediction expected if there is negative feedback at the level of GnRH synthesis (32). A recent comprehensive summary does not show systematic increases in GnRH synthesis following castration (33).

In dramatic contrast, there are some data implicating hormone-influenced GnRH alterations in positive feedback mechanisms. Indirectly, effects of estrogen at the pituitary level require constant pulses of GnRH for positive feedback to occur (34). Electron microscopically, ultrastructural features associated with protein synthesis suggest that GnRH synthesis is increasing from diestrous to proestrous (35). In monkeys as well, GnRH-releasing patterns did not change immediately after estrogen treatment in females or males, even though plasma LH fell rapidly, and later, estrogen treatment actually increased GnRH levels and pulse amplitude before plasma LH increased (36); these results fit the conclusion that an increase in GnRH secretion is associated with estradiol treatment and leads to the LH surge (37). This suggestion is constant across different macaque species (38).

Since castration of the male rat decreases the secretion of both GnRH and GAP under both basal and stimulated conditions (39), and since lowered estrogen levels were associated with decreased GnRH message (40) and lowered estrogen levels in diabetic animals were associated with decreased GnRH concentrations (41), the most reasonable conclusion, consistent with the *in situ* hybridization of Rothfeld *et al.* (5), is that under some conditions estrogen stimulates GnRH synthesis. Indeed, in chronically ovariectomized female rats, estrogen administration seems to enhance the overall activity of the GnRH pulse generator (42) and pregnanolone, a progesterone metabolite, can do so as well (43). It is important to remember that these stimulatory effects of a sex steroid on the GnRH message could be indirect, following GnRH release. Remembering that estradiol and progesterone do not directly address the cell nucleus of the GnRH neuron (15, 44), an indirect, sluggish mechanism is indicated. This type of mechanism is not consistent with rapid, negative feedback but rather with long-term stimulatory preparations for sudden release, with changes during seasons, and with reproductive behavior.

Future Directions

The work described here essentially consists of using labeled oligonucleotide probes to localize and quantitate GnRH mRNA under a variety of different physiological conditions. We have demonstrated that this type of probe can be used successfully to provide an estimate of relative mRNA levels in specific areas of the brain. Using these techniques, we have demonstrated that gonadal steroids maintain hypothalamic stores of GnRH while at the same time promoting the release of the peptide. We are currently extending these observations in several ways.

While the above observations are suggestive, more detailed time courses under a wide variety of conditions are necessary. In order to pursue these studies, we are investigating the use of riboprobes corresponding to the first exon of the GnRH gene synthesized in pt7t318u. These probes seem to have all the advantages of oligonucleotides in that they are single-stranded to reduce background and networking (potentially risky in quantitative studies), can be made a uniform and selectable size that can be optimized for specificity and tissue penetration, and require relatively little effort to maintain plasmid stocks and prepare labeled probe. In addition, they can easily be made longer than oligonucleotides, can be labeled uniformly and to a higher specific activity, and have the advantage of stronger binding of RNA–DNA hybrids. Their disadvantages to date are related to the sensitivity of RNA to degradation.

These probes will allow a more detailed investigation of low-level expression, and, by increasing the ease of the analysis, will make it possible to perform experiments requiring processing of larger numbers of samples. This will allow investigation of GnRH expression in additional areas of the brain and in tissues such as the testis and placenta. Finally, riboprobes are suitable for use in RNase protection assays which allow detection of low levels of mRNA in tissues. The results from such analyses would complement and confirm the results of the *in situ* hybridization studies. Together, these techniques promise to provide a clearer understanding of developmental and hormonal control of GnRH synthesis and the role it plays in reproductive function.

References

1. P. H. Seeburg and J. P. Adelman, *Nature (London)* **311,** 666 (1984).
2. J. P. Adelman, A. J. Mason, J. S. Hayflick, and P. H. Seeburg, *Proc. Natl. Acad. Sci. U.S.A.* **83,** 179 (1986).
3. B. D. Shivers, J. F. Hejtmancik, P. M. Conn, and D. W. Pfaff, *Endocrinology (Baltimore)* **118,** 883 (1986).
4. J. M. Rothfeld, J. F. Hejtmancik, P. M. Conn, and D. W. Pfaff, *Exp. Brain Res.* **67,** 113 (1987).
5. J. M. Rothfeld, J. F. Hejtmancik, P. M. Conn, and D. W. Pfaff, *Mol. Brain Res.,* in press (1988).
6. L. J. Standish, L. A. Adams, L. Vician, D. K. Clifton, and R. A. Steiner, *Soc. Neurosci. Abstr.* **12,** 1175 (1986).
7. R. T. Zoeller, P. H. Seeburg, and W. S. Young III, *Endocrinology (Baltimore)* **122,** 2570 (1988).
8. R. Guillemin, *Science* **202,** 390 (1978).
9. R. L. Moss and S. M. McCann, *Science* **181,** 177 (1973).
10. C. Bennet-Clarke and S. A. Joseph, *Cell Tissue Res.* **221,** 493 (1982).
11. M. Schwanzel-Fukuda and A. J. Silverman, *J. Comp. Neurol.* **191,** 213 (1980).
12. R. L. Goodman and E. Knobil, *Neuroendocrinology* **32,** 57 (1981).
13. B. Halasz and R. A. Gorski, *Endocrinology (Baltimore)* **80,** 608 (1967).

14. N. Barfield and J. J. Chen, *Endocrinology (Baltimore)* **101,** 1716 (1977).
15. B. D. Shivers, R. E. Harlan, J. I. Morrell, and D. W. Pfaff, *Nature (London)* **304,** 345 (1983).
16. B. D. Shivers, R. E. Harlan, J. I. Morrell, and D. W. Pfaff, *Neuroendocrinology* **36,** 1 (1983).
17. J. T. McCabe, J. I. Morrell, D. Richter, and D. W. Pfaff, *Front. Neuroendocrinol.* **9,** 149 (1987).
18. J. T. McCabe, J. I. Morrell, R. Ivell, H. Schmale, D. Richter, and D. W. Pfaff, *J. Histochem. Cytochem.* **34,** 45 (1986).
19. B. D. Shivers, B. S. Schachter, and D. W. Pfaff, *in* "Methods of Enzymology" (P. M. Conn, ed.), Vol. 124, p. 497. Academic Press, Orlando, Florida, 1986.
20. S. Hayashi, I. C. Gillam, A. D. Delaney, and D. M. Terner, *J. Histochem. Cytochem.* **26,** 677 (1978).
21. D. E. Mathews and V. T. Farewell, "Using and Understanding Medical Statistics," Vol. 2. Karger, Basel, 1988.
22. J. Roberts, *Mol. Brain Res.,* in press (1988).
23. Y. Park, S. D. Park, W. K. Cho, and K. Kim, *Brain Res.* **451,** 255 (1988).
24. J. E. Levine and V. D. Ramirez, *in* "Methods in Enzymology" (P. M. Conn, ed.), Vol. 124, p. 466. Academic Press, Orlando, Florida, 1986.
25. C. A. Wilson, H. J. Herdon, L. C. Baily, and R. N. Clayton, *J. Endocrinol.* **108,** 441 (1986).
26. J. E. Levine and V. D. Ramirez, *Endocrinology (Baltimore)* **111,** 1439 (1982).
27. J. E. Levine, D. G. Karhalios, M. B. Sholand, P. C. Fallest, and J. F. Azzarello, *Soc. Neurosci. Abstr.* **12,** 322.3 (1986) (Abstr.).
28. F. J. Strobl and J. E. Levine, *Endocrinology (Baltimore)* **123,** 622 (1988).
29. J. E. Levine and M. T. Duffy, *Endocrinology (Baltimore)* **122,** 2211 (1988).
30. M. D. Culler, M. M. Valenca, I. Merchenthaler, B. Flerko, and A. Negro-Vilar, *Endocrinology (Baltimore),* in press (1988).
31. R. M. Kream, A. N. Clancy, M. S. A. Kumar, T. A. Schoenfeld, and F. Macrides, *Neuroendocrinology* **46,** 297 (1987).
32. I. Merchanthaler, M. D. Culler, A. Negro-Vilar, and B. Flerko, *Endocr. Soc.,* 49 (1987) (Abstr.).
33. P. S. Kalra, C. P. Phelps, and S. P. Kalra, *Soc. Neurosci. Abstr.* **14,** 1069 (1988).
34. W.-S. A. Wun and I. H. Thorneycroft, *Mol. Cell. Endocrinol.* **54,** 165 (1987).
35. G. R. Seiler, P. G. Brunetta, and J. C. King, *Soc. Neurosci. Abstr.* **14,** 398 (1988) (Abstr. 161.9).
36. K.-Y. F. Pau, P. M. Gliessman, D. L. Hess, and H. G. Spies, *Brain Res.* **459,** 70 (1988).
37. J. E. Levine, R. L. Norman, P. M. Gliessman, T. T. Oyama, D. R. Bangsberg, and H. G. Spies, *Endocrinology (Baltimore)* **117,** 711 (1985).
38. J. E. Levine, C. L. Bethea, and H. G. Spies, *Endocrinology (Baltimore)* **16,** 431 (1985).
39. W. C. Wetsel, P. T. Walton, and M. G. Wisniewski, *Endocr. Soc.,* 24 (1988) (Abstr. 14).
40. M. V. Raynolds, K. E. Elkind-Hirsch, C. T. Valdes, C. Bond, and J. Adelman, *in* "Reproductive Neuroendocrinology" (J. Ladoski, ed.), in press, 1989.

41. C. T. Valdes and K. E. Elkind-Hirsch, *Endocr. Soc.*, 320 (1988) (Abstr. 1200).
42. D. E. Dluzen and V. D. Ramirez, *Neuroendocrinology* **43**, 459 (1986).
43. O. K. Park and V. D. Ramirez, *Brain Res.* **437**, 245 (1987).
44. S. Fox, B. Shivers, R. Harlan, and D. W. Pfaff, *Soc. Study Reprod., Annu. Meet., 19th* (1986) (Abstr.).

[14] Location of Gene Expression in Tissue Sections by Hybridization Histochemistry Using Oligodeoxyribonucleotide Probes

Jennifer D. Penschow, Jim Haralambidis,
Scott Pownall, and John P. Coghlan

The advent of molecular cloning has provided a new and expanding set of research tools which have been particularly well adapted to the neurosciences. In particular, RNA–DNA and RNA–RNA hybridization techniques are being used to investigate expression of particular neuropeptide genes either *in situ* (in intact cells within tissue sections) or in tissue extracts. In this chapter, we shall describe in detail the technique of hybridization histochemistry (1), whereby labeled nucleic acid probes are applied to tissue sections where they hybridize with intracellular complementary target mRNA sequences which have been preserved during the tissue preparation. The mRNA–DNA hybrids formed at sites of gene expression are located in the tissue by the probe label. Here we describe the synthesis, labeling, and use of oligodeoxynucleotides in the technique of hybridization histochemistry. We have chosen this type of probe as they may be tailor-made for a specific purpose. Where it is necessary to discriminate between closely homologous mRNAs, probes may be designed to exploit regions of maximum difference in mRNA sequences (Fig. 1). Oligodeoxynucleotides confer a high degree of consistency on a given set of experiments, as the product of one synthetic batch provides numerous aliquots of probe of equivalent

Methods in Neurosciences, Volume 1

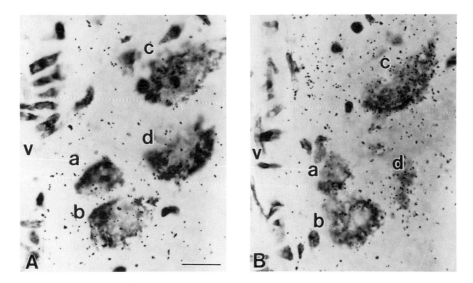

FIG. 1   Autoradiographs of adjacent 10-μm frozen sections of hypothalamus from a lactating ewe showing magnocellular neurons of the supraoptic nucleus after hybridization with discriminating ^{32}P-labeled oligodeoxynucleotide probes. The probes were complementary to nucleic acids 373–402 of bovine arginine vasopressin–neurophysin II (A) and oxytocin–neurophysin I (B) mRNAs [H. Land, M. Grez, S. Ruppert, H. Schmale, M. Rehbein, D. Richter, and G. Schutz, *Nature* (*London*) **302**, 342 (1983)]. With blood vessel (v) partly in the field as a landmark, four neuronal cell bodies labeled a, b, c, and d appear consecutively in both sections. b contains vasopressin mRNA, c and d contain oxytocin mRNA, and a does not contain either. Stain, Neutral red. Bar, 30 μm.

concentration and specific activity. The use of ^{32}P as a probe label permits X-ray film autoradiography of hybrids (2), which provides a rapid result and a convenient guide to subsequent exposures of liquid emulsion. The technique of hybridization histochemistry we have described is simple and convenient and has been used for several years for a variety of research topics and myriads of specimens (3, 4) with consistent success.

Materials

N,N-Diisopropyl-O-cyanoethyl nucleoside phosphoramidites, controlled-pore glass derivatized with protected nucleosides, dry acetonitrile for DNA synthesis (Applied Biosystems Inc., Melbourne, Australia)

Tetrazole gold label grade; 3-aminopropyltriethoxysilane (Aldrich Chemical Co., Milwaukee, WI)

Acetonitrile, ChromAR HPLC grade (Mallinckrodt Australia Pty Ltd., Clayton, Australia)

Acrylamide and bisacrylamide, Electran Grade (BDH Chemicals, Kilsyth, Australia)

T4 polynucleotide kinase, Sephadex G-25 fine [Pharmacia (Australia) Pty Ltd., North Ryde, Australia]

[γ-^{32}P]ATP, [α-^{35}S]dATP, polynucleotide kinase (Amersham Australia Pty Ltd., Melbourne, Australia)

[α-^{32}P]dATP, [α-^{32}P]dCTP (Bresa S.A. Pty Ltd., Adelaide, Australia)

OCT compound (Lab-Tek, Naperville, IL)

Glutaraldehyde, formamide, #4239,#9684, respectively, silica gel TLC sheets #5735 (Merck, Darmstadt, FRG)

Formaldehyde, ethylene glycol (Ajax Chemicals, Auburn, NSW, Australia)

Cacodylic acid, Ficoll type 70, bovine albumin fraction V, poly(vinylpyrrolidone)–40, DNA (degraded free acid) (Sigma Chemical Co., St. Louis, MO)

Ion-exchange resin #142-6425 (Bio-Rad, Richmond, CA)

Kodak XAR-5 X-ray film, X-ray developer, X-ray fixer (Eastman Kodak Co., Rochester, NY)

[Tyr^{11}] Somatostatin #8017 (Peninsula Laboratories Inc., Belmont, CA)

X-Ray cassettes, Dupont MRF-34 X-ray film (Dupont, Wilmington, DE)

Liquid emulsion, Ilford K5 and G5, "Hypam" fixer for emulsion (Ilford, Essex, UK)

Liquid emulsion, Kodak NTB-2 and NTB-3, D19 developer (Eastman Kodak Co., Rochester, NY)

Methodology

Probe Synthesis, Purification, and Labeling

Oligodeoxyribonucleotide Probe Synthesis

Oligodeoxyribonucleotides are routinely synthesized by the solid-phase method on an Applied Biosystems Inc. 380A DNA synthesizer, using phosphoramidite chemistry (5). The probes are assembled on a 0.2 μmol scale using *N,N*-diisopropyl-*O*-cyanoethyl nucleoside phosphoramidite monomers (6), in the "trityl off, auto" mode. The ammonia solution containing the probe is then treated at 50°C for 16 hr to remove the base-protecting groups, the solvent is removed *in vacuo,* and the residue redissolved in 2 ml of 0.2 mM EDTA. This solution is usually stable at −20°C indefinitely, and aliquots are purified as required.

Oligonucleotide Purification

The most convenient method for the routine purification of large numbers of oligonucleotides is polyacrylamide gel electrophoresis (PAGE). The purification of 120 μl of the crude sample gives approximately 20 μg of the pure probe, which is more than sufficient for most applications. The crude sample (20 μl of sample mixed with 10 μl of formamide for each well of 15 mm depth and 7 mm width) is loaded on a 10%, 0.8-mm-thick 20- × 20-cm polyacrylamide gel, and electrophoresed at constant power (10 W, ∼400 V) for 2–3 hr, depending on the length of the probe. A 30-mer runs at approximately half way between the bromphenol blue and xylene cyanole dyes, and the gel is electrophoresed till the fast dye (bromphenol blue) has reached the bottom of the gel. Dye tracks are run separately, and the gel has to be preelectrophoresed for at least 1 hr.

The gel plates are then prized apart, and the gel placed on a fluorescent TLC plate that has been wrapped in plastic wrapping. Upon illumination of this gel with a hand-held UV lamp (254 nm), the DNA appears dark on a fluorescent background. The product is usually the slowest moving major band, although a standard of known length is always run on an adjacent track for comparison. The band containing the probe is cut out with a razor blade without undue delay, the gel slices placed in an Eppendorf tube, and the DNA eluted by covering the slices with 0.2 mM EDTA and leaving at room temperature for 2 days. The solution is then dialyzed against water, the absorbance of the solution measured at 260 nm to determine the amount of DNA (1 OD_{260} unit ≈ 30 μg of single-stranded DNA), and then freeze-dried. It is then redissolved, when required, with 0.2 mM EDTA to a concentration of 50 ng/μl (∼5 μM for a 30-mer).

Oligonucleotide Labeling

There are two alternative methods using enzyme-catalyzed reactions which are commonly used for radioactive labeling of oligonucleotides. T4 polynucleotide kinase (7) catalyzes the phosphorylation of the 5′ end of an oligonucleotide using [γ-^{32}P]ATP as the radioactive phosphate donor. This method incorporates one radioactive phosphate per molecule of oligonucleotide. The other method utilizes terminal deoxynucleotidyltransferase, which catalyzes the polymerization of deoxynucleoside triphosphates (dNTPs) on the 3′ hydroxy thus extending the chain length of the oligonucleotide (8). Various labeled deoxynucleoside triphosphates ([α-^{35}S]-, [α-^{32}P]-,

[³H]dNTP or biotinylated dUTP) can be incorporated using this "tailing" method.

5'-End Labeling with T4 Polynucleotide Kinase

The following mixture is combined in an Eppendorf tube: the appropriate volume of oligonucleotide solution (from a 50 ng/μl stock), 4 μl of 10× denaturation buffer (0.2 M Tris-HCl, pH 9.5, 10 mM spermidine, 1 mM EDTA), and distilled H$_2$O to 40 μl. The tube is heated at 70°C for 5 min and then immediately chilled on ice. Five microliters of 10× kinase buffer [0.5 M Tris-HCl, pH 9.5, 0.1 M MgCl$_2$, 50 mM dithiothreitol (DTT), 50% glycerol] and 1 μl T4 polynucleotide kinase (PNK) (10 U, Pharmacia) are added. If a number of oligonucleotides are to be labeled in the one session, then the commercial stock of PNK (typically at 10 U/μl) can be diluted immediately before use with a dilution buffer (50 mM Tris-HCl, pH 7.5, 10 mM 2-mercaptoethanol, 0.05% DNase-free BSA) to a level of 5 U/μl and 1 μl of this solution is used. The contents of the tube are mixed by gently flicking it with a finger. Two molar equivalents of label are then added, i.e., 5 μl (50 μCi) of a 10 mCi/ml solution of [γ-³²P]ATP (5000 Ci/mmol) for 50 ng of a 30-mer oligonucleotide (average molecular weight is 9207). The tube is spun briefly in an Eppendorf centrifuge and then incubated at 37°C for 1 hr. The purification procedure is as described in *Purification of Labeled Probes*.

3' Labeling with Terminal Deoxynucleotidyltransferase

A typical tailing reaction is set up as follows: 1 μl of a 50 ng/μl oligonucleotide stock solution, distilled H$_2$O to give a final reaction volume of 50 μl, and 2.5 μl each of [α-³²P]dATP and [α-³²P]dCTP are combined in an Eppendorf tube. The cold nucleotides TTP and dGTP can be added to a final concentration of 1 μM each to minimize background. The tube is mixed by gently flicking it and then 5 μl of 10× tailing buffer (1 M potassium cacodylate, 250 mM Tris base, pH 7.6, 10 mM CoCl$_2$, 2 mM DDT) is added, followed by 1 μl of terminal deoxynucleotidyltransferase (TdT) (10 U/ml, Amersham). The tube is mixed as before and given a quick spin in a centrifuge. The mixture is incubated at 37°C for 1 hr. The tailed probes are spin column purified and ethanol precipitated as for the kinase end-labeled probes.

Care must be taken in preparing the 10× tailing buffer as the cobalt ions can be easily precipitated. The method of Roychoudhury and Wu (9) can be used to prepare this buffer. Cacodylic acid (1.38 g) and 0.3 g Tris base are suspended in 3.5 ml distilled water. The pH is adjusted to pH 7.6 by addition of solid KOH with constant mixing. The solution is then made up to 8.8 ml with distilled water and chilled on ice; 200 μl of 0.1 M DTT is mixed in and then 1 ml of 0.1 M CoCl$_2$ is added dropwise with constant mixing.

The resulting "tail" length from the TdT labeling reaction is influenced by the concentration of the enzyme, the duration of the incubation period, and the relative amounts of dNTPs to oligonucleotide. Pyrophosphate, a product of the transferase reaction, forms an insoluble precipitate with the cobalt cofactor. Thus, depletion of the cofactor can stop the reaction at high substrate concentrations.

The choice of radioisotope used for incorporation into the oligonucleotide depends on the experimental requirements, which are discussed later in this chapter.

Purification of Labeled Probes

To purify the labeled oligonucleotide probe from the free label, the sample can be either run through a conventional Sephadex G-25 gel filtration column or can be purified using a Sephadex G-25 spin column (10). Routinely, spin columns are used as they are more convenient to handle with a large number of samples. The following method is used to make and use the spin columns.

Sephadex G-25 Fine (6 g) is swelled in 40 ml of column buffer (10 mM Tris-HCl, pII 7.5, 1 mM EDTA, 0.1 M NaCl) for a minimum of 3 hr. A polyethylene frit (alternatively, sterile glass wool) is placed in the bottom of a 1-ml disposable syringe which is then placed in an uncapped 10-ml plastic tube. The Sephadex slurry is pipetted into the syringe barrel. Sufficient quantity of Sephadex is added such that it will bed down to the 0.9 ml mark of the syringe after a single spin in a bench centrifuge at 1500 rpm for 4 min.

Just before use, 190 μl of column buffer is added to the column and centrifuged as before to equilibrate the column, which is then transferred to a clean 10-ml tube. This tube is placed in a disposable 50-ml screw-cap tube. This outer tube is used to contain the radioactive material in the event of a spillage.

Finally, to purify the labeled oligonucleotide the reaction mixture, after incubation, is made up to a total volume of 190 μl with column buffer. This is applied to the top of the spin column which is then spun again for 4 min at 1500 rpm. The free label remains in the column and the oligonucleotide is eluted. The eluted oligonucleotide is transferred to an Eppendorf tube and ethanol precipitated overnight at $-20°C$ by adding 5 μl of 10 mg/ml tRNA, 0.1 volume of 3 M sodium acetate, and 2.5 vol of absolute ethanol. The sample is then centrifuged in an Eppendorf centrifuge for 15 min and supernatant decanted. It is then made up with the hybridization buffer used for probing tissue sections (see sections *Prehybridization* and *Hybridization*). A 1-μl sample should be taken at this stage for analysis on a 10% denaturing polyacrylamide gel (see Table I for an overview of *Methodology*).

TABLE I   Protocol for Hybridization Histochemistry

Probe synthesis, purification, and labeling
  Synthesize oligodeoxynucleotide using DNA synthesizer
  Purify oligonucleotide by PAGE
  Label oligonucleotide using T4 polynucleotide kinase or terminal
    deoxynucleotidyltransferase
  Purify labeled probe by gel filtration using drip or spin column
Tissue preparation, hybridization, and autoradiography
  Embed tissues in OCT compound and freeze in hexane/dry ice (prefix cell cultures or
    smears in acetone at 4°C)
  Cut sections of 5–10 μm with cryostat, thaw onto coated slides, and leave on dry ice
  Fix sections (and cell cultures or smears) in glutaraldehyde at 4°C, rinse in buffer
  Prehybridize sections or cells in hybridization buffer at 40°C, rinse in ethanol
  Dilute labeled probe to 400 ng/ml in hybridization buffer, heat for 3 min at 90–100°C
    (oligonucleotides or cDNA) or at 70°C (RNA probes), apply to sections or cells, overlay
    with coverslip, and incubate for 1 to 3 days
  Dislodge coverslip in 4× SSC, transfer slide to 2× SSC, wash in 1× SSC at 40–50°C for
    45 min, rinse in ethanol
  Tape slides in backing sheet in lightproof cassette and overlay with fast X-ray film.
    Expose for 24 hr at RT, develop, and fix. Evaluate results. Reexpose to high-resolution
    film if required
  Estimate exposure for liquid emulsion. Dip slides in emulsion, expose for 1–20 days
    (for ^{32}P) at RT. Develop and fix emulsion, harden with formaldehyde, wash, stain, and
    mount

Tissue Preparation, Hybridization, and Autoradiography

Freezing Fresh Tissue or Preparing Cells

Molds of heavy-duty aluminum foil are prepared slightly larger than the intended specimen. A small quantity of OCT compound at 4°C is added to the mold followed by the specimen of fresh tissue. After the tissue is orientated, the mold is filled with sufficient OCT at 4°C to cover the specimen. The mold is lowered into a bath of hexane containing dry ice at −78°C that is of sufficient volume to ensure that the temperature of the freezing bath is not raised by addition of the specimen. The surface of the OCT compound is held above the freezing mixture to permit expansion of the specimen during freezing, thereby reducing the risk of cracking. For very large specimens (>25 mm^3) it is preferable to first freeze the tissue in hexane/dry ice, then freeze-embed as described. The frozen embedded tissues are sealed in plastic and stored at −20°C for short periods (3 months) or −80°C for longer periods.

  Cell cultures or smears are washed in serum-free medium, fixed in acetone at 4°C for 1 min, and allowed to dry. The next step for these preparations is described in *Fixation*.

Sectioning

Frozen sections are cut at 6–10 μm (thicker sections are avoided due to poor resolution in liquid emulsion autoradiographs) using a conventional cryo-microtome at −12 to −20°C and then mounted on treated dry slides kept at room temperature (RT). [Clean slides are precoated by immersion in 2% 3-aminopropyltriethoxysilane in acetone followed by two acetone and water rinses, then drying at 42°C (11).] Slides carrying sections are laid immediately on dry ice to freeze the section rapidly, thereby reducing the risk of mRNA degradation by tissue ribonucleases. Sections retained for routine histology are air dried at RT.

Fixation

Slides for hybridization are removed directly into fixative at 4°C. Fixative is 4% glutaraldehyde in 0.1 M phosphate buffer at pH 7.2, containing 20% ethylene glycol. After 5 min fixation, slides are rinsed in two changes of hybridization buffer (see *Prehybridization*) at room temperature, then at 40°C. Sections for routine histology are fixed for 10 sec in 75% ethanol containing 10% formaldehyde, rinsed in water, and dried.

Acetone-prefixed cell cultures or smears are fixed as above and subsequently treated as for sections.

Prehybridization

Slides are soaked in hybridization buffer at 40°C for up to 4 hr, then rinsed in three changes of absolute ethanol and allowed to dry. Hybridization buffer is 600 mM sodium chloride, 50 mM sodium phosphate buffer, pH 7.0, 5.0 mM EDTA, 0.02% Ficoll, 0.02% bovine serum albumin, 0.02% poly(vinylpyrrolidone), 0.1% degraded DNA, and 40% formamide (deionized by adding 3 g/liter ion-exchange resin and filtered). Solutes are dissolved in distilled water with gentle heating, the solution filtered, and the formamide added. The buffer is designed to encourage specificity of hybridization and stability of hybrids (12). Sections may be stored at this stage over absolute ethanol, at 4°C for short periods (days) or −20°C for some months.

Hybridization

The labeled probe is diluted in hybridization buffer (10 mM DTT is included for ^{35}S-labeled probes) to approximately 40 nM (400 ng/ml for a 30-mer; higher probe concentrations may cause nonspecific binding). DNA probes are heated for 3 min at 90–100°C (or SP6 RNA to 70°C) to dissociate any base pairing, mixed by vortex, and centrifuged. A drop of probe is applied to a clean glass coverslip (approximately 20 μl is sufficient for the 22- $\times$ 22-mm size; the quantity varies with the section thickness) and the coverslip applied to the sections. Slides are laid on a plastic grill in a chamber humidified by hybridization buffer. The chamber is sealed and incubated at a temperature appropriate for the probe length (usually 40°C for DNA probes larger than 25 nucleotides—see *Discussion of Method*—or 60–70°C for RNA). However, an overnight incubation is sufficient for detecting abundant mRNA transcripts; up to 3 days is recommended for greater sensitivity.

Washing

After hybridization, slides are placed vertically in a beaker of 4$\times$ SSC (standard saline–citrate, 4$\times$ SSC is 0.6 M sodium chloride and 0.06 M sodium citrate in distilled water) until coverslips dislodge. Slides are transferred to 2$\times$ SSC at RT, then soaked in 1$\times$ SSC for 45 min at 40°C with occasional agitation, rinsed in three changes of absolute ethanol, and allowed to dry at RT.

Autoradiography: X-Ray Film for ^{32}P- or ^{35}S-Labeled Hybrids

The dry slides are placed side-by-side and taped to a sheet of heavy paper in an X-ray cassette. A sheet of fast X-ray film (Kodak XAR-5) is laid over the sections, and the cassette is sealed and left at RT for 24 hr (for ^{32}P) to expose (intensifying screens are not used because of the resulting poor resolution). The film is developed for 2 min, rinsed, and fixed (developer and fixer are prepared according to the manufacturer). For subsequent exposures within the half-life of the isotope, approximately five times longer than the Kodak XAR-5 exposure will be required to obtain an equivalent signal if high-resolution films such as Dupont MRF-34 are used. These films are very convenient for mapping.

Liquid Emulsion Autoradiography

Where resolution to single cells or groups of cells is required, sections are coated with liquid emulsion following the fast X-ray film exposure, using the signal intensity on the film as a guide to estimate exposure times for individual slides. As a rough guide, for ^{32}P-labeled probes a test section coated in emulsion should be developed after 10 times the duration of the Kodak XAR-5 exposure which gave a dark gray image. Due to the short half-life of ^{32}P, slides should be dipped as soon as possible after the Kodak XAR-5 exposure.

Ilford K5 or Kodak NTB-2 emulsion is diluted 1 : 1 with distilled water (G5 or NTB-3 with larger silver grain size may be used for greater sensitivity) and heated to 40°C until homogeneous and then maintained at this temperature. Slides are dipped in emulsion and placed vertically in slide racks. The filled racks are placed over dry silica gel in a light-proof, air-tight tin at RT to expose. When the correct exposure time has been established by developing extra slides, the remainder are developed in Kodak D19 for 2 min at RT, rinsed in water, fixed for 1 to 5 min, rinsed in water, and the emulsion hardened by immersion for 1 min in 4% formaldehyde in 0.1 M phosphate, pH 7.2. After thorough rinsing, slides can be stained, with due caution not to dislodge the emulsion layer or to use acid solutions which may cause dissolution of developed silver grains. For detailed information on autoradiography refer to Ref. 13.

Discussion of Method

Hybridization Temperature

The temperature for hybridization of sections with oligodeoxynucleotides is related to the probe length, specificity of the probe for the target mRNA, and the formamide and salt concentration of the hybridization buffer (14). Raised temperature and formamide and lowered salt concentrations are inhibitory to hybridization, thus lower temperatures (and/or formamide) are necessary for hybridization of short sequences. This also reduces specificity, thereby generating an increase in background. We prefer to vary only the temperature, according to the probe length and specificity, while maintaining the salt concentration constant at 0.6 M and formamide at 40%. For homologous systems, the following temperatures may be used as a guide: RT for 15- to 18-mer, 30°C for 19- to 25-mer, 40°C for probes longer than 25-mer. Higher temperatures are indicated where cross-hybridization is a potential problem, otherwise 40°C is preferred. For nonhomologous systems, lower temperatures usually will be necessary. For such experiments it is preferable to hybridize multiple samples at different temperatures.

For SP6 RNA probes (15), temperatures of 70°C have been recommended as optimal, as the melting temperature of the RNA–RNA hybrids is higher than for RNA–DNA; however, temperatures above 60°C may reduce the quality of sections, or cause dislodgement from slides if the coating is inappropriate.

Posthybridization Washing

In our experience, hybrids formed *in situ* are extremely stable to low-salt/high-temperature washes (4), and nonspecific interactions which may have occurred during hybridization remain through the most stringent of washes.

It is therefore essential for minimum background to have probes which are not contaminated by shorter sequences or unincorporated label.

Controls

There are several types of controls which should be included with each hybridization reaction. Where possible, control tissues with abundant target mRNA and tissues with none should be sectioned and hybridized along with the tissues of interest.

One or more control probes of the same type and length as the test probes but with no specificity whatsoever for the tissue of interest should be prepared at the same specific activity and concentration as the test probes. By hybridizing control and test probes to identical sets of sections, sites of nonspecific binding in tissues may be identified.

Another specificity control is pretreatment of sections with ribonuclease A which should abolish or greatly reduce the hybridization signal, the degree of reduction depending on the abundance of mRNA in the tissue and the extent of the treatment. For this procedure, sections are fixed as usual then rinsed three times in 4× SSC and incubated at 37°C for 30 min in 20 μg/ml ribonuclease A in 0.1 M phosphate buffer at pH 7.2. A control set of slides is incubated without the ribonuclease. Following the incubation, slides are rinsed at 37°C in one change of 0.1 M phosphate buffer, pH 7.2, and two changes of 4× SSC and then prehybridized and hybridized according to the method.

Quantitation

Relative levels of mRNA in tissue sections may be determined by densitometry of autoradiographs using automated image analyzers which can provide color-coded images indicating the relative intensity of signal in X-ray film autoradiographs (16). Automated or manual grain counts of liquid emulsion autoradiographs may provide similar data at higher resolution. It is important to remember that the quantity of mRNA present in a tissue may be the result of high-level transcription in a small number of cells or lower levels of transcription in a larger group of cells, both of these instances providing the same net result. Thus densitometric measurements of hybridized sections without adequate sampling of tissue may not reflect accurately the total tissue mRNA level. Indeed, there is evidence of recruitment of additional cell populations to transcription of specific mRNAs in situations of high demand for the translation product (17). This is an important consideration in the interpretation of densitometric data from hybridized sections. Measurements of extracted mRNA by dot-blot, Northern blot, or solution hybridization can be undertaken in parallel with hybridization histochemistry to measure relative tissue mRNA levels (18).

Comparison of Methods

Tissue Preparation

Some methods (19) employ perfusion fixation of brains and other tissues for hybridization histochemistry, which provides good morphology and facilitates antibody staining, although it may result in suboptimal hybridization signals (20). Alternatively, the use of fresh frozen tissue permits maximal hybridization signals and the freezing method is portable and universally applicable. Specific binding studies (21) may be carried out on adjacent sections of unfixed tissue, an example of which is illustrated in Fig. 2. We find that glutaraldehyde-fixed frozen sections are morphologically superior to those fixed with formaldehyde or ethanol-based fixatives. Although glutaraldehyde-fixed tissues may hinder the penetration of long probes (22), we find no reduction in hybridization signals where oligodeoxynucleotides are used when compared to tissues fixed by other methods.

Probes and Labels

The selection of types of probes and labels largely depends on the desired result. ^{32}P-Labeling is applicable to all probe types at high specific activity and permits rapid results on X-ray film and on liquid emulsion, with resolution to single cells in some cases (Figs. 1 and 2), or to groups of cells. ^{35}S is similarly applicable, with higher resolution than ^{32}P but requiring longer exposure times and with greater potential for background, even in the presence of reducing agents. ^{3}H label enables high resolution of signals but with longer exposure times than for the other isotopes. Extensive microscopic survey of sections is usually necessary to detect ^{3}H-labeled hybrids, as X-ray film exposures are impractical due to the low energy and long half-life of this isotope.

Nonradioactive probe labels are now being compared in a number of different systems, with conflicting reports of sensitivity but with single-cell resolution (23, 24).

Types of probes commonly used for hybridization histochemistry include cDNA, oligodeoxyribonucleotide, and single-stranded RNA probes trans-

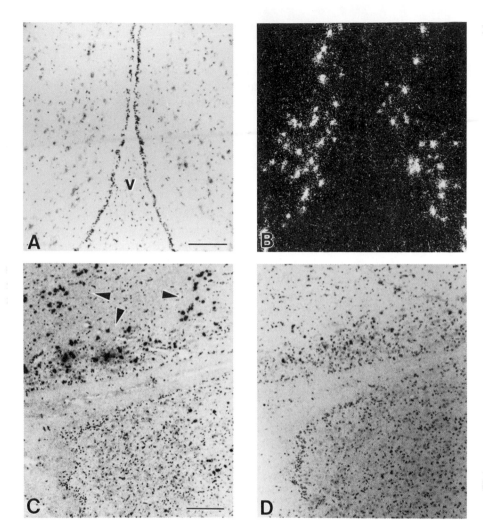

FIG. 2 Liquid emulsion autoradiographs of 8-μm coronal frozen sections of ovine anterior hypothalamus. (A and B) Bright-field and dark-field photomicrographs of the same field. This section was hybridized with a ^{32}P-labeled 30-mer probe complementary to rat preprosomatostatin mRNA [R. H. Goodman, D. C. Aron, and B. A. Roos, *J. Biol. Chem.* **258,** 5570 (1983)]. Labeled neurons in the periventricular area adjacent to the third ventricle (v) can be seen clearly in B. (C and D) Adjacent sections, which are close to A, have been incubated with 1 nm (1.2×10^6 cpm/ml) of ^{125}I-labeled [Tyr^{11}] somatostatin ligand and the control section (D) with an additional 100 nmol of unlabeled somatostatin in the incubation mixture. Specific binding to groups of neurons (arrowheads) in the supraoptic nucleus can be seen in C (magnocellular neurons have not stained clearly in these treated sections). The same field in specificity control (D) shows that the binding has been blocked. Stain, Thionin. Bar, A and B, 0.6 mm; C and D, 0.5 mm.

cribed in the SP6 vector system (25). cDNAs were the original recombinant probes and suffer from the disadvantage of being double-stranded, hybridization efficiency being markedly reduced by the presence of a competing DNA strand, although this is partly compensated by the network-forming potential of these long probes. Probe efficiency is increased significantly by cloning the cDNA insert into the SP6 vector. In this way, large amounts of single-stranded cRNA probe may be produced from added substrate ribonucleotides in the presence of SP6 polymerase. The specific activity of the probe produced may be maximized by incorporation of all four component ribonucleotides as labeled bases instead of the usual one or two. However, such "hot" probes are very expensive to produce and may be liable to degradation by radiolysis and/or RNase. The SP6 system has been recently adapted to generate RNA copies of oligodeoxynucleotides (26) which have been used for hybridization histochemistry.

Oligodeoxynucleotides also have the advantage of being single-stranded. These may be labeled as we have described, at the 5′ end with ^{32}P or at the 3′ end by addition of a number of deoxyribonucleotides carrying conventional radioactive or nonradioactive labels. The specific activity of labeled probes varies for different sequences and probe lengths. To optimize the 5′ end-labeling reaction and avoid excess residual unlabeled probe, the quantity of labeled nucleotide must match the length and quantity of oligodeoxynucleotide. The specific activity of a ^{32}P-end-labeled 25-mer probe can be adequate for the detection of low-abundance mRNA transcripts such as corticotropin-releasing hormone (CRH) in hypothalamic neurons (Fig. 3). Oligodeoxynucleotides are particularly valuable for the specificity which may be conferred by the probe design, as it is possible to prepare probes which encompass discriminating regions of closely homologous mRNAs. This facility is indispensable for studies of multigene families or where no recombinant DNA is available. The simplicity of labeling oligodeoxynucleotides permits their use where access to molecular biology facilities is limited.

Conclusion

The technique of hybridization histochemistry may be used in conjunction with immunohistochemistry for the investigation of transcriptional regulation of neuroendocrine peptides and identification of the peptide product(s). Once sites of expression of neuropeptide genes have been located by hybridization histochemistry, it is possible to measure cellular and regional levels of gene expression in varying physiological states by quantitation of specific RNA–DNA hybrids in sections and in RNA extracts of tissues. Products of translation may then be determined by immunohistochemistry

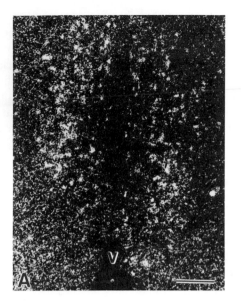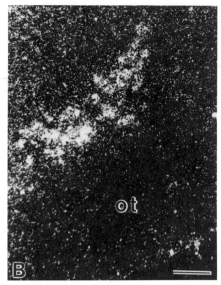

F IG. 3 Liquid emulsion autoradiographs of coronal 10-μm frozen sections of hypothalamus from a stressed sheep after hybridization with a 25-mer oligodeoxynucleotide complementary to ovine corticotropin-releasing hormone mRNA [H. Ohkubo, R. Kageyama, M. Ujihara, T. Hirose, S. Inayama, and S. Nakanishi, *Proc. Natl. Acad. Sci. U.S.A.* **80,** 2196 (1983)]. Photomicrographs by dark-field illumination show labeled neurons of the paraventricular nucleus in A and of the supraoptic nucleus of B. v, Third ventricle; ot, optic tract. Bar, A, 0.6 mm; B, 0.2 mm.

using specific antibodies. These may be region-specific, designed to target products of posttranslational processing from larger precursor molecules. Hybridization histochemistry provides an important adjunct also to studies where specific receptor sites are located by peptide ligand binding or by antibodies directed to receptor proteins. By a combination of these techniques, sites of gene expression and target cells for the translation products may be identified in the one tissue or organism.

The new wave of molecular techniques are integral to the elucidation of neuroendocrine regulatory systems and the location of gene expression is central to this approach.

Acknowledgments

We thank Dr. Geoffrey Tregear for valuable support and advice, Ms. Paula Darling and Ms. Tiina Oldfield for excellent technical assistance, and Ms. Zena Roslan for typing the manuscript. This work was supported by grants in aid from the National Health and Medical Research Council of Australia, the Myer Family Trusts, the Ian Potter Foundation, the Howard Florey Biomedical Foundation, and by Grant HD11908 from the National Institutes of Health.

References

1. P. Hudson, J. D. Penschow, J. Shine, G. Ryan, H. D. Niall, and J. P. Coghlan, *Endocrinology (Baltimore)* **108,** 353 (1981).
2. J. D. Penschow, J. Haralambidis, P. Aldred, G. W. Tregear, and J. P. Coghlan, *in* "Methods in Enzymology" (P. M. Conn, ed.), Vol. 124, p. 534. Academic Press, Orlando, Florida, 1986.
3. J. P. Coghlan, P. Aldred, J. Haralambidis, H. D. Niall, J. D. Penschow, and G. W. Tregear, *Anal. Biochem.* **149,** 1 (1985).
4. J. D. Penschow, J. Haralambidis, P. E. Darling, I. A. Darby, E. M. Wintour, G. W. Tregear, and J. P. Coghlan, *Experientia* **43,** 741 (1987).
5. S. L. Beaucage and M. H. Caruthers, *Tetrahedron Lett.* **22,** 1859 (1981).
6. N. D. Sinha, J. Biernat, and H. Koster, *Tetrahedron Lett.* **24,** 5843 (1983).
7. A. M. Maxam and W. Gilbert, *in* "Methods in Enzymology" (L. Grossman and K. Moldave, eds.), Vol. 65, p. 499. Academic Press, New York, 1980.
8. K.-I. Kato, J. Moura Concalves, G. E. Harts, and F. J. Bollum, *J. Biol. Chem.* **242,** 2780 (1967).
9. R. Roychoudhury and R. Wu, *in* "Methods in Enzymology" (L. Grossman and K. Moldave, eds.), Vol. 65, p. 43. Academic Press, New York, 1980.
10. T. Maniatis, E. F. Fritsch, and J. Sambrook, "Molecular Cloning: A Laboratory Manual." Cold Spring Harbor Laboratory, Cold Spring Harbor, New York, 1982.
11. M. Rentrop, B. Knapp, H. Winter, and J. Schweizer, *Histochem. J.* **18,** 271 (1986).
12. D. T. Denhart, *Biochem. Biophys. Res. Commun.* **23,** 641 (1966).
13. A. W. Rogers, "Techniques of Autoradiography," 3rd Ed. Elsevier, Amsterdam, 1979.
14. M. Smith, *in* "Methods of RNA Sequencing" (S. M. Weissman, ed.), pp. 182–187. Praeger, New York, 1982.
15. K. H. Cox, D. V. De Leon, L. M. Angerer, and R. C. Angerer, *Dev. Biol.* **101,** 485 (1984).
16. C. Goochee, W. Rasband, and L. Sokoloff, *Ann. Neurol.* **7,** 359 (1985).
17. L. G. Davis, R. Arentzen, J. M. Reid, R. W. Manning, B. Wolfson, K. L. Lawrence, and F. Baldino, Jr., *Neurobiology* **83,** 1146 (1986).
18. B. van Leeuwen, J. D. Penschow, J. P. Coghlan, and R. I. Richards, *EMBO J.* **6,** 1705 (1987).
19. C. E. Gee, C.-L. C. Chen, J. L. Roberts, R. Thompson, and S. J. Watson, *Nature (London)* **306,** 374 (1983).
20. B. D. Shivers, B. S. Schachter, and D. W. Pfaff, *in* "Methods in Enzymology" (P. M. Conn, ed.), Vol. 124, p. 497. Academic Press, Orlando, Florida, 1986.

21. M. Millan, G. Aguilera, P. C. Wynn, F. A. O. Mendelsohn, and K. J. Catt, *in* "Methods in Enzymology" (P. M. Conn, ed.), Vol. 124, p. 590. Academic Press, Orlando, Florida, 1986.
22. J. B. Lawrence and R. H. Singer, *Nucleic Acids Res.* **13,** 1777 (1985).
23. G. V. Childs, J. M. Lloyd, G. Unabia, S. D. Gharib, M. E. Wierman, and W. W. Chin, *Mol. Endocrinol.* **1,** 926 (1987).
24. A.-F. Guittcny, B. Fouque, C. Mougin, R. Teoule, and B. Bloch, *J. Histochem. Cytochem.* **36,** 536 (1988).
25. D. A. Melton, P. A. Kreig, M. R. Rebagliati, T. Maniatis, K. Zinn, and M. R. Green, *Nucleic Acids Res.* **12,** 7035 (1986).
26. P. Denny, Q. Hamid, J. E. Krause, J. M. Polak, and S. Legon, *Histochemistry* **89,** 481 (1988).

[15]   *In Situ* mRNA Hybridization: Standard Procedures and Novel Approaches

C. Anthony Altar, Susan Ryan, Mary Abood, and James H. Eberwine

Introduction

The technique of *in situ* hybridization (ISH) is an elegant synthesis of molecular biology and histology. Hybridization is a process whereby two single-stranded nucleic acid chains bind together by hydrogen bonding of complementary base pairs. ISH takes advantage of the ability of mRNA within a cell to hybridize with exogenously applied RNA or DNA molecules (Goodman and Spiegelman, 1971). This interaction is visualized by labeling the applied nucleic acid (probe) with a detectable molecule. The greatest strength of this technique is the capacity to localize cytosolic and nuclear messenger RNA (mRNA) to the single-cell level in thin tissue sections. As a result, ISH has expanded the study of neuronal structure, metabolism, and transmission. As more DNA sequences encoding neuronal proteins are

Methods in Neurosciences, Volume 1

discovered (Sutcliffe, 1988), ISH will be in greater demand to aid in their characterization. This chapter is a review of current methods and a discussion of future applications for this method, including *in situ* transcription (IST) and a novel strategy for the *in situ* quantitation of mRNA.

ISH has yielded valuable information regarding the distribution and regulation of mRNAs in discrete neural systems because it localizes mRNA within the cell body. This is possible because mRNA is present only in the cell soma and is not transported along the axon of neurons as compared to its protein products, which can be found throughout the neuron. One can therefore establish the distribution of mRNA synthesis in individual cells and within cell groups. ISH can also be used to examine changes in steady-state mRNA levels at the single cell (microscopy) or regional (film autoradiography) level.

ISH can also be combined with other histological methods, including immunohistochemistry, receptor autoradiography, lesioning, and pathway tracing techniques. This provides information regarding the function of individual cells, nuclear groups, and chemically or anatomically distinct pathways (Watts and Swanson, this volume [7]). The following paragraphs will provide specific examples of the benefit to be gained from using ISH and combining it with other histological techniques. Table I gives numerous examples of ISH use over the last 10 years.

One of the most pressing questions after detection of mRNA within a cell is whether the mRNA is translated into protein. Immunocytochemistry and pathway tracing have been used with ISH to examine proopiomelanocortin (POMC) mRNA in the arcuate nucleus of the hypothalamus (Wilcox *et al.*, 1986). In this study, immunoreactive POMC and POMC mRNA was colocalized within the same arcuate nucleus cells. Using the retrograde transport of fast blue, these same neurons have been shown to project to the preoptic area (Wilcox *et al.*, 1986). Such an analysis shows where a neuromodulator is made, as well as the range of tissue where it presumably exerts biological activity.

Aside from its use in mapping mRNAs, ISH is also useful as a way of expanding upon the information gained from receptor autoradiography studies. For instance, the expression of the γ-aminobutyric acid (GABA$_A$) receptor gene is most concentrated in cell bodies of the thalamus, olfactory bulb, and hippocampus (Sequier *et al.*, 1988a). GABA$_A$ immunoreactivity with the bd-17 monoclonal antibody and receptor autoradiography with [^{3}H]flumazenil show that GABA receptors are also found in these same brain areas but are more broadly distributed in cell body and dendritic regions.

ISH can be coupled to more standard neuroanatomical manipulations such as lesioning techniques to examine regulatory aspects of mRNA production. For example, the dopamine receptor antagonist haloperidol

TABLE I Probes for Peptide Precursors, Enzymes, Receptors, Other Proteins, and Viruses[a]

Probe name	Probe type[b]	Label[c]	Species and tissue	Reference
Probes for Peptide Precursors				
Oxytocin	oligo(20) kinase	p	r br	Jirikowski et al. (1988)
Oxytocin	oligo(48) tail	s	r br	Lightman and Young (1987)
Oxytocin	sscDNA(M13)	s	r hy	Burbach et al. (1987)
Oxytocin	oligo(25) kin, tail	p, h	r br	Kawata et al. (1988)
Oxytocin	oligo(48) kin, tail	s	r br	Young et al. (1986a)
Oxytocin	nt cDNA	h	r scn	McCabe et al. (1986a)
Vasopressin	oligo(24) tail	i, s	r br	Card et al. (1988)
Vasopressin	oligo(24) klen ext, kin	i, p	r br	Lewis et al. (1986b)
Vasopressin	oligo(48ex, 42int, 42int) kin, tail	s	r br	Young et al. (1986b)
Vasopressin	oligo(22) kin	p	r hy	Nojiri et al. (1985)
Vasopressin	oligo(15) kin	p	r hy	Fuller et al. (1985)
Vasopressin	oligo(8,11,15,19,24,45, 75,45kfi) kin, 40kfi	p, h, s	r hyp	Uhl et al. (1985)
Vasopressin	nt cDNA	h	r br	McCabe et al. (1986b)
Vasopressin	oligo(26) tail, kin	p, h	r br	Sherman et al. (1986a)
Vasopressin	oligo(45,35) 5' link, tail	b (ap, bio-AB, per)	r br, h car	Guitteny et al. (1988)
Vasopressin	oligo(26) tail	s	r br	Sherman et al. (1986b)
Vasopressin	oligo(48) tail	s	r br	Lightman and Young (1987)
Vasopressin	nt cDNA, gene	s	r hy	McCabe et al. (1986a)
Vasopressin	oligo(24) tail	i	r br	Baldino et al. (1988)
Growth hormone	nt cDNA	p, h	r br, pit	Gossard et al. (1987)
Vasoactive intestinal polypeptide	oligo(29) tail	i, s	r scn	Card et al. (1988)
Peptide histidine isoleucine	oligo(33) tail	i, s	r scn	Card et al. (1988)
Somatostatin	oligo(39) tail	i, s	r scn	Card et al. (1988)
Somatostatin	riboprobe	h, p	r br	Hoefler et al. (1986)
Somatostatin	oligos(22,24,lig46) kin	p	r hy	Fuller et al. (1985)
Somatostatin	oligo(39) tail	s	r hy	Werner et al. (1988)
Somatostatin	riboprobe	s	r br	Rogers et al. (1987)
Insulin	oligo(46) kin	p	r br	Arentzen et al. (1985)
Insulin	oligo(48) tail	s	r br	Young et al. (1986a)
IGF-I, IGF-II	oligo(II-30,I-30) kin	p	r emb	Beck et al. (1987)
IGF-I	nt cDNA	p	GH$_3$, c	Fagin et al. (1987)
Insulin-related mRNA	nt cDNA	h, p	cul r, h, m pit	Budd et al. (1986)
Enkephalin	oligo(30) kin	p	r str	Angulo et al. (1987)

Enkephalin	nt cDNA	p	r br	Morris et al. (1988)
Enkephalin	oligo(48) tail	s	r fbr	Young et al. (1986b)
Enkephalin	nt cDNA	p	b, ham, gp adr	Bloch et al. (1985a)
Enkephalin	nt cDNA	s, p	r br, adr	Bloch et al. (1986)
Enkephalin	riboprobe	s	r br	Siegal and Young (1985)
Enkephalin	nt cDNA	p	b adr, pri cul	Bloch et al. (1984a)
Enkephalin	oligo(45) kfi	s	r br	Nishimori et al. (1988)
Enkephalin	nt cDNA, riboprobe	s	r br	Normand et al. (1988)
Enkephalin	oligo(48) tail	s	r br	Lightman and Young (1987)
Enkephalin	nt cDNA	h	r br	Harlan et al. (1987)
Enkephalin	nt cDNA	p, h	r br	Romano et al. (1987)
Substance P	oligo(33)	p	r str	Angulo et al. (1987)
Substance P	oligo(48) tail	s	r fbr	Young et al. (1986b)
Substance P	oligo(48) tail	s	r br	Warden and Young (1988)
Neurokinin B	oligo(48) tail	s	r br	Warden and Young (1988)
Substance P	riboprobe	s	r, m br	Chesselet et al. (1987)
Glucagon	oligo(20) kin	p	r br	Han et al. (1986)
Osteonectin (SPARC)	riboprobe	s	m emb	Holland et al. (1987)
GnRH	riboprobe	s	m br (trans)	Mason et al. (1986a)
GnRH	oligo(48,48) tail	s	m br	Mason et al. (1986b)
GnRH-like mRNA	oligo(59) kin, tail	p, h	r fbr	Shivers et al. (1986b)
GnRH	oligo(48) tail	s	r br	Zoeller et al. (1988)
GAP	oligo(48) tail	s	r br	Zoeller et al. (1988)
GnRH	oligo(59) kin	p	r fbr	Rothfeld et al. (1987)
Calcitonin	oligo(45) 5' link, tail	b (ap, bio-AB, per)	r br, h car	Amara et al. (1985)
CGRP-a,b	riboprobe	p	r br	Amara et al. (1985)
CGRP	oligo(45) 5' link, tail	b (ap, bio-AB, per)	r br, h car	Guitteny et al. (1988)
Dynorphin	oligo(100) klen ext	p	r br	Morris et al. (1988)
Dynorphin	oligo(48) tail	s	r br	Ruda et al. (1988)
Dynorphin	oligo(48) tail	s	r fbr	Young et al. (1986b)
Dynorphin	oligo(30) tail	s	r br	Sherman et al. (1986a)
Dynorphin	oligo(45) kfi	s	r br	Nishimori et al. (1988)
Dynorphin	oligo(48) tail	s	r br	Lightman and Young (1987)
POMC	riboprobe, nt cDNA	s, h	r pit	Chronwall et al. (1987)
POMC	oligo(24) tail	h, b (ap)	r, m pit	Larsson et al. (1988)
POMC	nt cDNA	h	r pit	Shivers et al. (1986b)
POMC	nt cDNA	p	h, b, c, r, p pit	Bloch et al. (1985b)
POMC	oligo(24) kin, tail	p	r pit	Lewis et al. (1986a)

(continued)

TABLE I (continued)

Probe name	Probe type[b]	Label[c]	Species and tissue	Reference
POMC	nt cDNA	p	r pit	Kelsey et al. (1986)
POMC	nt cDNA	h	r pit	Gee et al. (1983)
POMC	riboprobe	s	r pit	Chronwall et al. (1987)
TRH	riboprobe	p	r br	Segerson et al. (1987a)
TRH	riboprobe	s	r hy	Segerson et al. (1987b)
TRH	oligo(48) tail	s	r br	Koller et al. (1987)
Prolactin	1st strand cDNA, rt	h	r pit	Pochet et al. (1981)
Prolactin	nt cDNA	h	r pit	Hogami et al. (1985)
Prolactin	nt cDNA	h	r pit	Yamamoto et al. (1986)
Prolactin	riboprobe	s	r pit	Stell et al. (1988)
NPY	nt gene	s	r lung	Ericsson et al. (1987)
CRF	oligo(48) tail	s	r br	Palkovits et al. (1987)
CRF	oligo(48) tail	s	r br	Lightman and Young (1987)
CRF	oligo(48) tail	s	r pvn	Kovacs and Mezey (1987)
Cholecystokinin	riboprobe	s	r br	Siegel and Young (1985)
Cholecystokinin	nt cDNA	p	r br	Bonnemann et al. (1987)
Angiotensinogen	oligo(42) kin, riboprobe	p	r br	Lynch et al. (1987)
Galanin	oligo(48) tail	s	r hy	Rokaeus et al. (1988)
Probes for Enzymes, Receptors, and Other Proteins				
EGF	oligo(30) kin	p	m sal gl	van Leeuwan et al. (1987)
Transforming growth factor α	riboprobe	s	m br	Wilcox and Derynck (1988)
Nicotinic acetylcholine receptor, α 2,3,4	riboprobe	s	r br	Wada et al. (1988)
GABA$_A$ receptor	riboprobe	s	r br	Sequier et al. (1988b)
Neurofilament	nt cDNA	b (avi-gold)	r br	Leissi et al. (1986)
Glutamate decarboxylase	riboprobe	s	m cer	Wuenschell et al. (1986)
Glutamate decarboxylase	riboprobe	s	m cer	Wuenschell et al. (1986)
Glutamate decarboxylase	nt cDNA	s	rb	Julien et al. (1987)
Glutamate decarboxylase	riboprobe	s	r, m br	Chesselet et al. (1987)
Tyrosine monooxygenase	nt cDNA	s	r br	Berod et al. (1987a)
Tyrosine monooxygenase	oligo(34) kin	p	r br, adr	Han et al. (1987)
Tyrosine monooxygenase	oligo(48) tail	s	r fbr	Young et al. (1986a)
Tyrosine monooxygenase	oligo(48) tail	s	r br	Young et al. (1987)
Tyrosine monooxygenase	riboprobe	s	r, m br	Chesselet et al. (1987)

Tyrosine monooxygenase	riboprobe	s	r br, adr	Schalling et al. (1986)
Tyrosine monooxygenase	riboprobe	s	r br, adr	Schalling et al. (1986)
Odorant-binding protein	riboprobe	s	r nas epi	Pevsner et al. (1988)
G-protein	ds oligo(46) klen ext	s	r br	Largent et al. (1988)
Chromogranin A	riboprobe	s	b adr, pit, br	Siegel et al. (1988)
PNMT	oligo(48) tail	s	b adr	Siegel et al. (1988)
PNMT	oligo(48) tail	p	r br, adr	Schalling et al. (1986)
Estrogen receptor	oligo(72) kinase	s	r pit	Pelletier et al. (1988)
Homeobox Hox-1.5	riboprobe	s, h	m emb	Gaunt (1987)
Glial fibrillary acidic protein	riboprobe	s	r br, pri cul	Holmes et al. (1988)
Glial fibrillary acidic protein	nt cDNA	b (dab-per)	r astro cul	Eng et al. (1986)
Glial fibrillary acidic protein	nt cDNA	s	r br	Lewis and Cowan (1985)
Glycerol-phosphate dehydrogenase	riboprobe	s	r br, pri cul	Holmes et al. (1988)
Myelin basic protein	riboprobe	s	r br, pri cul	Holmes et al. (1988)
Myelin basic protein	cDNA (tail)	s	dev r br	Kristensson et al. (1986)
Vimentin	nt cDNA	b (dab-per)	r astro cul	Eng et al. (1986)
Actin	nt cDNA	b (dab-per)	r astro cul	Eng et al. (1986)
Tublin, α-, β-	nt cDNA	b (dab-per)	r astro cul	Eng et al. (1986)
Tublin, α-	nt cDNA	h	r cer	Ginzburg et al. (1986)
Nerve growth factor	riboprobe, oligo(18) kin	s	r br	Bandtlow et al. (1987)
Nerve growth factor	nt cDNA	p	m sal gl, r ir	Wilson et al. (1986)
Nerve growth factor	riboprobe	p	m br	Rennert and Heinrich (1986)
Calcium/calmodulin-dependent protein kinase	riboprobe	s	r br	Lin et al. (1987)
Na$^+$,K$^+$-ATPase A1, A2, A3	riboprobe	s	r br, emb	Schneider et al. (1988)
Ribosomal RNA	nt cDNA	h	r br	McCabe et al. (1986c)
Human neuror-specific protein	cDNA (tail)	s	dev r br	Kristensson et al. (1986)
Keratin	nt cDNA	s	m tongue	Rentrop et al. (1986)
Amyloid	rp cDNA	s	m br	Bencotti et al. (1988)
Renin	nt cDNA	s	r pit, adr	Deschepper et al. (1986)
Mouse brain-specific mRNAs	nt cDNA	p, s	m br	Branks and Wilson (1986)
Kallikrein	nt cDNA	p	r pit	Clements et al. (1986)
Kallikrein	oligo(30) kin	p	m sal, gland	van Leeuwen et al. (1987)
Opsin	oligo(48) tail	s	b retina	Brarn and Young (1986)
Transducin	oligo(48) tail	s	b retina	Brarn and Young (1986)

(continued)

243

TABLE I (continued)

Probe name	Probe type[b]	Label[c]	Species and tissue	Reference
Transthyretin (albumin)	nt cDNA	s	r br	Stauder et al. (1986)
Transferrin	nt cDNA	p	r br	Jirikowski et al. (1988)
LH, β-	rp cDNA	b (ap)	p pit	Liu et al. (1988)
Transferrin	nt cDNA	p, s	r br	Bloch et al. (1987)
Calbindin, D28	riboprobe	s	r br	Sequier et al. (1988a)
Synapsin	riboprobe	s	r cer	Haas and DeGennaro (1988)
Probes for Viruses				
Lymphocytic choriomeningitis virus (l, s)	nt cDNA	p	r emb	Southern et al. (1984)
Theillors virus	nt DNA	h	rab, m br	Stroop et al. (1982)
Theillors virus	nt cDNA	h	r sc	Brahic et al. (1984)
Herpes simplex virus II	nt cDNA	h	vc, gp tg	Tenser et al. (1982)
Herpes simplex virus I, II	nt cDNA	h	m br	Stroop et al. (1984); Stroop and Schaefer (1987)
Vesicular stomatitis virus	nt cDNA	h	m br	Fournier et al. (1988)
Measles virus	nt cDNA	h	m br	Haase et al. (1981)
Visna virus	nt DNA	h	m br	Stowring et al. (1985)

[a] Data are from many of the ISH papers published between 1977–1988 that presented data from neural or endocrine tissue. When designing ISH experiments, list probe name, probe type (the specific probe used in the study), label (the atom or molecule used to label the probe), tissue (the tissue examined in the study), and the reference. This table shows how ISH has been used to examine mRNAs in brain and to provide a ready reference for ISH methods for a specific class of mRNA.

[b] ex, Exon probe; int, intron probe; oligo, oligonucleotide; kinase, kin, oligo was kinased; kfl, klen ext, oligo was hybridized to a oligonucleotide region complementary to the original oligonucleotide and this oligo served to prime the polymerase activity of Klenow (large fragment of DNA polymerase); lig, two oligos were ligated together and used as a probe; nt, nick-translated probe; riboprobe, RNA probe; rp, random-primed probe; rt, reverse transcriptase used to make cDNA; tail, oligo was labeled with terminal transferase; ( ), nucleotide length of oligo.

[c] p, 32P; s, 35S; h, 3H; i, 125I; b, biotin; ap, alkaline phosphatase detection of b; bio–AB, antibody detection of biotin; per, peroxidase detection of biotin; avi–gold, avidin–gold complex used to detect biotin; dab–per, diaminobenzidine peroxidase reaction to detect biotin.

[d] b, Bovine; c, cat; gp, guinea pig; h, human; m, mouse; r, rat; rab, rabbit; adr, adrenal; astro cul, astrocyte culture; br, brain; car, c, carcinoid; cer, cerebellum; dev, developing; emb, embryo; fbr, fibroblast; GH3, GH3 cells; hy, hypothalamus; ir, iris; nas epi, nasal epithelium; pit, pituitary; pri cul, primary culture; pvn, paraventricularnucleus; sal gl, salivary gland; sc, spinal cord; scn, suprachiasmatic nucleus; str, striatum; (trans), transgenic animal; tg, trigeminal ganglion; vc, Vero cells.

markedly elevates enkephalin mRNA levels in the caudate putamen examined by Northern blot analysis and ISH (Harlan *et al.*, 1987; Mocchetti *et al.*, 1985; Young *et al.*, 1986a; Angulo *et al.*, 1986). The dependence of this effect on dopamine receptor antagonism, and not other receptor actions of haloperidol, is supported by selective lesions of the nigrostriatal dopamine pathway, which also elevate enkephalin mRNA. One area of great potential for ISH is in the study of the human brain (Higgins and Mah, this volume [11]), where ISH is likely to have a major impact on the understanding of the etiology and treatment of neurological impairments. One example is the identification of mRNA for preprotachykinin in the caudate nucleus and putamen using a ^{35}S-labeled RNA probe (Chesselet and Affolter, 1988). Procedures developed for the use of postmortem human tissues (Tourtellote *et al.*, 1987) will aid future efforts to help determine potential alterations in diseases such as Alzheimer's (Goedert, this volume [23]) and schizophrenia (Sherrington *et al.*, 1988).

In Situ Hybridization: Theoretical Considerations

ISH involves the same general molecular biological principles as those used in solution hybridization or Northern blot analysis. However, ISH presents some challenges due to the combination of molecular biology and histology. First, *in situ* analysis demands that hybridization be carried out in a heterogeneous, and consequently less favorable, environment composed of the protein, lipid, and nucleic acid components of the cell, all of which are either cross-linked or precipitated by a fixative. While Northern analysis allows hybridization to purified RNA, cells within a tissue section contain many other polar molecules which may interfere with or change conditions of hybridization. Second, cell membranes have been extracted from the preparation prior to Northern analysis or solution hybridization, while intact membranes present a diffusion barrier to the ISH probe. Third, a message in low abundance can be concentrated for Northern blot or solution hybridization analysis, but must be detected at the endogenous levels of single cells for ISH.

These challenges point out the four important elements in an ISH experiment: (1) characterization of the mRNA of interest, (2) selection of probe, (3) preparation of tissue, and (4) optimization of hybridization conditions. The investigator has some control over each of these except the characteristics of the mRNA in question (message abundance, nucleic acid content, and secondary structure). The remaining components must be adjusted to maximize localization and abundance of the mRNA signal.

Probe Selection

The three types of probes most generally used are RNA, cDNA, and oligonucleotide probes. The mRNA in question will dictate, to some extent, the choice of probe type. For example, visualization of a low-abundance message may require a probe labeled to a very high specific activity, and this is possible with a RNA or cDNA probe. On the other hand, if the mRNA is a member of a highly homologous family of RNAs with similar distributions, specificity of the probe may be a concern. Probes which hybridize to only the unique portions of the message are the most appropriate probe choice. In addition, new techniques for hybridization are becoming available (Table I).

Tissue Preparation

Tissue preparation will depend on the use of tissue sections or intact cells, the methods one chooses to fix the tissues, and the mRNA and probes to be used. That is, heavy fixation tends to lower the signal and raise background; this may be tolerated better by a high-abundance message. Also, if the probe itself is large and bulky, permeabilization becomes a more important consideration. Specific fixation, tissue digestion, and permeabilization treatments will be discussed below.

Hybridization Conditions

Hybridization buffers and stringency conditions must be customized to suit the mRNA, the tissue conditions, and the probe type. Other than method of fixation, the most important parameters which can be manipulated to produce a good ISH signal are those of the hybridization conditions. These must be varied in such a manner as to promote the interaction of the probe with the mRNA of interest (Wetmur and Davidson, 1968). When this interaction occurs in solution it can be characterized by a R_0t (RNA concentration × time) equation from which the time necessary to achieve any percentage of hybridization can be calculated:

$$t_{1/2} = N \ln 2/3.5 \times 10^5 L^{0.5} C \tag{1}$$

In Eq. (1) $t_{1/2}$ is the time required to hybridize one-half of the probe, N is the complexity of the RNA being hybridized (total number of unique base pairs), L is the base-pair length of the probe, and C is the molar probe concentration. Other factors such as the pH and ionic strength of the hybridization buffer are important factors in using this equation and are discussed in detail by Meinkoth and Wahl (1984). These equations hold well when both the probe and the mRNA being detected are chemically pure and freely diffusible, as in a solution hybridization assay (Britten *et al.,* 1974; Casey and Davidson, 1977). The equations do not strictly hold when they are applied to a mRNA bound to a solid support in a semipermeable matrix (as is the case of mRNA in a fixed tissue section). However, the R_0t equation can be used to determine approximate hybridization times or the minimum probe concentration necessary to saturate the mRNA. *In situ* experiments are most informative when performed in probe excess so that all of the mRNA within a section can be hybridized.

It is important to consider other factors which affect the stability of hybrids and which may be manipulated to suit each unique situation. Hybrids are held together by noncovalent forces, such as hydrogen bonding and base stacking. These forces are sensitive to temperature changes and to other interventions such as changes in formamide or ionic strength. The following equation (from Thomas and Dancis, 1973) defines the relationship between these variables and the melting temperature (T_m; °C) which predicts dissociation of one-half of all hybrids at equilibrium:

$$T_m = 81.5°C + 16.61(\log M) + 0.41(\%GC) \\ - 820/L - 0.6(\%F) - 1.4(\% \text{ mismatch}) \tag{2}$$

where M refers to the ionic strength of the hybridization solution in mol/liter, %GC refers to mol % of GC base pairs in the probe, L refers to probe length in base pairs, %F refers to % formamide, and % mismatch refers to the percentage of noncomplementary base pairs between hybridizing strands. Thus, three of these factors relate to the probe and mRNA characteristics, and three relate to the hybridization environment.

The probe and mRNA characteristics which affect stability are the %GC content, the probe length, and the percentage base-pair mismatch. A higher GC content will mean greater stability since GC base pairs are stabilized by three hydrogen bonds, and AT/AU base pairs by only two bonds. Likewise, the longer the probe, the greater the number of hydrogen bonds which can form and the greater the maximal hybrid stability. This relationship suggests that very short oligonucleotide probes may be problematic. In fact, probes below about 20 base pairs, depending on GC content, are relatively unstable. Furthermore, probe and mRNA base-pair mismatches will disrupt hybrid stability.

The environmental factors which govern hybridization, also referred to as stringency factors, include temperature, formamide concentration, and salt concentration. Higher temperature and higher formamide concentration will disrupt hydrogen bonding, and thus destabilize hybrids. Conversely, a higher salt concentration will strengthen hydrogen bonds and encourage hybrid formation. For a more detailed consideration of factors governing hybridization, the reader is referred to additional discussions (Lewis and Cowan, 1985; Tecott *et al.*, 1987).

The information contained in the R_0t and the T_m equations provides a starting point for optimizing hybridization conditions. It has been empirically determined that hybridization proceeds best at 25°C below the T_m. However, it is best to consider this information and then experimentally determine the hybridization conditions that produce optimal signal-to-noise ratios in each system. One should also keep in mind that stringency can be adjusted at several points in the hybridization procedure, including posthybridization washes. Last, since the main goal of ISH is localization of mRNA to the cellular level, one must be careful to select hybridization parameters that maintain the integrity of cellular morphology.

Controls for Hybridization Specificity

The multiplicity of mRNA species within a cell and the availability of other cell constituents for nonspecific retention of the labeled probe necessitate the use of controls to prevent false-positives. The choice of appropriate controls for ISH experiments is somewhat controversial. We will discuss the general aims of controls and suggest several approaches. For a more extensive range of suggestions, the reader is directed to Tecott *et al.* (1987) and Watson *et al.* (1988).

The determination of hybridization specificity involves several issues. The first concern is whether the probe hybridizes to mRNA or binds to other cell constituents. Second, to what extent is the hybridization specific for the mRNA under consideration? The first question is most easily answered. Tissue can be pretreated with RNase. This should eliminate the mRNA hybridization signal and leave non-RNA binding relatively undisturbed. The second issue is more difficult to address with one particular control. Instead, one may depend on corroborating evidence from several control strategies. (1) The thermal stability, defined by the T_m equation, can be predicted for a particular probe–mRNA hybrid. Therefore, analysis of hybrid stability as a function of temperature ("melting curve determination") should yield an empirical value close to the predicted T_m if the hybrid is specific. (2) One may also use competition between labeled probe and excess cold probe. This control makes the assumption that specific hybridization is of limited capacity and nonspecific hybridization is relatively unlimited. This control indicates specific hybridization to the mRNA sequence from which the probe is derived. However, since the cold probe used for the displacement contains the identical nucleic acid sequence to the labeled probe, this control does not verify the identify of the mRNA to which the labeled probe is hybridized.

Other controls may be used to address the hybridization identity issue more appropriately. We believe that the best controls in this regard are (1) the use of multiple oligonucleotide probes which hybridize to different regions of the same mRNA. An anatomically overlapping hybridization signal indicates an mRNA-specific labeling. This control strategy is especially important when examining an mRNA that is thought to be derived from a gene family. (2) The combination of *in situ* transcription with gel electrophoresis (see *In Situ Transcription* section of this chapter), which identifies the mRNA molecules that served as a template for the *in situ* transcription reaction.

General Methods

Experimental Animal Treatments

Transcriptional, translational, and posttranslational modification of neuro-transmitters, enzymes, receptors, and receptor-associated proteins are all candidates for change as a result of experimental manipulation (see Diagram 1). Not all of these potential modifications will be elucidated by ISH, however. For example, haloperidol increases the levels of enkephalin peptide and preproenkephalin mRNA, while fenfluramine increases enkephalin peptide content without causing a change in steady-state mRNA levels (Mocchetti *et al.*, 1985). Also, the time between the detection of changes in levels of a specific mRNA and the actual change in its nuclear precursor (HnRNA) may vary depending on the experimental treatment (Eberwine *et al.*, 1987; Birnberg *et al.*, 1983). Experimentally induced changes in steady-state mRNA levels have been observed within several hours (Chen *et al.*, 1984) to several days (Barinaga *et al.*, 1985). The experimenter should be aware, therefore, that a change could be missed simply by looking at the wrong time after treatment. For example, POMC in the rat pituitary gland can respond differentially to acute and chronic stressors. In one study, transcriptional regulation followed chronic disturbances but not relatively acute perturbations (Shiomi *et al.*, 1986).

Tissue Fixation

Tissue fixation is necessary for retention of cellular RNA. The tissue may be fixed by perfusing the whole animal, or after sectioning in a cryostat (Tecott

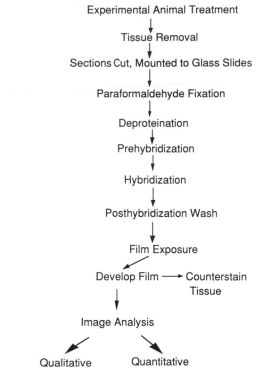

Experimental Animal Treatment

↓

Tissue Removal

↓

Sections Cut, Mounted to Glass Slides

↓

Paraformaldehyde Fixation

↓

Deproteination

↓

Prehybridization

↓

Hybridization

↓

Posthybridization Wash

↓

Film Exposure

↓

Develop Film ⟶ Counterstain
Tissue

↓

Image Analysis

Qualitative   Quantitative

DIAGRAM 1   Flow chart of *in situ* hybridization procedures.

et al., 1987; Watson *et al.,* 1988; Young, 1988; Schachter, 1987). Several fixatives are routinely used, including paraformaldehyde and formaldehyde. Tissue is generally fixed in 3% paraformaldehyde immediately following sectioning. This method produces a better ISH signal-to-noise ratio than does whole animal perfusion (Tecott, 1986). Sections are allowed to dry at room temperature on the slides for 5–20 min. Tissue is then fixed in 3% paraformaldehyde (pH 7.2) for 5 min followed by several 1-min washes in PBS. Tissue is dehydrated through graded ethanols (70, 95, 100%) and then air dried. Sections are stored at −80°C. Diethyl pyrocarbonate (DEPC) treatment (0.02%) of the solutions is employed to protect against RNA degradation. Perfusion fixation can be used for combined ISH/ immunocytochemistry when the whole animal is perfused with paraformaldehyde or glutaraldehyde which helps fix peptides within the tissue section. If combined ISH and immunocytochemistry is desired, then protocols for this combination of techniques should be consulted for their recommendations regarding fixation and sequential processing (Shivers *et al.,* 1986a; Griffin, 1987; Watts and Swanson, this volume [7]).

Collecting Tissue

It is common to remove the tissue from the animal and freeze it in isopentane (2-methylbutane, Mallinkrodt). The isopentane is kept in a hood and cooled to $-15°C$ with dry ice. Tissue extraction and blocking do not differ from any standard histological techniques. For ISH, immunocytochemistry, or both, the time between tissue extraction, blocking, and freezing should be minimized. Furthermore, tissue should be frozen as quickly as possible in isopentane, liquid nitrogen, cryoquick, or on dry ice. Tissue should be stored at $-70°C$ prior to sectioning in a cryostat, and should not be thawed before cutting. See Herkenham and Pert (1982) and Altar (1988) for other procedures in the cutting, storing, and processing of brain sections for autoradiography.

Section Thickness

Thin sections (4–12 μm) increase the number of sections derived from a given tissue. Thin sections also enhance the autoradiographic resolution of high-energy isotopes such as ^{32}P and ^{125}I by more closely limiting the sources of emitted particle to a plane. The increased surface area-to-volume ratio of thin sections also increases the likelihood of delivering the cDNA or cRNA probes to the mRNAs of interest, especially within the nucleus (Angerer *et al.,* 1987). The preparation of thin tissue sections that remain attached to glass slides is essential for the lengthy procedures of ISH. Advances in cryostat technology, a greater variety of coatings for adhering sections to glass, and the use of unfixed, fresh-frozen tissue make it easier to prepare thin sections with these advantages. Thin brain sections also produce relatively stronger hybridizations following fixation in 4% paraformaldehyde (Schachter, 1987).

Slide Subbing

Subbing is a procedure whereby glass microscope slides are coated with a material that (1) promotes section adherence and (2) decreases nonspecific probe binding. Several procedures are commonly used for this aspect of ISH. Clean glass slides are dipped for 10 sec in a solution of gelatin (300 Bloom; 5 g/liter; Sigma) and chromium potassium sulfate (0.5 g/liter; Sigma), poly(L-lysine periodate) (Sigma, 50 μg/ml in 10 mM Tris-HCl, pH 8.0), or their combination (Pintar, 1988), silane derivatives (1% TESPA in dimethylformamide (Dawes and Neve, cited in Pintar, 1988), or Denhardt's (1966) solution [0.02% Ficoll, poly(vinylpyrrolidone), and BSA; Griffin, 1987]. There are no published reports that directly compare these methods.

Cutting Sections

Sections are cut at 10–15°C at a thickness of 4–12 μm. Each section is thaw-mounted onto a subbed slide. It is important to keep the slide only slightly warmer than the section (e.g., by 5–10°C) that is transferred from the cryostat blade to the subbed slide. This slight temperature difference creates a thermal gradient that helps move the section to the slide but also minimizes the condensation of water onto the slide. Condensed water that freezes between the section and coating on the slide will tend to dislodge the section during incubations. The slides are placed in a slide box which is wrapped in aluminum foil, sealed in an air-tight plastic bag, and stored at −70°C.

Brain matrix autoradiography (Altar, 1988) employs sequential mounting and cutting of up to five brain hemispheres or other tissues on a single cryostat chuck. This procedure is especially helpful in conserving the use of labeled probe, increasing the uniformity of conditions employed between tissues, and in decreasing the effort and materials required for the generally detailed *in situ* procedures.

Hybridization Methods

The procedures involved in ISH are illustrated in Fig. 1. Figure 1 and the following steps are primarily for the use of [35]S- or ^{32}P-labeled oligonucleotide probes. For protocols better suited to cRNA or cDNA probes see Angerer *et al.* (1987) and Watson *et al.* (1987).

Tissue Permeabilization

In some cases, particularly when tissue has been heavily fixed, the RNA may remain unavailable to the probe. Tissue deproteination prior to hybridization may increase probe access. Two methods are widely used: proteinase K deproteination (Brahic and Haase, 1983; Cox *et al.,* 1983) and HCl deproteination (John *et al.,* 1977; Brahic and Haase, 1983). Proteinase K is a much harsher treatment than HCl, but may be necessary with heavier fixation or with a rarer mRNA. Allow frozen tissue sections to come to room temperature for at least 15 min prior to either treatment.

HCl Deproteination

Sections are dipped in 0.2 *N* HCl for 20 min at room temperature and then washed in 2× SSC for 10 min (Watson *et al.,* 1988). Sections may be dehydrated through graded ethanols and air dried for later processing or may be immediately used in the prehybridization step. If ethanols were not used in the fixation procedure, they may be used here as a mild delipidation step.

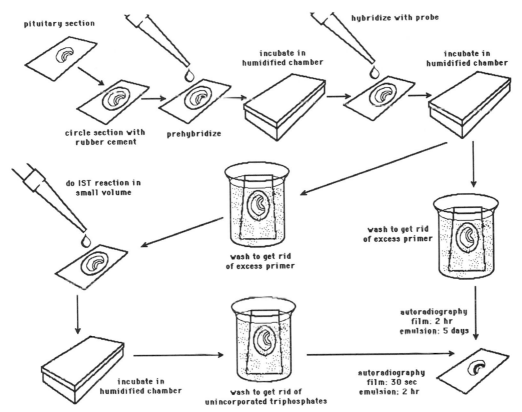

FIG. 1   The steps involved in performing an ISH or an IST reaction are depicted for a rat pituitary section. A positive hybridization signal with a POMC oligonucleotide is illustrated by the dark intermediate lobe.

Proteinase K Deproteination

A concentration of 1 μg of proteinase K per milliliter of 100 mM Tris-HCl, pH 8, 50 mM EDTA may be used. Depending on the size of the tissue section, cover the slides in 40–125 μl of the solution for 30 min at 37°C. Wash in water followed by 0.1 M triethanolamine (TEA) at pH 8, each for 1 min (at room temperature). Place sections in fresh 0.1 M TEA and add 0.25% (v/v) acetic anhydride (to stop proteinase K activity and decrease charged amino groups on proteins) with stirring (Watson *et al.*, 1988). Continue to stir for 10 min. Wash in 2× SSC for 5 min, and either dehydrate through ethanols or move to the prehybridization step.

Prehybridization

Prehybridization is optional, but we find that it enhances the signal-to-noise ratio with some probes. If cost of the prehybridization buffer is not a limiting factor, sections can be preincubated in buffer contained in a staining dish or Coplin-type slide jar. Otherwise, sections are covered with the buffer and are placed in a humidified chamber. We incubate the tissue sections at room temperature for about 2 hr in a prehybridization buffer which includes 0.6 M NaCl, 10 mM Tris (pH 7.5), 0.02% Ficoll, 0.02% poly(vinylpyrrolidone), 0.02% bovine serum albumin, 1 mM EDTA, 0.005% tRNA, 0.05% salmon sperm or herring sperm DNA, 0.05% NaPP$_i$, 5 μM each of dATP, dCTP, dGTP, and dTTP, 50% formamide, and water (adapted from Shivers *et al.*, 1986a; Shivers *et al.*, 1988). 2-Mercaptoethanol (40 mM) must be added when using ^{35}S probes. We apply droplets of 50 μl/pituitary, 85 μl/cross section, and 120 μl/sagittal section of brain.

Hybridization

Tissue sections are briefly dipped in 2× SSC and dried. At this point, the probe is dissolved in the buffer and applied to the tissue. The duration of hybridization should be 2–3 times the $t_{1/2}$ or usually 12–36 hr, which is calculated according to Eq. (1). The optimal hybridization temperature needs to be determined empirically, but a good starting temperature is 37°C. The buffer includes all ingredients mentioned above plus 10% dextran sulfate and labeled probe in a final concentration of 10,000 to 1,000,000 counts per microliter. The dextran sulfate greatly decreases the time necessary for complete hybridization. Increasing the number of counts beyond 1,000,000 per microliter may generate an unacceptably low signal-to-noise ratio.

Posthybridization Washes

The buffer–probe solution is poured off the sections prior to immersion in the wash buffers. The ionic concentration and temperature of the washes will be determined by the stringency desired for each situation. However, we find the following wash sequences to be a good protocol with which to begin. When the need to increase stringency arises, there are several options. We suggest that raising the temperature be avoided, and that the first modifications be an increase in either the wash duration or the percentage of formamide in the hybridization, solution ionic concentration of the washes, or hybridization duration. Cellular morphology is better preserved by maintaining temperatures below 50°C and by keeping formamide concentrations below 60%.

The sections are washed for 20 min in 2× SSC and 0.1% sodium pyrophosphate at room temperature. The solution is changed after 10 min. Next, the sections are washed in 0.5× SSC overnight at about 40°C. The solution is changed at some time in this period. 2-Mercaptoethanol (14 m*M*) is added to each of these washes for ³⁵S probes. The sections are then dehydrated through a series of ethanols (70, 95, 100%) or thoroughly by a stream of room temperature air. Ethanols may be diluted from 300 m*M* ammonium acetate instead of water to reduce hybrid loss. Sections may then be apposed to film (Kodak XAR; ³H-Hyperfilm) or may be dipped in emulsion (Kodak NTB-2 diluted 1 : 1 with water). Vasopressin mRNA in the hypothalamus has been visualized in the same section by both methods for comparison (see Fig. 2; see also Sherman *et al.*, 1984).

In Situ Transcription

A new technique termed *in situ* transcription (IST) has recently been described (Tecott *et al.*, 1988a; Tecott and Eberwine, 1988; Zangger *et al.*,

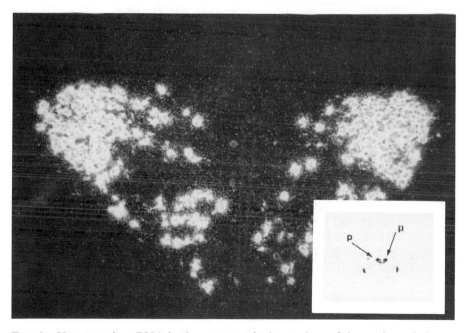

FIG. 2   Vasopressin mRNA in the paraventricular nucleus of the rat hypothalamus (p) was detected by an oligonucleotide probe labeled with ³⁵S-dCTP. The same section was first exposed to X-ray film (inset) and then dipped in photographic emulsion (Kodak NTB-2). The larger photograph is a dark-field photomicrograph taken after a 2-month exposure.

1989). IST offers some advantages over the standard ISH technique (see Fig. 1). IST requires the hybridization of a primer to the tissue section (*in situ*), followed by extension of this primer into cDNA with the enzyme reverse transcriptase (transcription) (Baltimore and Smoler, 1971; Houts *et al.,* 1979; Temin and Baltimore, 1971). This reaction takes place directly on the section. Unlike ISH, IST allows a specific cDNA to be synthesized, *in situ,* labeled to a very high specific activity, isolated from the section, and analyzed using gel electrophoresis.

An IST reaction consists of the following steps: (1) hybridize the primer to the endogenous mRNA, (2) wash the nonhybridized primer off of the section, (3) perform the IST reaction, (4) wash the sections to stop the reverse transcription reaction and to remove the unincorporated labeled triphosphates from the section, and (5) perform either film autoradiography or emulsion autoradiography.

1. The primer is hybridized as described for ISH, except that the hybridization buffer is minimal in composition (50% formamide, 6× SSC, 1× Denhardt's). For a 36-base-long POMC oligonucleotide (Drouin *et al.,* 1985), 2.5 ng/μl of the oligonucleotide primer is added to the hybridization buffer. This concentration is approximately 250,000 times that of POMC mRNA in an 11-μm-thick section of the rat pituitary. The hybridization proceeds for 1.5 days to generate adequate hybridization of the POMC primer.

2. The sections are washed in 2× SSC for 4 hr followed by a wash in 0.5× SSC for 1 hr at 40°C. This is followed by a wash with transcription buffer. These washing steps remove nonhybridized oligonucleotide (which may contribute to background signals) as well as hybridization buffer so that cDNA synthesis can occur in a buffer of appropriate composition.

3. The reverse transcriptase reaction consists of transcription buffer [50 mM Tris-HCl (pH 8.3), 6 mM MgCl$_2$, 120 mM KCl, 7 mM dithiothreitol] plus 250 μM each of dATP, dGTP, and TTP, 50 nM [^{32}P]dCTP, 0.12 unit of RNasin/μl, and 1.0 unit of reverse transcriptase/μl. The sections are incubated at 37°C for 60 min in a humidified chamber. The volume for this reaction is determined by the amount of solution required to cover the sections. Typically, we use a volume of 20 μl per 3 mm^2 for sections. This volume can be reduced considerably if the sections are protected from evaporation by placing coverslips over the sections during the reaction. The quality of the reverse transcriptase enzyme is important in obtaining strong IST signals. We recommend using reverse transcriptase produced by Seikakagu, Inc. (St. Petersburg, FL). The reverse transcriptase extends the oligonucleotide which remains hybridized to the mRNA (Tecott *et al.,* 1988a).

4. IST sections require extensive washing to remove unincorporated

nucleotide triphosphates from the sections. Otherwise, the signal produced by unincorporated nucleotides will obscure the specific signal generated by the synthesized cDNA. Sections are washed in $2\times$ SSC for 30 min at room temperature followed by washing in $0.5\times$ SSC, 3 mM NaPP$_i$ for 8 hr at 42°C. This is sufficiently stringent to remove most of the unincorporated triphosphates, yet will not destabilize the cDNA–mRNA hybrids. Higher temperatures may further reduce the background and hence improve the signal-to-noise ratio. However, such treatment may also decrease the integrity of cellular morphology.

5. IST sections are visualized by autoradiography using either film autoradiography or liquid emulsion. Autoradiographic techniques are described later in this chapter. Exposure times for IST sections must be empirically determined for each system because of the dramatic increase in signal intensity produced by this technique. The signals generated by POMC and poly(T)oligonucleotides in the rat pituitary are presented in Fig. 3 as an example of IST film autoradiography.

The IST-derived cDNA transcripts can be removed from the sections and analyzed by gel electrophoresis (Tecott *et al.*, 1988a) to determine the specificity of the cDNA signal produced (see Fig. 4). This is possible because a banding pattern is generated that is specific to the mRNA transcribed into cDNA by the IST procedure. A discussion of this phenomenon and its implications for verification of ISH signals will be presented by Tecott *et al.* (1989).

The background labeling in tissue sections is a drawback to the use of IST for cellular localization studies (Eberwine *et al.*, 1988). Endogenous double-stranded nucleic acid complexes contribute to the background. These serve as primer–template complexes for the activity of reverse transcriptase. If the mRNA that is being detected with the IST technique is of low abundance, then its cellular visualization may be obscured by the background signal. The advantage of IST over the Northern solution hybridization is its greater sensitivity and localization to specific cell types. Many approaches can be taken to reduce background. One technique has been to dissociate the endogenous double-stranded complexes by incorporating a denaturation step (heating of sections in $0.5\times$ SSC at 85°C for 5 min) into the IST procedure prior to hybridization of the specific primer to the tissue. Future improvements in reducing the endogenous background will undoubtedly make the IST technique more widely useful in the study of low-abundance mRNAs.

A future application of IST may be the quantitation of mRNA levels within a tissue. The approach involves the hybridization of two oligonucleotides, separated from one another by 50–100 bases, to the mRNA of interest. The oligonucleotide positioned at the 5′ end of the mRNA molecule can be

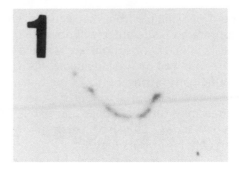

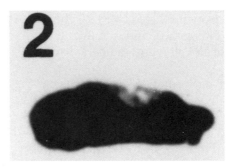

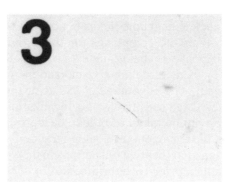

FIG. 3   These X-ray film autoradiograms show the ^{35}S IST signal produced in the rat pituitary using (1) POMC oligonucleotide primer, (2) poly(T)primer, and (3) tyrosine hydroxylase (TH) oligonucleotide primer. Since TH is not present in the rat pituitary, 3 shows the experimental background in this section. Background signals will vary depending on the tissue being examined. [Data were first presented in Tecott *et al.* (1988b).]

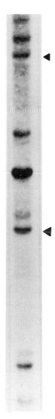

FIG. 4   ^{32}P-Labeled POMC-primed IST transcripts were removed from a rat pituitary section and electrophoresed on a 5% polyacrylamide-urea denaturing gel. This banding pattern (arrowheads) is specific for rat POMC. See Tecott *et al.* (1988a) for appropriate controls and specificity of hybridization.

blocked with a dideoxynucleotide, so that it cannot be extended with reverse transcriptase into cDNA. Specific cDNA synthesis initiated at the 3'-oligonucleotide will be terminated by the 5'-oligonucleotide (Tecott *et al.*, 1989) and labeled cDNA will be derived from that region of the mRNA between the two primers. In this reaction, the distance between the two primers, the time of the reaction, the specific activity of the labeled deoxynucleotide triphosphate, the sequence, and the cold : hot nucleotide ratio are known. Thus, the percentage of the synthesized cDNA that is labeled can be calculated. A rate equation should be derived which will permit the determination of the amount of cDNA that was synthesized. This quantitation technique requires the removal of the transcripts from the section. The free transcripts can either be counted in a scintillation counter or run on a sequencing gel. However, once a standard curve is generated (see the section *Quantitation with Sense Standards* below), quantitation can also proceed in hybridized sections via image analysis of the film autoradiograms or by grain counting of emulsion-dipped sections. The caveat of this approach is that it depends on the efficiency of hybridization of two oligonucleotides to the mRNA and the length of the IST-derived cDNA transcripts. Thus, this technique will provide a lower limit on the amount of mRNA within a tissue section.

Production of Labeled Probes

The level of required resolution in each particular study is one of the most important considerations in the selection of the type of radionucleotide. Film autoradiography may be sufficient if one needs to localize the probe only to a tissue, and not to a single cell. Either a ^{125}I-, ^{32}P-, or ^{35}S-labeled probe followed by film autoradiography is appropriate for this level of resolution (Coghlan *et al.*, 1987). If cellular resolution is required, then ^{35}S- or ^{3}H-labeled probes should be used followed by emulsion dipping of the hybridized sections. There also are techniques that allow both tissue and cellular localization that do not rely on radioactivity, but rather the detection of modified probes, e.g., biotinylated DNA probes, using enzymatic antibody techniques (McGadey, 1970; Singer *et al.*, 1987; Unger *et al.*, 1986) (see Table I). The most commonly used labeling procedures are detailed in the next few sections. Tritium is a more weakly penetrating β emitter and therefore yields a finer spatial resolution than a primary γ emitter such as ^{32}P.

Nick Translation

Nick translation (NT) was the first method developed for incorporating radiolabeled nucleotides into DNA (Rigby *et al.*, 1977) (see Fig. 5). *Escherichia coli* DNA polymerase (Pol I) will add deoxynucleotide triphosphates (dNTPs) to the 3'-hydroxyl terminus that is created when one strand of a DNA molecule is nicked (the phosphodiester bond between two nucleotides is broken). The labeling procedure (Meinkoth and Wahl, 1987) is as follows: the cDNA of interest (0.1–1.0 μg in 19 μl of NT buffer) is nicked with DNase I (1 μl of a 40 pg/μl stock diluted in 50 mM Tris, pH 7.4, 10 mM MgCl$_2$, 1 mg/ml DNase-free BSA). NT buffer is 5 mM Tris, pH 7.4, and 20 μM each of unlabeled dNTP omitting the labeled nucleotides and 50–300 μCi of deoxynucleotide 5'-[α-^{32}P]triphosphate, usually, dCTP (3000 Ci/mmol, 10 μCi/μl). Other isotopes, such as ^{35}S or ^{3}H can also be used. This reaction is incubated at room temperature for 2 min, and a 0.5-μl

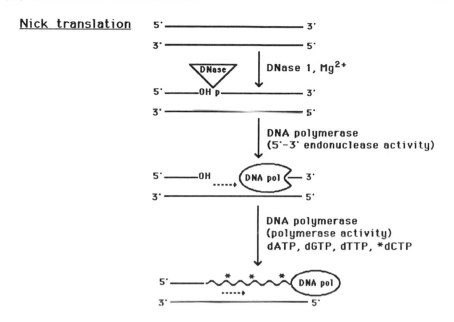

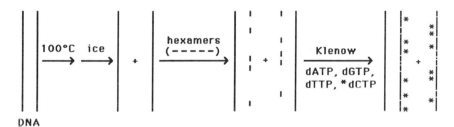

FIG. 5   Schematic of the nick translation and random priming procedures for labeling of ISH probes with radioactive DCTP. See the text for further details.

aliquot is removed for trichloroacetic acetic acid incorporation. Pol I is added (1 μl of 0.8 U/μl) and incubated at 15°C for 30–150 min. The reaction is terminated by the addition of 2 μl of 2% SDS, 250 m*M* EDTA. Unincorporated nucleotides can be removed by ethanol precipitation with 2 vol of 95% ethanol, 0.5 *M* NaCl, and 20 μg of glycogen as carrier. Two precipitations should be done for ISH, as each gets rid of about 90% of the free dNTPs. The incorporation of [^{32}P]dNTPs before and after the reaction is determined by TCA precipitation, by spotting a 0.5-μl aliquot of the reaction on Whatman GF/B filter paper (2.4 mm circle), drying the filter at room temperature, and then placing it for 5 min in 25 ml of 5% TCA. This is repeated twice and the filter is air dried and counted by adding liquid scintillation fluid and counting in the appropriate channel. The specific incorporation can be calculated by subtracting the counts on the filter prior to the addition of polymerase from those obtained after the polymerase reaction.

The optimal NT fragments are 50–500 nucleotides long. In order to achieve this length, it is necessary to titrate the DNase I reaction, by setting up several tubes with DNase I from 1–10 pg/μl final concentration and sizing an aliquot of each completed reaction. This is done by removing 2×10^5 cpm of probe from each reaction, The sample is heated to 100°C for 5 min and quickly cooled on ice to denature the probe. To the probe is added 0.2 vol of 50% glycerol and 0.5% bromphenol blue. The sample is loaded onto a 2% agarose gel with the appropriate denatured markers. The gel is run at 50 V until the bromphenol blue has migrated two-thirds of the way down the gel and is then stained with 0.1% ethidium bromide, photographed, and exposed to film. A "good" probe migrates as a smear from 50–500 bp. For hybridization to a section, the probe is heated to 100°C for 5 min to denature the strands and is cooled on ice to prevent reannealing of the complementary strands.

This NT technique is limited by several factors. (1) DNase I may be inhibited by "contaminants" in the DNA such as agarose. To prevent this, DNA which has been CsCl purified (Maniatis *et al.*, 1982) is recommended. (2) The NT reaction has to be monitored (as described above) since the reaction product is unstable due to the 5′–3′ exonuclease activity in Pol I. (3) The maximum labeling using a single nucleotide that can be achieved with NT is 10^8 cpm/μg of DNA, whereas 10 times greater specific activity can be achieved with RNA probes and randomly primed DNA probes.

An advantage of NT probes and random-primed probes is the possibility of probe: probe mRNA hybridization, i.e., if there are sequences on these relatively long probes that are not hybridized to mRNA they can hybridize to a complimentary sequence on another probe molecule. This is also a potential disadvantage if these probes reanneal in solution and thereby reduce the amount of single-stranded probe that hybridizes to the mRNA within the section. The smaller DNA fragments may also hybridize less specifically to tissue mRNA.

Random Priming

The random-priming reaction (Fig. 5) allows the radiolabeling of double-stranded or single-stranded DNA to high specific activity (up to 10^9 cpm/μg). This method was developed by Feinberg and Vogelstein (1983). Random oligonucleotides are used as primers, so that priming can start at several sites on the DNA. The large fragment of Pol I [Klenow (Bethesda Research

Laboratories, Gaithersburg, MD)] is used for extending the initial priming sites. Double-stranded DNA is heated to 100°C for 5 min to denature the strands, then placed on ice. Usually 100 ng–1 μg of DNA is used in the reaction. To the DNA is added 11.5 μl of LS (labeling solution) buffer (see below) along with 1 μl of 5 mg/ml BSA, 30 μCi of [α-^{32}P]dCTP (10 μCi/μl, 400 Ci/mmol), and 2.5 U of Klenow. A 0.5-μl aliquot of the reaction is removed before adding the Klenow reagent for the counting of unincorporated label. The reaction is incubated for 45 min at 30°C, extracted with an equal volume of phenol–chloroform, and precipitated by ethanol (95%). The incorporated label should be determined by TCA precipitation prior to using the probe for ISH. The LS buffer is made as follows: (1) make DTM = 100 μM each of dATP, dGTP, TTP, in 250 mM Tris, 25 mM MgCl$_2$, 50 mM 2-mercaptoethanol, pH 8; (2) make OL = 1 mM Tris, 1 mM EDTA, pH 7.5, to which 90 optical density units per milliliter of oligodeoxynucleotides have been added using Pharmacia hexamers; (3) mix 250 μl DTM, 250 μl HEPES, pH 6, and 70 μl OL = LS; (4) store in 11.5-μl aliquots at −20°C.

The random primed product is stable, since the Klenow fragment of Pol I lacks the 5′–3′ exonuclease activity which can degrade the labeled product, so the reaction can also be allowed to proceed overnight to achieve a larger amount of radiolabeled DNA. Prior to using a random primed probe, it is heated to 100°C for 5 min to denature the strands. It is not necessary to use DNA which has been purified over a CsCl gradient for this procedure. DNA isolated by a standard minipreparation procedure is adequate. Any radioisotope or biotin-labeled deoxynucleotide could be used in this reaction. Furthermore, any size DNA can be random primed. However, for ISH, smaller probes (50–500 bases) are thought to diffuse into sections better than longer probes.

RNA Probes

RNA probes (Angerer and Angerer, 1981) are made by *in vitro* transcription of template DNA by an RNA polymerase which initiates RNA synthesis at specific binding sites called promoters (see Fig. 6). There are several commercially available plasmid vectors with the SP6, T3, or T7 promoters separated by a multiple cloning site (e.g., Promega's pGEM-3 plasmid) into which the DNA of interest is cloned. The protocol to be described is by Angerer *et al.* (1987). The plasmid template (0.2–0.5 mg/ml) is linearized by a restriction endonuclease that cuts once downstream of the insert sequence, but not elsewhere between the insert and promoter. The buffer is removed by dialysis of the DNA at room temperature for 30 min against 5 mM Tris, pH 8.0, by placing 25–100 μl of the sample on the shiny hydrophobic side of a VMWP small-pore nitrocellulose filter (Millipore) on top of the dialyzate. The reaction is set up as follows: (1) dry the radioac-

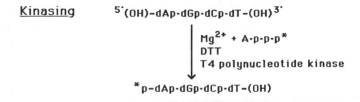

Kinasing

$5'(OH)-dAp-dGp-dCp-dT-(OH)^{3'}$

Mg^{2+} + A-p-p-p*
DTT
T4 polynucleotide kinase

$^*p-dAp-dGp-dCp-dT-(OH)$

Tailing

$5'(OH)-dAp-dGp-dCp-dT-(OH)^{3'}$

Co^{2+}(or Mn^{2+}) + n(α^*P)dCTP
terminal deoxynucleotide transferase

$5'(OH)-dAp-dGp-dCp-dT-dCp^*-dCp^*-dCp_n^* + nPP_i$

RNA probes

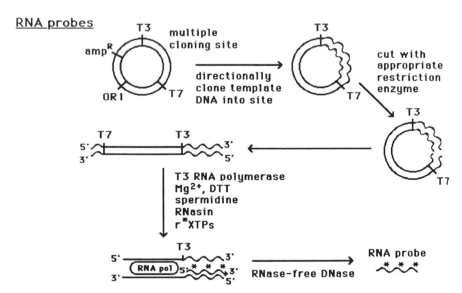

FIG. 6 Schematic of the kinasing, 3'-tailing, and RNA probe labeling of ISH oligonucleotide probes. See the text for further details.

tively labeled ribonucleotides in a microcentrifuge tube under vacuum (for a 10–100 μM final concentration); (2) add 20 μl of a solution containing 40 mM Tris, pH 7.5, 6 mM MgCl$_2$, 10 mM DTT, 100 μM unlabeled NTPs, 2 mM spermidine, and 100 U/ml placental RNase inhibitor (Promega Biotech); (3) add the template DNA (100 μg/ml) to the tube, mix quickly (to avoid precipitation of the DNA by the spermidine); (4) add 1200–1800 U/ml of the appropriate RNA polymerase. Incubate the reaction at 37 to 41°C for 60 min.

Measure incorporation of the nucleotides by TCA precipitation. The probe is purified by removing the DNA template with a 30-min digestion at 37°C with RNase-free DNase I (50 μg/ml in 50 mM Tris, pH 7.4, 10 mM MgCl$_2$). The probe is then extracted with an equal volume of phenol/ chloroform and ethanol precipitated with 0.2 M ammonium acetate and 2.5 vol of ethanol.

RNA probes have the advantage of using known "sense" and "anti-sense" strands for hybridization to the mRNA of interest and for the control of background hybridization. The "antisense" sequence is complementary to the RNA sequence and will hybridize to the mRNA. The "sense" sequence is the same as the mRNA. Either probe is single-stranded, so reannealing of the probe in solution is not a problem, and thus they can be labeled to high specific activity. One disadvantage is that RNA is very sensitive to degradation by RNase, so precautions must be taken to avoid degradation, such as autoclaving all the solutions and wearing gloves. Another problem is that RNA probes are "sticky," in that they adhere to more than just their complementary RNA. These nonspecific associations are lessened by treating sections with RNase following ISH. This reaction should be done in 0.5 M NaCl to prevent the RNase from digesting the RNA–RNA hybrids.

Oligonucleotide Probes

Kinasing Reaction

Oligonucleotides are single-stranded DNA molecules that are synthesized with a free 5'-hydroxyl. They can thus be labeled by transfer of [^{32}P]phosphate from γ-ATP with T4 polynucleotide kinase (Maniatis *et al.,* 1982) (see Fig. 6). The kinase reaction is set up as follows: to 100 ng of oligonucleotide in 1 μl are added 0.5 μl of 10× kinase buffer, 3 μl of [γ-^{32}P]ATP (10 μCi/μl, 5000 Ci/mmol), and 0.5 μl of T4 polynucleotide kinase (6 units; Boehringer-Mannheim). The 10× kinase buffer consists of 0.5 M Tris, pH 8, 100 mM MgCl$_2$, and 100 mM DTT. The reaction is terminated by ethanol precipitation with 2.5 vol ice-cold 95% ethanol, 0.5 M ammonium acetate, and 20 μg glycogen as carrier. The amount of ^{32}P incorporated can be determined by TCA precipitation as previously described.

Tailing Technique

Oligonucleotides can also be radiolabeled with terminal deoxynucleotide transferase (BRL) (Bollum, 1974) (see Fig. 6). This enzyme catalyzes the addition of deoxynucleotides ([^{3}H]-, [^{35}S]-, [^{32}P]dNTPs or biotinylated dUTP) to the 3' end of oligonucleotides (Lewis *et al.,* 1986a; Maniatis *et al.,*

1982), allowing labeled nucleotides to be added sequentially (tailed). A typical tailing reaction consists of 100 ng of oligonucleotide, 2 mM CoCl$_2$, 0.5 mM DTT, 30 μCi of [α-^{35}S]dCTP (400 Ci/mmol), and 20 U of terminal deoxynucleotide transferase (Tdt) in 100 mM potassium cacodylate, pH 7.2, incubated for 30 min at 37°C. The reaction is terminated by phenol–CHCl$_3$ extraction and ethanol precipitation. The amount of nucleotide added in the tail can be determined by running an aliquot of the reaction products (dissolved in 99% formamide, 0.3% xylene cyanol, 0.3% bromphenol blue) on a 20% polyacrylamide gel and exposing the gel to film.

The tailing reaction can use a single nucleotide as just described, forming a homopolymeric tail, or with a mixture of nucleotides, resulting in a heteropolymeric tail. A potential disadvantage of the homopolymeric tail is that it may hybridize to homopolymeric stretches of nucleotides in an mRNA population. An obvious example of this shortcoming would be tailing an oligonucleotide with T, generating a homopolymer-dT tail which will hybridize to all polyadenylated mRNAs within a tissue section. The best way to circumvent this problem is to limit the time of the tailing reaction (to be determined empirically) so that only four or five dC, dG, or dA bases are added to the oligonucleotide. Such a small homopolymeric tail should not interact with any homopolymeric regions of the mRNA in a manner that will survive the washing steps. This titration is an important aspect of optimization of this reaction. There are several features of this reaction that can be manipulated, such as temperature, time, enzyme amount, and nucleotide concentration. Additionally, Tdt is a metalloenzyme that requires a divalent cation in the reaction mix. This cation is usually either Co^{2+}, Mn^{2+}, or Mg^{2+}, with cobalt being the most active of the three metals. Usually, the supplier of the Tdt (BRL) will send a concentrated, cobalt-containing buffer with the enzyme for ease of use. The concentration of DTT will be relatively high in the reaction mix with the use of ^{35}S-labeled nucleotides.

The tailing technique has the advantage over the kinasing reaction because multiple labels are added and isotopes other than ^{32}P can be used. Both types of oligonucleotide probes are single stranded, so reannealing of the probe in solution is not a problem. Oligonucleotide probes are small (20–40 base pairs are typical), so tissue penetration is not a problem. It is important to confirm that the oligonucleotide recognizes the correct message by Northern blot or Southern blot analysis. In Fig. 7, we kinased a 36-nucleotide chain corresponding to rat enkephalin and probed a Northern blot of striatal mRNA prepared from rats treated with haloperidol and bromocriptine. The band seen at 1.5 kb is the expected size of rat enkephalin mRNA (Yoshikawa *et al.*, 1984). The increase in intensity following haloperidol treatment is also as reported (Mocchetti *et al.*, 1985). The oligonucleotide used for the Northern analysis was also used to generate the ISH emulsion exposure shown in Fig. 8.

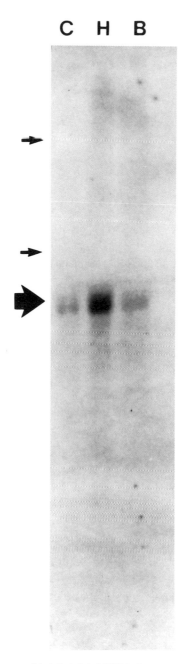

C H B

Fig. 7 Twenty micrograms of total striatal RNA from control (C), haloperidol (H), or bromocriptine(B)-treated rats was separated on a 1.25% formaldehyde–agarose gel, stained with ethidium bromide to visualize the 18 S and 28 S rRNA (small arrows), and transferred to nitrocellulose. The large arrow indicates the 1.5-kb message that was seen with the same 36-base-long oligonucleotide probe which was used in Fig. 8.

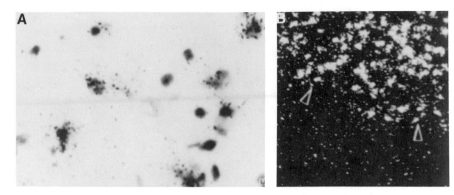

FIG. 8   The enkephalin oligonucleotide used to probe the Northern blot shown in Fig. 7 was used for ISH of enkephalin mRNA in the caudate putamen of the rat. The sections were dipped in NTB-2 emulsion and then developed using Kodak D-2 developer. The bright-field image is shown in A, while the dark-field image is shown in B. The arrowheads in the dark-field image show the border of the corpus callosum and the caudate. The perinuclear localization of the positive enkephalin ISH signal is clear from the bright-field image.

Autoradiography

The autoradiography of radiolabeled tissue sections has been optimized during the last two decades [see Rogers (1979) and Herkenham (1988) for reviews]. The quantitation of radioligand binding or [^{14}C]glucose uptake with autoradiographs is exposed with radiolabel-containing standards (Penny *et al.*, 1981; Unnerstall *et al.*, 1982; Alexander *et al.*, 1981) revealed several shortcomings of the receptor mapping technique. Subsequent improvements include the reduction or correction of regional differences in tissue quenching of radioemissions (Herkenham and Sokoloff, 1983; Geary and Wooten, 1985; Lidow *et al.*, 1988), increases in resolution (Herkenham and Pert, 1982; Herkenham, 1988), radioactivity standard calibration (Unnerstall *et al.*, 1982), and quantitative imaging of receptors using computer-assisted image analyzers [Altar *et al.*, 1984; see volumes by Boast *et al.* (1986) and Leslie and Altar (1988) for extensive reviews of these topics]. Many of these same challenges will confront the technique of ISH when quantitative analysis is achieved. At that time, the same autoradiography techniques that are the mainstay for visualizing ligand binding to tissue sections are likely to be used with ISH.

Dry Film

Direct exposure of the radiolabeled tissue can be achieved with dry, uncoated film such as Hyperfilm (Amersham) or XAR (Kodak). This procedure is simple and rapid (all sections are exposed to one piece of film). The slide-mounted sections are exposed to the film in an X-ray cassette (e.g., Spectroline or Wolf). The approximate duration of exposure can be calculated if one knows the number of disintegrations per minute (dpm) per brain section. This can be determined by swabbing a rinsed section with a GF/B filter disk and counting the radioactivity. Sections preincubated with an excess of unlabeled antisense probe can also be counted to approximate the specificity of hybridization. If measurable label is expected on about half the area of the section, then 15,000 dpm in a 15-μm-thick section will require about 48 hr to produce a well-exposed image with high contrast. The film is developed at 22°C with D-19 (4 min), indicator stop bath (30 sec), and rapid fixer (4 min) (all from Kodak). The film is washed in cool water for 5 min and will air dry within 15 min.

The dry film technique is used for macroscopic imaging in relatively low (≥ 50 μm) resolution conditions. If greater (cellular) resolution is required (e.g., 50–500× magnification), sections need to be exposed to hardened emulsion that has been coated onto an apposed coverslip or coated directly onto the section.

Emulsion Coatings

A liquid emulsion coating with Kodak NTB-2 is best for β emitters (^{3}H, ^{14}C, ^{35}S, or ^{32}P), whereas NTB-3 is recommended for γ emitters (^{125}I) (Eastman-Kodak, 1986, 1987). Under darkroom illumination, a dipping emulsion such as Kodak NTB-2 is diluted 50% with water at 40–42°C. The thickness of the resulting emulsion layer increases with lesser dilution, lower temperatures, a slower rate of slide withdrawal from the emulsion, and a horizontal position of the slide while the emulsion is drying (Eastman-Kodak, 1987). Typically, the slides are withdrawn from the emulsion bath over a couple of seconds and are dried vertically at room temperature for 2–3 hr. Exposure is achieved at 4–8°C in a sealed and light-tight slide box containing desiccant. The development of the exposed emulsion is acheived either immediately or 3 hr after removing the box from the refrigerator to prevent water condensation of room temperature air on a cold emulsion. D-19 (4 min), water (10 sec; not acid stop bath, which can bubble the emulsion layer), and Kodak fixer (5 min; not rapid fixer) are used to develop the silver grains. The slides are washed in water for 30 min and dried as described above for the dry film technique.

Counterstaining the Labeled Section

The dry film or coverslip emulsion techniques present no special problem for counterstaining, since the loss of label is inconsequential for the already developed hybridization image. However, with the dipping emulsion technique, the sections should be dehydrated in ascending (50, 70, 95, 100%) concentrations of ethanol containing 0.3 M ammonium acetate and dried in a vacuum desiccator before being coated with NTB2 emulsion (Shivers *et al.*, 1986c). Thereafter, the cells can be counterstained with hematoxylin and eosin.

Image Analysis

Microscopy of Emulsion-Based Images

The slides are coverslipped with 20% glycerol. The hybridization grains are easily viewed and photographed under bright-field or dark-field illumination The stained cells are best viewed under visible light.

Computer-Assisted Image Analysis

The distinct advantages of hybridizing nucleic acid probes to mRNA *in situ* include sensitivity and anatomical localization (e.g., identifying mRNA in a single cell body or nucleus and colocalizing the mRNA with other markers). The first advantage is best realized with ^{3}H-labeled probes, while the second is more fully derived with the use of radiolabels with highspecific activity (^{125}I, ^{32}P). The use of internal sense standards, to be discussed below, may also afford quantitation through the use of computer-assisted image analyzers. The use of these tools may allow an enhanced and highly resolved visualization of specific probes densities.

Choice of Labels

Radionucleotides, such as ^{32}P and ^{125}I, and biotin-labeled fluorescent probes (Singer and Ward, 1982; Brigati *et al.*, 1983) are two commonly used ways of visualizing hybridization to mRNA by RNA and DNA probes. Preferred features of radiolabels include high specific activity ($>$1000 Ci/mmol), lower isotope emission energy ($<$30 keV), and ease of attachment to nucleic acids [see Rogers (1979) or Herkenham (1988) for reviews].

Quantitation with Sense Standards

External Standards (Radioactivity Standards)

The quantitation of any bioassay is typically achieved in one of two ways. With the "external standard" method, the amount of signal produced by the detection system is determined over a wide concentration range of the material to be measured. The resulting "standard curve" is used to determine by interpolation the amount of unknown in the biological sample. However, accurate quantitation by the external standard technique necessitates that the signal generated by the unknown is produced with the same molar efficiency as by the external standards. This is rare, however, because of differences in the responses of the unknown in the biological sample and the authentic standard (e.g., differences in sample oxidation, conversion, recovery, extraction, etc.). Thus, a more common alternative is the use of an "internal standard." The internal standard is added to surplus biological samples. It is chemically similar to the unknown but can be resolved from it by chemical means (e.g., deuteration, radiolabeling) or merely by subtraction of the signal obtained by the biological sample alone. Thus, the signals produced by a range of internal standards added to biological material are used to calculate a standard curve that more closely approximates assay conditions.

The quantitation of optical densities by autoradiography has only been accomplished with the external standard technique. For example, the quantitation of receptor densities by autoradiography is typically achieved with tissue mash standards that have been mixed with various concentrations of the same isotope incorporated by the radioligand (Unnerstall *et al.*, 1982). Frozen cylinders of the mash are cut to the same thickness as the labeled tissue sections and are coexposed with them to autoradiography film or an emulsion coating. The tissue standards allow a calibration of film optical density as a function of isotope per milligram of tissue or tissue protein [Goochee *et al.*, 19880; see Boast *et al.* (1986) for a review]. This "external standard" scheme has also been applied to the quantitation of ISH studies (Young, 1986; Young *et al.*, 1986b). However, as already discussed, the amount of antisense probe which hybridize to its complimentary mRNA sequence depends on many procedural variables, including tissue fixation, probe penetration, prehybridization, hybridization, and complex washing procedures, and loss of mRNA during tissue processing. Each of these steps is likely to vary the amount of signal that is detected between experiments.

Internal Sense Standards

The between-experiment variation and the above variables in the hybridization process have suggested to us the utility of using internal standards which contain mRNA or cDNA sense strands that are recognized by the antisense probe. Unlike external standards used for receptor autoradiography, the signal produced by internal "sense standards" might be expected to vary depending on the many procedural variables that determine the efficiency of probe–mRNA hybridization. This would afford a quantitative measure of mRNA density in the tissue section that is more independent of these procedural variations.

We are presently testing this proposal. Sense standards have been produced by estimating the range of tissue densities for the mRNA to be measured. Unlabeled riboprobes or cDNA sense probes are synthesized from plasmids or by synthetic means, respectively. The probe of choice is added to the tissue mash in amounts sufficient to achieve a concentration of 0.1–40 times that expected in the average region of tissue. Four brains can be minced and homogenized with an inhibitor of endogenous RNase using a Teflon–glass mortar–pestle. Aliquots (0.5 g) of mash are then mixed with amounts of sense probe to acheive 0.1, 0.4, 1, 4, 10, and 40 times the approximate endogenous mRNA density. The six mash aliquots are forced into autoclaved cylindrical plastic molds centrifuged for 0.2 min at 50 *g* to remove air bubbles, and frozen on dry ice at −70°C. The wall of each mold containing the frozen mash is briefly warmed. The frozen cylindrical mash is pushed out and mounted on a cryostat chuck. Sections are cut to the same thickness as the tissue sections and thawed onto microscope slides coated exactly as those used with tissue sections. The slides are stored at −70°C. Thereafter, slides (one per piece of dry film to be used or three per experiment using liquid emulsion) are to be processed for ISH in parallel with the tissue samples.

Image Conversion

1. The use of sense standards might reveal the relationship between optical density and the concentration of hybridized probe. It should thus be possible to have an image processor convert the ISH images to quantitative images which reflect concentration as a linear function of image darkness. Image linearization enables a subtraction of nonspecific labeling from total labeling (Altar *et al.*, 1984, 1985) and should afford an illustration of specific hybridization at the macroscopic level.

2. A second way to determine hybridization specificity by image processing is the use of two nonhomologous probes for a single mRNA or DNA target (Pintar *et al.*, 1987; Watson *et al.*, 1987). For example, adjacent sections can be labeled with two probes, each of which hybridizes to separate regions of the same mRNA. Autoradiographic grains of the images can be color coded (e.g., one image converted to green and the other red), spatially superimposed, and the colors of overlapping pixels added. The confirmation of specificity is indicated by the prevalence of yellow-coded (red + green) versus red- or green-coded regions. The specificity of hybridization can be quantified by dividing the number of yellow pixels by the number of yellow + red + green pixels.

Emerging Techniques

The potentials of *in situ* hybridization and transcription are becoming increasingly clear. As described above, accurate quantitation of mRNA copies per cell or per tissue area may be possible with sense standards. Quantitation might allow the statistical between-group analysis of treatment effects on mRNA levels. The conversion of hybridization images to quantitative mRNA maps may allow mRNA hybridization levels to be visualized through an entire brain section. We anticipate that these quantitative advances will improve the value and afford objective scrutiny of *in situ* hybridizations, as they have for receptor autoradiography (Boast *et al.*, 1986; Leslie and Altar, 1988).

Major advances in sensitivity, the ability to quantitate mRNA, and in the ease of ISH are likely to appear as new labeling and detection methods are developed. Certainly, the ability to use fluorescently tagged probes for ISH (Baldino and Lewis, this volume [16]) promises to be one improvement over the use of radiolabeled probes.

One of the most important challenges facing the neurobiologist is discerning the link between the molecular biology of the cell and cellular physiology. With the advent of ISH it has been possible to localize mRNAs to single cells within the nervous system. This has permitted the defining of the chemical anatomy of the brain beyond that attainable with immunochemical and ligand autoradiographic studies. Knowing that a specific mRNA is present within a certain cell does not by itself demonstrate whether this mRNA is translated and processed into functional protein, nor does it directly show how this mRNA functions within that cell. To answer these questions, it will be important to complement ISH with other techniques such as immunocytochemistry and receptor autoradiography on the same or adjacent tissue sections. In the future, examinations of single-cell gene function from mRNA to protein may become a rudimentary analysis in the central nervous system. With this information, the neurobiologist can better answer questions concerning the link between molecular biology and the physiology of a single cell.

Acknowledgments

We gratefully acknowledge the enthusiasm and support of Jack Barchas. Larry Tecott and Karen Valentino collaborated with us in the production of Fig. 8. The work described in this chapter was supported in part by grants MH23861 and DA05010 and by a generous gift of the Watis Foundation to Jack Barchas.

References

G. M. Alexander, R. J. Schwartzman, R. D. Bell, J. Yu, and A. Renthal, *Brain Res.* **223,** 59 (1981).

C. A. Altar, *in* "Receptor Localization: Ligand Autoradiography" (F. M. Leslie and C. A. Altar, eds.), p. 191. Liss, New York, 1988.

C. A. Altar, R. J. Walter, K. A. Neve, and J. F. Marshall, *J. Neurosci. Methods* **10,** 173 (1984).

C. A. Altar, S. O'Neil, R. J. Walter, and J. F. Marshall, *Science* **228,** 597 (1985).

S. G. Amara, J. L. Arriza, S. E. Leff, L. W. Swanson, R. M. Evans, and M. G. Rosenfeld, *Science* **229,** 1094 (1985).

L. M. Angerer and R. C. Angerer, *Nucleic Acids Res.* **9,** 2819 (1981).

L. M. Angerer, M. H. Stoler, and R. C. Angerer, *in* "*In Situ* Hybridization: Applications to Neurobiology" (K. L. Valentino, J. H. Eberwine, and J. D. Barchas, eds.), p. 42. Oxford Univ. Press, London and New York, 1987.

J. A. Angulo, L. G. Davis, R. A. Burkhart, and G. R. Christoph, *Eur. J. Pharmacol.* **130,** 341 (1986).

J. A. Angulo, G. R. Christoph, R. W. Manning, B. A. Burkhart, and L. G. Davis, *Adv. Exp. Med. Biol.* **221,** 385 (1987).

R. Arentzen, F. Baldino, Jr., L. G. Davis, G. A. Higgins, Y. Lin, R. W. Manning, and B. Wolfson, *J. Cell. Biochem.* **27,** 415 (1985).

F. Baldino, Jr., M. O'Kane, S. Fitzpatrick-McElligott, and B. Wolfson, *Science* **241,** 978 (1988).

D. Baltimore and D. F. Smoler, *Proc. Natl. Acad. Sci. U.S.A.* **68,** 1507 (1971).

C. E. Bandtlow, R. Heumann, M. E. Schwab, and H. Thoenen, *EMBO J.* **6,** 89 (1987).

M. Barinaga, L. Bilezikjian, W. W. Vale, M. G. Rosenfeld, and R. M. Evans, *Nature (London)* **314,** 279 (1985).

F. Beck, N. J. Samani, J. D. Penschow, B. Thorley, G. W. Tregear, and J. P. Coghlan, *Development* **101,** 175 (1987).

C. Bendotti, G. L. Forloni, R. A. Morgan, B. F. O'Hara, M. L. Oster-Granite, R. H. Reeves, J. D. Gearhart, and J. T. Coyle, *Proc. Natl. Acad. Sci. U.S.A.* **85,** 3628 (1988).

A. Berod, N. F. Biguet, S. Dumas, B. Block, and J. Mallet, *Neurology* **84,** 1699 (1987a).

A. Berod, N. F. Biguet, S. Dumas, B. Bloch, and J. Mallet, *Proc. Natl. Acad. Sci. U.S.A.* **84,** 1699 (1987b).

N. C. Birnberg, J. C. Lissitzky, M. Hinman, and E. Herbert, *Proc. Natl. Acad. Sci. U.S.A.* **80,** 6982 (1983).

B. Bloch, R. J. Milner, A. Baird, U. Gubler, C. Reymond, P. Bohlen, D. Le Guellec, and F. E. Bloom, *Regul. Pept.* **8,** 345 (1984).

B. Bloch, D. Le Guellec, and Y. De Keyzer, *Neurosci. Lett.* **53,** 141 (1985a).

B. Bloch, T. Popovici, M. J. Levin, D. Tuil, and A. Kahn, *Proc. Natl. Acad. Sci. U.S.A.* **82,** 6706 (1985b).

B. Bloch, T. Popovici, S. Chouham, and C. Kowalski, *Neurosci. Lett.* **64,** 29 (1986).

B. Bloch, T. Popovici, S. Chouham, M. J. Levin, D. Tuil, and A. Kahn, *Brain Res. Bull.* **18,** 573 (1987).

C. Boast, E. Snowhill, and C. A. Altar, "Quantitative Receptor Autoradiography." Liss, New York, 1986.

F. J. Bollum, *in* "The Enzymes" (P. D. Boyer, ed.), Vol. 10. Academic Press, New York, 1974.

C. Bonnemann, P. Giraud, L. E. Eiden, and D. K. Meyer, *Neurochem. Int.* **10,** 521 (1987).

M. Brahic and A. T. Haase, *Proc. Natl. Acad. Sci. U.S.A.* **75,** 6125 (1978).

M. Brahic, A. T. Haase, and E. Cash, *Proc. Natl. Acad. Sci. U.S.A.* **81,** 5445 (1984).

P. L. Branks and M. C. Wilson, *Mol. Brain Res.* **1,** 1 (1986).

M. R. Brann and W. S. Young III, *FEBS Lett.* **200,** 275 (1986).

R. J. Britten, E. D. Graham, and B. R. Neufel, *in* "Methods in Enzymology" (L. Grossman and K. Moldave, eds.), Vol. 29, p. 363. Academic Press, New York, 1974.

G. C. Budd, B. Pansky, and B. Cordell, *J. Histochem. Cytochem.* **34,** 673 (1986).

J. P. H. Burbach, T. A. M. Voorhuis, H. H. M. van Tol, and R. Ivell, *Biochem. Biophys. Res. Commun.* **145,** 10 (1987).

J. P. Card, S. Fitzpatrick-McElligott, I. Gozes, and F. Baldino, Jr., *Cell Tissue Res.* **252,** 307 (1988).

J. Casey and N. Davidson, *Nucleic Acids. Res.* **4,** 1539 (1977).

J. L. Casey, M. W. Hentze, D. M. Koeller, S. W. Caughman, T. A. Rouault, R. D. Klausner, and J. B. Harford, *Science* **240,** 924 (1988).

C. L. Chen, F. T. Dionne, and J. L. Roberts, *Proc. Natl. Acad. Sci. U.S.A.* **80,** 2211 (1984).

M. F. Chesselet and H.-U. Affolter, *Brain Res.* **410,** 83 (1988).

M. F. Chesselet, L. Weiss, C. Wuenschell, A. J. Tobin, and H.-U. Affolter, *J. Comp. Neurol.* **262,** 125 (1987).

B. M. Chronwall, W. R. Millington, W. S. T. Griffin, J. R. Unnerstall, and T. L. O'Donohue, *Endocrinology (Baltimore)* **120,** 1201 (1987).

J. A. Clements, P. J. Fuller, M. McNally, I. Nikolaidis, and J. W. Funder, *Endocrinology (Baltimore)* **119,** 268 (1986).

J. P. Coghlan, J. D. Penschow, J. R. Fraser, P. Aldred, J. Maralambidis, and G. W. Tregear, *in* "*In Situ* Hybridization: Applications to Neurobiology" (K. L. Valentino, J. H. Eberwine, and J. D. Barchas, eds.). Oxford Univ. Press, London and New York, 1987.

K. H. Cox, D. V. DeLeon, L. M. Angerer, and R. C. Angerer, *Dev. Biol.* **100,** 197 (1983).

C. F. Deschepper, S. H. Mellon, F. Cumin, J. D. Baxter, and W. F. Ganong, *Proc. Natl. Acad. Sci. U.S.A.* **83,** 7552 (1986).

J. Drouin, M. Chamberland, J. Charron, L. Jeanotte, and M. Nemer, *FEBS Lett.* **193,** 54 (1985).

Eastman-Kodak Co., "Autoradiography of Macroscopic Specimens," Kodak Tech. Bull. M3-508. Eastman-Kodak, Rochester, New York, 1986.

Eastman-Kodak Co., "Kodak Products for Light Microscope Autoradiography," Kodak Tech. Bull. P-64. Eastman-Kodak, Rochester, New York, 1987.

J. H. Eberwine, J. A. Jonassen, M. J. Q. Evinger, and J. L. Roberts, *DNA* **6,** 483 (1987).

J. H. Eberwine, I. Zangger, and L. H. Tecott, *Soc. Neurosci. Abstr.* **14,** 69 (1988).

L. F. Eng, E. Stöcklin, Y.-L. Lee, R. A. Shiurba, F. Coria, M. Halks-Miller, C. Mozsgai, G. Fukayama, and M. Gibbs, *J. Neurosci. Res.* **16,** 239 (1986).

A. Ericsson, M. Schalling, K. R. McIntyre, J. M. Lundberg, D. Larhammar, K. Seroogy, T. Hokfelt, and H. Persson, *Proc. Natl. Acad. Sci. U.S.A.* **84,** 5585 (1987).

A. P. Feinberg and B. Vogelstein, *Anal. Biochem.* **132,** 6 (1983).

J. G. Fournier, O. Robain, I. Cerutti, I. Tardevel, F. Chany-Fournier, and C. Chany, *Acta Neuropathol.* **75,** 554 (1988).

P. J. Fuller, J. A. Clements, and J. W. Funder, *Endocrinology (Baltimore)* **116,** 2366 (1985).

C. R. Gallistel, C. T. Piner, T. O. Allen, T. Adler, R. Yadin, and M. Negin, *Neurosci. Biobehav. Rev.* **6,** 409 (1982).

S. J. Gaunt, *Development* **101,** 51 (1987).

W. A. Geary and G. F. Wooten, *Brain Res.* **336,** 334 (1985).

C. E. Gee, C.-L. C. Chen, and J. L. Roberts, *Nature (London)* **306,** 374 (1983).

I. Ginzburg, A. Teichman, W. S. T. Griffin, and U. Z. Littauer, *FEBS Lett.* **194,** 161 (1986).

C. Gooche, W. Rasband, and M. D. Sokoloff, *Ann. Neurol.* **7,** 359 (1980).

N. D. Goodman and D. Spiegelman, *Proc. Natl. Acad. Sci. U.S.A.* **68,** 2203 (1971).

F. Gossard, F. Dihl, G. Pelletier, P. M. Dubois, and G. Morel, *Neurosci. Lett.* **79,** 251 (1987).

S. T. Griffin, *in* "*In Situ* Hybridization: Applications to Neurobiology" (K. L. Valentino, J. H. Eberwine, and J. D. Barchas, eds.), p. 97. Oxford Univ. Press, London and New York, 1987.

A.-F. Guitteny, B. Fouque, C. Mougin, R. Teoule, and B. Bloch, *J. Histochem. Cytochem.* **36,** 563 (1988).

C. A. Haas and L. J. DeGennaro, *J. Cell Biol.* **106,** 195 (1988).

A. T. Haase, P. Ventura, C. J. Gibbs, and W. W. Tourtellotte, *Science* **212,** 672 (1981).

V. K. M. Han, M. A. Hynes, C. Jin, A. C. Towle, J. M. Lauder, and P. K. Lund, *J. Neurosci. Res.* **16,** 97 (1986).

V. K. M. Han, J. Snouweart, A. C. Towle, P. K. Lund, and J. M. Lauder, *J. Neurosci. Res.* **17,** 11 (1987).

R. E. Harlan, B. D. Shivers, G. J. Romano, R. D. Howells, and D. W. Pfaff, *J. Comp. Neurol.* **258,** 159 (1987).

M. Herkenham, *in* "Receptor Localization: Ligand Autoradiography" (F. M. Leslie and C. A. Altar, eds.), p. 37. Liss, New York, 1988.

M. Herkenham and C. B. Pert, *J. Neurosci.* **2,** 1129 (1982).

M. Herkenham and L. Sokoloff, *Soc. Neurosci. Abstr.* **9,** 329 (1983).

H. Hoefler, H. Childers, M. R. Montminy, R. M. Lechan, R. H. Goodman, and H. J. Wolfe, *Histochem. J.* **18,** 597 (1986).

H. Hogami, F. Yoshmura, A. J. Carrillo, Z. D. Sharp, and P. J. Sheridan, *Endocrinol. Jpn.* **32,** 625 (1985).

P. W. H. Holland, S. J. Harper, J. H. McVey, and B. L. M. Hogan, *J. Cell Biol.* **105,** 473 (1987).

E. Holmes, G. Hermanson, R. Cole, and J. de Vellis, *J. Neurosci. Res.* **19,** 389 (1988).

G. E. Houts, M. Miyagi, D. Ellis, D. Beard, and J. W. Beard, *J. Virol.* **29,** 517 (1979).

G. F. Jirikowski, F. Ramalho-Ortigao, and H. Seliger, *Mol. Cell. Probes* **2,** 59 (1988).

H. A. John, M. Patrinou-Georgoulas, and K. W. Jones, *Cell* **12,** 501 (1977).

E. G. Jones, S. H. C. Hendry, P. Isackson, and R. A. Bradshaw, *in* "*In Situ* Hybridization: Applications to Neurobiology" (K. L. Valentino, J. H. Eberwine, and J. D. Barchas, eds.), Appendix B, p. 229. Oxford Univ. Press, London and New York, 1987.

J.-F. Julien, F. Legay, S. Dumas, M. Tappaz, and J. Mallet, *Neurosci. Lett.* **73,** 173 (1987).

M. Kawata, J. T. McCabe, and D. W. Pfaff, *Brain Res. Bull.* **20,** 693 (1988).

J. E. Kelsey, S. J. Watson, S. Burke, H. Akil, and J. L. Roberts, *J. Neurosci.* **6,** 38 (1986).

K. J. Koller, R. S. Wolff, M. K. Warden, and R. T. Zoeller, *Proc. Natl. Acad. Sci. U.S.A.* **84,** 7329 (1987).

K. J. Kovacs and E. Mezey, *Neuroendocrinology* **46,** 365 (1987).

K. Kristensson, N. K. Zeller, M. E. Dudois-Dalcq, and R. A. Lazzarini, *J. Histochem. Cytochem.* **34,** 467 (1986).

B. L. Largent, D. T. Jones, R. R. Reed, R. C. A. Pearson, and S. H. Snyder, *Proc. Natl. Acad. Sci. U.S.A.* **85,** 2864 (1988).

L.-I. Larsson, T. Christensen, and H. Dalboge, *Histochemistry* **89,** 109 (1988).

F. M. Leslie and C. A. Altar (eds.), "Receptor Localization: Ligand Autoradiography." Liss, New York, 1988.

M. E. Lewis, R. Arentzen, and F. Baldino, Jr., *J. Neurosci. Res.* **16,** 117 (1986a).

M. E. Lewis, T. G. Sherman, S. Burke, H. Akil, L. G. Davis, R. Arentzen, and S. J. Watson, *Proc. Natl. Acad. Sci. U.S.A.* **83,** 5419 (1986b).

S. A. Lewis and N. I. Cowan, *J. Neurochem.* **45,** 913 (1985).

M. S. Lidow, P. S. Goldman-Rakic, P. Rakic, and D. W. Gallager, *Brain Res.* **459,** 105 (1988).

P. Liessi, J.-P. Julien, P. Vilja, F. Grosveld, and L. Rechardt, *J. Histochem. Cytochem.* **34,** 923 (1986).

S. L. Lightman and W. S. Young III, *J. Physiol. (London)* **394,** 23 (1987).

C. R. Lin, M. S. Kapiloff, S. Durgerian, K. Tatemoto, A. F. Russo, P. Hanson, H. Schulman, and M. G. Rosenfeld, *Proc. Natl. Acad. Sci. U.S.A.* **84,** 5962 (1987).

Y. C. Liu, Y. Kato, K. Inoue, S. Tanaka, and K. Kurosumi, *Biochem. Biophys. Res. Commun.* **154,** 80 (1988).

K. R. Lynch, C. L. Hawelu-Johnson, and P. G. Guyernet, *Mol. Brain Res.* **2,** 149 (1987).

J. T. McCabe, J. I. Morrell, R. Ivell, H. Schmale, D. Richter, and D. W. Pfaff, *J. Histochem. Cytochem.* **34,** 45 (1986a).

J. T. McCabe, J. I. Morrell, R. Ivell, H. Schmale, D. Richter, and D. W. Pfaff, *Neuroendocrinology* **44,** 361 (1986b).

J. T. McCabe, J. I. Morrell, and D. W. Pfaff, *in "In Situ* Hybridization in Brain" (G. R. Uhl, ed.), p. 73. Plenum, New York, 1988.

J. McGadey, *Histochimie* **23,** 180 (1970).

T. Maniatis, E. F. Fritsch, and J. Sambrook, "Molecular Cloning: A Laboratory Manual." Cold Spring Harbor Laboratory, Cold Spring Harbor, New York, 1982.

A. J. Mason, J. S. Hayflick, R. T. Zoeller, W. S. Young III, H. S. Phillips, K. Nikolics, and P. H. Seeburg, *Science* **234,** 1366 (1986a).

A. J. Mason, S. L. Pitts, K. Nikolics, E. Szonyi, J. N. Wilcox, P. H. Seeburg, and T. A. Stewart, *Science* **234,** 1372 (1986b).

J. Meinkoth and G. Wahl, *Anal. Biochem.* **138,** 267 (1984).

J. Meinkoth and G. Wahl, *in* "Methods in Enzymology" (S. L. Berger and A. R. Kimmel, eds.), Vol. 152, p. 91. Academic Press, Orlando, Florida, 1987.

I. Mocchetti, J. P. Schwartz, and E. Costa, *Mol. Pharmacol.* **28,** 86 (1985).

B. J. Morris, K. J. Feasey, G. Bruggencate, A. Herz, and V. Hollt, *Proc. Natl. Acad. Sci. U.S.A.* **85,** 3226 (1988).

T. Nishimori, M. A. Moskowitz, and G. R. Uhl, *J. Comp. Neurol.* **274,** 142 (1988).

H. Nogami, F. Yoshimura, A.-J. Carrillo, Z. D. Sharp, and P. J. Sheridan, *Endocrinol. Jpn.* **32,** 625 (1985).

H. Nojiri, M. Sato, and A. Urano, *Neurosci. Lett.* **85,** 101 (1985).

E. Normand, T. Popovici, B. Onteniente, D. Fellmann, D. Piatier-Tonneau, C. Auffray, and B. Bloch, *Brain Res.* **439,** 39 (1988).

M. Palkovits, C. Léránth, T. Görcs, and W. S. Young III, *Proc. Natl. Acad. Sci. U.S.A.* **84,** 3911 (1987).

G. Pelletier, N. Liao, N. Follea, and M. V. Govindan, *Mol. Cell. Endocrinol.* **56,** 29 (1988).

J. B. Penny, H. S. Pan, A. B. Young, K. A. Frey, and G. W. Dauth, *Science* **214,** 1036 (1981).

J. Pevsner, P. M. Hwang, P. B. Sklar, J. C. Venable, and S. H. Snyder, *Proc. Natl. Acad. Sci. U.S.A.* **85,** 2383 (1988).

J. E. Pintar, *in "In Situ* Hybridization and Related Techniques to Study Cell-Specific Gene Expression in the Nervous System" (J. Roberts, ed.), p. 94. Society for Neuroscience, Toronto, Ontario, Canada, 1988.

J. E. Pintar and D. I. Lugo, *in "In Situ* Hybridization: Applications to Neurobiology" (K. L. Valentino, J. H. Eberwine, and J. D. Barchas, eds.), Chap. 10. Oxford Univ. Press, London and New York, 1987.

R. Pochet, H. Brocas, G. Vassart, G. Toubeau, H. Seo, S. Refetoff, J. E. Dumont, and J. L. Pasteels, *Brain Res.* **211,** 433 (1981).

P. D. Rennert and G. Heinrich, *Biochem. Biophys. Res. Commun.* **138,** 813 (1986).

M. Rentrop, B. Knapp, H. Winter, and J. Schweizer, *Histochem. J.* **18,** 271 (1986).

P. W. J. Rigby, M. Dieckmann, C. Rhodes, and P. Berg, *J. Mol. Biol.* **113,** 237 (1977).

A. W. Rogers, "Techniques of Autoradiography," 3rd Ed. Elsevier, Amsterdam, 1979.

K. V. Rogers, L. Vician, R. A. Steiner, and D. K. Clifton, *Endocrinology (Baltimore)* **121,** 90 (1987).

Å. Rökaeus, W. S. Young III, and E. Mezey, *Neurosci. Lett.* **90,** 45 (1988).

G. J. Romano, B. D. Shivers, R. E. Harlan, R. D. Howells, and D. W. Pfaff, *Mol. Brain Res.* **2,** 33 (1987).

J. M. Rothfeld, J. F. Hejtmancik, P. M. Conn, and D. W. Pfaff, *Exp. Brain Res.* **67,** 113 (1987).

M. A. Ruda, M. J. Iadarola, L. V. Cohen, and W. S. Young III, *Proc. Natl. Acad. Sci. U.S.A.* **85,** 622 (1988).

B. S. Schachter, *in* "*In Situ* Hybridization: Applications to Neurobiology" (K. L. Valentino, J. H. Eberwine, and J. D. Barchas, eds.), p. 111. Oxford Univ. Press, London and New York, 1987.

M. Schalling, T. Hökfelt, B. Wallace, M. Goldstein, D. Filer, C. Yamin, and D. H. Schlesinger, *Proc. Natl. Acad. Sci. U.S.A.* **83,** 6208 (1986).

M. Schalling, A. Dagerlind, S. Brene, R. Petterson, S. Kvist, M. Brownstein, S. E. Hyman, L. Mucke, H. M. Goodman, T. H. Joh, M. Goldstein, and T. Hokfelt, *Acta Physiol. Scand.* **131,** 631 (1987).

J. W. Schncider, R. W. Mercer, M. Gilmore-Hebert, M. F. Utset, C. Lai, A. Greene, and E. J. Benz, Jr., *Proc. Natl. Acad. Sci. U.S.A.* **85,** 284 (1988).

T. P. Segerson, H. Hoefler, H. Childers, H. J. Wolfe, P. Wu, I. M. D. Jackson, and R. M. Lechan, *Endocrinology (Baltimore)* **121,** 98 (1987a).

T. P. Segerson, J. Kauer, H. C. Wolfe, H. Mobtaker, P. Wu, I. M. D. Jackson, and R. M. Lechan, *Science* **238,** 78 (1987b).

J.-M. Séquier, W. Hunziker, and G. Richards, *Neurosci. Lett.* **86,** 155 (1988a).

J.-M. Séquier, J. G. Richards, S. Mathews, and H. Mohler, *Proc. Natl. Acad. Sci. U.S.A.* **85,** 7815 (1988b).

T. G. Sherman, S. J. Watson, E. Herbert, and H. Akil, *Soc. Neurosci. Abstr.* **10,** 359 (1984).

T. G. Sherman, O. Civelli, J. Douglass, E. Herbert, S. Burke, and S. J. Watson, *Fed. Proc., Fed. Am. Soc. Exp. Biol.* **45,** 2323 (1986a).

T. G. Sherman, J. F. McKelvy, and S. J. Watson, *J. Neurosci.* **6,** 1685 (1986b).

R. Sherrington, J. Brynjolfsson, H. Petursson, M. Potter, K. Dudleston, B. Barraclough, J. Wasmuth, M. Dobbs, and H. Gurling, *Nature (London)* **336,** 164 (1988).

H. Shiomi, J. W. Stanley, J. E. Kelsey, and H. Akil, *Endocrinology (Baltimore)* **119,** 1793 (1986).

B. D. Shivers, R. E. Harlan, J. F. Hejtmancik, P. M. Conn, and D. W. Pfaff, *Endocrinology (Baltimore)* **118,** 883 (1986a).

B. D. Shivers, R. E. Harlan, D. W. Pfaff, and B. S. Schachter, *J. Histochem. Cytochem.* **34,** 39 (1986b).

B. D. Shivers, B. S. Schachter, and D. W. Pfaff, *in* "Methods in Enzymology" (P. M. Conn, ed.), Vol. 124, p. 497. Academic Press, Orlando, Florida, 1986c.

B. D. Shivers, R. E. Harlan, G. J. Romano, R. D. Howells, and D. W. Pfaff, *in* "*In Situ* Hybridization in Brain" (G. R. Uhl, ed.), p. 3. Plenum, New York, 1988.

R. E. Siegel and W. S. Young III, *Neuropeptides* **6,** 573 (1985).

R. E. Siegel, A. Iacangelo, J. Park, and L. E. Eiden, *Mol. Endocrinol.* **2,** 368 (1988).

R. H. Singer and D. C. Ward, *Proc. Natl. Acad. Sci. U.S.A.* **79,** 7331 (1982).

R. H. Singer, J. B. Lawrence, and R. N. Rashtchian, *in* "*In Situ* Hybridization: Applications to Neurobiology" (K. L. Valentino, J. H. Eberwine, and J. D. Barchas, eds.), Chap. 4. Oxford Univ. Press, London and New York, 1987.

P. J. Southern, P. Blount, and M. B. A. Oldstone, *Nature* (*London*) **312,** 555 (1984).

A. J. Stauder, P. W. Dickson, A. R. Aldred, G. Schreiber, F. A. O. Mendelsohn, and P. Hudson, *J. Histochem. Cytochem.* **34,** 949 (1986).

J. H. Steel, Q. Hamid, S. Van Noorden, P. Jones, P. Denny, J. Burrin, S. Legon, S. R. Bloom, and J. M. Polak, *Histochemistry* **89,** 75 (1988).

W. G. Stroop and D. C. Schaefer, *Acta Neuropathol.* **74,** 124 (1987).

W. G. Stroop, H. Brahic, and J. R. Baringer, *Infect. Immun.* **37,** 763 (1982).

W. G. Stroop, D. L. Rock, and N. W. Fraser, *Lab. Invest.* **51,** 27 (1984).

L. Stowring, A. T. Haase, G. Petursson, P. Georgsson, P. Palsson, R. Lutlgy, R. Roos, and S. Szuchet, *Virology* **141,** 311 (1985).

J. G. Sutcliffe, *Annu. Rev. Neurosci.* **11,** 157 (1988).

L. Tecott, Ph.D. Thesis, Stanford University, Stanford, California, 1986.

L. Tecott and J. Eberwine, *Soc. Neurosci. Abstr.* **12,** 27 (1988).

L. H. Tecott, J. H. Eberwine, J. D. Barchas, and K. L. Valentino, *in* "*In Situ* Hybridization: Applications to Neurobiology" (K. L. Valentino, J. H. Eberwine, and J. D. Barchas, eds.), p. 3. Oxford Univ. Press, London and New York, 1987.

L. H. Tecott, J. D. Barchas, and J. H. Eberwine, *Science* **240,** 166 (1988a).

L. Tecott, D. Newell, J. Eberwine, and A. Hoffman, *Abstr. Meet. Endocr. Soc. 70th* (1988b).

L. Tecott, J. D. Barchas, I. Zangger, and J. H. Eberwine, "Template Specific Termination of *in Situ* Transcription." Submitted for publication (1989).

H. M. Temin and D. Baltimore, *Adv. Virus. Res.* **17,** 129 (1971).

R. B. Tenser, M. Dawson, S. J. Ressel, and M. E. Dunstan, *Ann. Neurol.* **11,** 285 (1982).

C. A. Thomas and B. M. Dancis, *J. Mol. Biol.* **77,** 44 (1973).

W. W. Tourtellote, R. Thomsen, I. Rosario, and P. Shapshak, *in* "*In Situ* Hybridization in Brain" (G. R. Uhl, ed.), p. 288. Plenum, New York, 1987.

G. R. Uhl and S. M. Reppert, *Science* **231,** 390 (1986).

G. R. Uhl, H. H. Zingg, and J. F. Habener, *Proc. Natl. Acad. Sci. U.S.A.* **82,** 5555 (1985).

E. R. Unger, H. T. Budgeon, D. Myerson, and D. J. Brigati, *Am. J. Surg. Pathol.* **10,** 1 (1986).

J. R. Unnerstall, D. L. Niehoff, M. J. Kuhar, and J. M. Palacios, *J. Neurosci. Methods* **6,** 59 (1982).

B. H. van Leeuwen, J. D. Penschow, J. P. Coghlan, and R. I. Richards, *EMBO J.* **6,** 1705 (1987).

K. Wada, M. Ballivet, J. Boulter, J. Connolly, E. Wada, E. S. Deneris, L. W. Swanson, S. Heinemann, and J. Patrick, *Science* **240,** 330 (1988).

M. K. Warden and W. S. Young III, *J. Comp. Neurol.* **272,** 90 (1988).

S. J. Watson, T. G. Sherman, J. E. Kelsey, S. Burke, and H. Akil, *in* "*In Situ* Hybridization: Applications to Neurobiology" (K. L. Valentino, J. H. Eberwine, and J. D. Barchas, eds.), p. 126. Oxford Univ. Press, London and New York, 1987.

S. Watson, P. Patel, S. Burke, J. Herman, M. Schafer, and S. Kwak, *in* "*In Situ* Hybridization and Related Techniques to Study Cell-Specific Gene Expression in the Nervous System" (J. Roberts, ed.), pp. 4–29. Society for Neuroscience, Toronto, Ontario, Canada, 1988.

H. Werner, Y. Koch, F. Baldino, Jr., and I. Gozes, *J. Biol. Chem.* **263,** 7666 (1988).

J. G. Wetmur and N. Davidson, *J. Mol. Biol.* **31,** 349 (1968).

J. N. Wilcox and R. Derynck, *J. Neurosci.* **8,** 1901 (1988).

J. N. Wilcox, J. L. Roberts, B. M. Chronwall, J. F. Bishop, and T. O. O'Donohue, *J. Neurosci. Res.* **16,** 89 (1986).

P. A. Wilson, J. Scott, J. Penschow, J. Coghlan, and R. A. Rush, *Neurosci. Lett.* **64,** 323 (1986).

C. W. Wuenschell, R. S. Fisher, D. L. Kaufman, and A. J. Tobin, *Proc. Natl. Acad. Sci. U.S.A.* **83,** 6193 (1986).

N. Yamamoto, H. Seo, N. Suganuma, N. Matsui, T. Nakane, A. Kuwayama, and N. Kageyama, *Neuroendocrinology* **42,** 494 (1986).

K. Yoshikawa, C. Williams, and S. L. Sabol, *J. Biol. Chem.* **259,** 14301 (1984).

W. S. Young III, *Neuropeptides* **8,** 93 (1986).

W. S. Young III, *in* "*In Situ* Hybridization and Related Techniques to Study Cell-Specific Gene Expression in the Nervous System" (J. Roberts, ed.), pp. 30–39. Society for Neuroscience, Toronto, Ontario, Canada, 1988.

W. S. Young III and M. J. Kuhar, *in* "*In Situ* Hybridization in Brain" (G. R. Uhl, ed.), pp. 243–248. Plenum, New York, 1988.

W. S. Young III, T. I. Bonner, and M. R. Brann, *Proc. Natl. Acad. Sci. U.S.A.* **83,** 9827 (1986a).

W. S. Young III, E. Mezey, R. E. Siegel, *Mol. Brain Res.* **1,** 231 (1986b).

W. S. Young III, M. Warden, and E. Mezey, *Neuroendocrinology* **46,** 439 (1987).

I. Zangger, L. Tecott, J. Barchas, and J. Eberwine, submitted for publication (1989).

R. T. Zoeller, P. H. Seeburg, and W. S. Young III, *Endocrinology (Baltimore)* **122,** 2570 (1988).

[16] Nonradioactive *in Situ* Hybridization Histochemistry with Digoxigenin–Deoxyuridine 5′-Triphosphate-Labeled Oligonucleotides

Frank Baldino, Jr., and Michael E. Lewis

Introduction

In situ hybridization histochemistry has become a powerful tool to study the regulation of selected mRNA species in various regions of the central nervous system (CNS). Several laboratories have successfully used this technology to localize relatively rare mRNAs within the cytoplasm of individual neurons (1–4). The localization of these transcripts to single cells has allowed, for the first time, the identification of the neurons which actually synthesize a given enzyme, protein, or neuropeptide. In addition, refinement of this hybridization technology has yielded insights into the regulation of neuropeptides, enzymes, and other CNS-related proteins at the level of single neurons.

The use of synthetic oligodeoxyribonucleotide (oligonucleotide) probes to detect mRNA sequences provides significant advantages for *in situ* hybridization studies. Unlike cloned cDNA probes, oligonucleotides are single stranded, unique for a particular sequence of mRNA, and are easily labeled on either the 3′ or 5′ end with a variety of markers. The relatively short size of these probes (usually 20–50 bases) renders them less susceptible to many of the methodological limitations often associated with long DNA or RNA sequences. Melting temperatures of the hybrids formed with these oligonucleotides can be easily determined *in situ* to assess the specificity of hybridization accurately (2, 5, 6).

Oligonucleotide probes penetrate the cell in fixed tissue sections and thus have a high probability of forming stable DNA–RNA hybrids. Although high-resolution autoradiographic images have been successfully produced with radiolabeled probes, the sensitivity, level of background, and the prolonged autoradiographic exposure time (10–15 weeks) required with ^{35}S- and ^{3}H-labeled probes have limited their utility. In addition, simultaneous detection of multiple mRNA species within a single neuron in the same tissue section has only been achieved by one laboratory (7) using an elegant but complicated chemical process with color photographic emulsions.

Nonradioactive Detection Systems

In recent years, several nonradioactive markers have been developed to detect specific nucleotide sequences under a variety of hybridization conditions. These nonradioactive markers are particularly useful for *in situ* hybridization studies, where they have overcome several limitations inherent to the use of radiolabeled sequences as probes. The prolonged exposure required with low-energy radionuclides (e.g., ^{35}S and ^{3}H) on emulsion-coated slides has been cumbersome, costly, and difficult to reproduce, as the time of exposure is a function of the degree of hybridization. Furthermore, with the exception of the technology reported by Haase *et al.* (7), it is impossible to detect multiple species of mRNAs within a single neuron or tissue section with radiolabeled DNA probes. More critical is the high level of nonspecific background which is often associated with the use of radiolabeled probes. Even the use of relatively low-energy β-particle emitters (e.g., ^{35}S or ^{3}H) produces a degree of background which often precludes the detection of very rare mRNA species. Furthermore, with nonradioactive markers, the degree of cellular resolution, a prime requisite for *in situ* hybridization, is significantly improved over that normally achieved with autoradiography. Last, the use of these nonradioactive probes avoids the biohazards normally associated with the use of radioisotopes.

Biotinylated Probes

Complexing biotin with nucleotides has been particularly useful for hybridization studies. Biotin can be complexed with nucleotides by several methods. Direct labeling can be achieved with either a photoactivatable analog of biotin called photobiotin, or biotin hydrazide. These methods have been previously reviewed (8, 9). Alternatively, biotinylated nucleotides (e.g., biotin-11–dUTP or biotin-21–dUTP) can be incorporated enzymatically into a cDNA by nick translation, or an oligonucleotide by primer extension or serial addition to the 3′ end with terminal deoxynucleotidyl-transferase. Although each of these labeling methods produces biotinylated probes, the sensitivity of detection has been shown to be dependent on the position of the biotin molecule within the nucleotide sequence. Cook *et al.* (10) have shown that biotin labels at the ends of the probe provide for more sensitive detection than internal biotin labels.

A few laboratories have successfully used biotinylated cDNA probes to detect relatively abundant DNA or RNA immobilized on nitrocellulose (11) or with *in situ* hybridization (12–15). However, positive results with biotinylated oligonucleotides for *in situ* hybridization have only recently been demonstrated (16, 17).

Enzyme/Hapten-Conjugated Probes

Several different classes of enzymes or haptens can be directly conjugated to nucleotides. Histochemical studies have focused on the use of alkaline phosphatase or horseradish peroxidase for the detection of antigen and hybridization signals. One laboratory has published a method which chemically incorporates modified bases with functionalized "linker arms" into synthetic oligonucleotides (18, 19). These linker arms can be conjugated to several different enzymes. Although this approach offers precise control over the location and number of labeling sites within the oligonucleotide, the sensitivity of these probes is limited by the addition of only a single alkaline phosphatase into the nucleotide sequence. Moreover, it is not a routine procedure to conjugate alkaline phosphatase to nucleotides by this method.

Recently, a new method has been developed which incorporates digoxigenin–dUTP (Dig–dUTP) into a probe sequence (Boehringer Mannheim). This Dig–dUTP labeled probe is subsequently detected with an alkaline phosphatase-conjugated IgG which is highly specific for the digoxigenin molecule. Unlike the direct conjugation of a single-enzyme molecule to the probe, this new methodology offers the advantge of adding multiple labels to the probe sequence, thus amplifying the hybridization signal. In addition, IgG detection also provides the advantage of using "bridging" antibody techniques to further amplify the signal. Thus, a certain degree of amplification is an intrinsic feature of the digoxigenin detection system. We have recently developed the Dig–dUTP detection system for *in situ* hybridization histochemistry with synthetic oligonucleotides. The purpose of this chapter is to provide a detailed guide to enable the reader to use this high-resolution methodology to preform nonradioactive *in situ* hybridization histochemistry in neural tissue.

Digoxigenin–dUTP

Synthetic oligonucleotide probes are labeled on their 3′ end with Dig–dUTP. The dUTP is linked via an 11-atom spacer arm to the steroid hapten digoxigenin (Fig. 1; Boehringer Mannheim). The size of the hapten and its conjugation of dUTP does not interfere with the 3′ serial addition of Dig–UTPs by terminal transferase. Dig–dUTP also lends itself readily to random priming of cDNA restriction fragments with the Klenow fragment of DNA polymerase I (Boehringer Mannheim). DNA probes labeled in this manner are stable for extended periods of time when stored at −20°C.

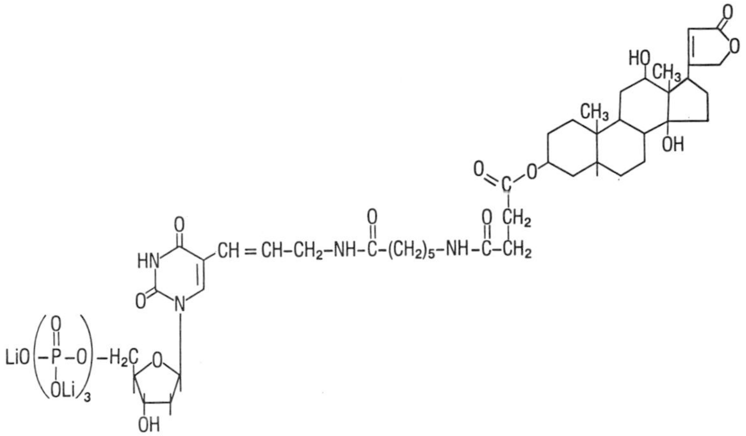

FIG. 1 Structure of digoxigenin-11–dUTP. (Figure provided courtesy of Boehringer Mannheim.)

Labeling Reaction

3′-End labeling is accomplished with a dNTP mixture containing Dig–dUTP or Dig–dUTP alone (Boehringer Mannheim) and terminal deoxynucleotidyltransferase (Boehringer Mannheim). The labeling reaction is as follows.

To a sterile 1.5 ml Eppendorf tube, add
  2.5 μl 10× reaction buffer (1.4 mM potassium cacodylate, pH 7.2, 300 mM Tris base, 10 mM CoCl$_2$, 1 mM dithiothreitol)
  18.0 μl HPLC-grade sterile water
  1.0 μl oligonucleotide (0.005 OD$_{260}$)
  2.5 μl dNTP labeling mixture (Boehringer Mannheim) or digoxigenin-11–dUTP (Boehringer Mannheim)
  1.0 μl terminal transferase (25 U; Boehringer Mannheim)
The reactants are mixed gently, briefly microfuged, and incubated at 37°C for 1.5 hr.

In Situ Hybridization

The protocol used to detect mRNA *in situ* was developed from previously published methods in our laboratory (3, 4). This protocol also considered the methodologies to detect RNA and DNA on Northern and Southern blots with a nonradioactive DNA labeing kit (#1093 657, Boehringer Mannheim). The following is a protocol for performing hybridization with the digoxigenin-11–dUTP-labeled probes on tissue sections obtained from adult rats.

Tissue Preparation

1. Freeze tissue in powdered dry ice and mount on cryostat chuck with Lipshaw M-1 embedding matrix (Lipshaw, Detroit, MI).
2. Section tissue at 20μm in a cryostat at $-18°$C and thaw-mount on subbed (gelatin-coated) slides at room temperature (RT). Place slides in slide box in dry ice during cutting and then store at $-70°$C.

Prehybridization

1. Tissue sections are quickly dried and warmed to RT with a blow dryer set on "cool."
2. The sections are then fixed in buffered 3% paraformaldehyde for 5 min at RT and rinsed three times in phosphate-buffered saline (PBS) at RT (with shaking).
3. Incubate for 10 min in $2\times$ SSC at RT.
4. Excess $2\times$ SSC is removed and slides are placed in a Nunc tissue culture dish (Thomas Scientific, Swedesboro, NJ; #3488-H90) lined with wetted filter paper backing (Bio-Rad, Richmond, CA; #165-0921).
5. Five hundred microliters of prehybridization buffer is pipetted onto each slide covering the sections (e.g., 3–6 brain sections/slide). The culture dish lid is replaced and the slides are permitted to incubate at RT for 1 hr.

Hybridization

1. The digoxigenin-labeled probe is diluted with prehybridization buffer, allowing 250 μl of buffer per slide. The required concentration of probe will depend on mRNA abundance and must be determined experimentally. To conserve probe, the volume can be reduced (e.g., to 30 μl/section) by covering the sections with a Parafilm coverslip.
2. Excess prehybridization buffer is removed from the slides (by decanting onto the filter paper backing) and the glass surrounding the tissue is carefully dried with a paper towel. The digoxigenin-labeled probe is then

applied at 250 μl per slide, or 30 μl per section if Parafilm coverslips are used. The culture dish is carefully placed in the incubator (37°C) overnight.

Posthybridization

1. The slides are washed (with gentle shaking on a rotary shaker) as follows.
   a. 2× SSC for 1 hr at RT
   b. 1× SSC for 1 hr at RT
   c. 0.5× SSC for 0.5 hr at 37°C
   d. 0.5× SSC for 0.5 hr at RT

Immunological Detection

1. Wash slides for 1 min in 200 ml of buffer 1 in a Wheaton dish at RT.
2. Cover sections with 2% normal sheep serum (Sigma S-2382) plus 0.3% Triton X-100 (Sigma T-6878) (in buffer 1) for 30 min at RT.
3. Dilute antidigoxigenin antibody–alkaline phosphatase conjugate (1 : 500, Boehringer Mannheim) with buffer 1 containing 1% normal sheep serum and 0.3% Triton X-100.
4. Pipette diluted antibody–enzyme conjugate (100 μl/section) onto sections and incubate at RT for 2 hr in a Nunc culture dish with wetted filter paper backing.
5. Wash slides twice for 15 min each in 200 ml of buffer 1 in a Wheaton dish at RT.
6. Incubate slides for 2 min in 200 ml of buffer 3 in a Wheaton dish at RT.
7. Incubate slides with 500 μl/slide of color solution. Slides are placed in light-tight boxes on buffer-wetted filter backing. Slides must be kept in the dark during incubation (0.5–24 hr), but can be checked periodically for color development.
8. Reaction can be stopped in 200 ml of buffer 4 in a Wheaton dish.
9. Tissue is dehydrated in a fume hood as follows:
   a. Distilled H$_2$O   10 dips
   b. 70% ethanol*   10 dips
   c. 95% ethanol   2 min (×2)
   d. 100% ethanol   2 min (×2)
   e. Xylenes   2 min (×4)

---

* Only absolute ethanol should be used.

10. Slides are coverslipped using mounting medium (e.g., Eukit Ealatt; Calibrated Inst., Inc., Ardsley, NY), allowed to dry, and examined with a microscope.

Solutions

In general, solutions should be prepared using sterile, double-distilled H_2O and stored in autoclaved containers.

1. Paraformaldehyde (3%, v/v) in phosphate-buffered saline: On day of use, warm 150 ml of water (40–50°C), add 6 g paraformaldehyde (Fisher, T-353) while stirring, and add 1–2 drops 10 N NaOH to clear solution. Turn off heat and add 50 ml of 4× PBS (1 bottle of Sigma #1000-3 dissolved in 250 ml water). Let cool to RT, and adjust pH to 7.2–7.4 with dilute HCl. Filter through a 0.22-μm filter to sterilize.
2. 1× phosphate-buffered saline (PBS), pH 7.4
    120 mM NaCl
    2.7 mM KCl
    1.36 g/liter KH_2PO_4
    Alternatively, dissolve one bottle of prepared PBS buffer (Sigma #1000-3) in 1 liter of H_2O.
3. 20× SSC
    175.32 g NaCl (Sigma S-9625)
    88.23 g sodium citrate (Sigma C-7254)
    1 liter H_2O final volume
    Stir to dissolve, then autoclave. Alternatively, 20× stock may be purchased from Sigma (S6639).
4. 50× Denhardt's solution
    1 g Ficoll (Sigma F-9378)
    1 g poly(vinylpyrrolidone) (Sigma PVP260)
    1 g BSA fraction V (Sigma A7906)
    100 ml H_2O
    Stir until dissolved, then sterile filter. Alternatively, 50× stock may be purchased from Sigma (D 2532).
5. Deionized formamide (BRL, Gaithersburg, MD; 5515UB): Mixed bed ion-exchange resin (Bio-Rad AG501-X8, 20–50 mesh). Stir formamide for 30 min with resin (5 g per 50 ml) at RT. Filter through Whatman #1 filter paper. Aliquot and store at −20°C.
6. Salmon sperm DNA (Sigma D1626): Dissolve DNA (Sigma type III sodium salt) in sterile H_2O, 10 mg/ml. Stir for 2–4 hr at RT. Shear DNA by passing it through a sterile 18-gauge hypodermic needle several

times. Heat in boiling water, aliquot, and store at $-20°C$. Alternatively, 10 mg/ml stock may be purchased from Sigma (D 9156).

7. Yeast tRNA (BRL 5401SA): Dissolve tRNA in 10 mg/ml of sterile water, aliquot, and freeze at $-20°C$.

8. $2\times$ SSC: 25 ml $20\times$ SSC + 225 ml H_2O
   $1\times$ SSC: 12.5 ml $20\times$ SSC + 237.5 ml H_2O
   $0.5\times$ SSC: 6.25 ml $20\times$ SSC + 243.75 ml H_2O

9. Prehybridization/hybridization buffer
   5 ml deionized formamide
   2 ml $20\times$ SSC
   0.2 ml $50\times$ Denhardt's solution
   0.5 ml 10 mg/ml salmon sperm DNA
   0.25 ml 10 mg/ml yeast tRNA
   2 ml dextran sulfate, probe grade, 50% solution (cat # 54030 Oncor Inc., Gaithersburg, MD)

10. Buffer 1
    100 mM Tris-HCl, pH 7.5 (20°C)
    150 mM NaCl

11. Buffer 3
    100 mM Tris-HCl, pH 9.5 (20°C)
    100 mM NaCl
    50 mM $MgCl_2$

12. Buffer 4
    100 mM Tris-HCl, pH 8.5 (20°C)
    1 mM EDTA

13. Color solution
    45 μl NBT solution (Boehringer Mannheim)
    35 μl X-phosphate solution (Boehringer Mannheim)
    2.4 mg levamisole (Sigma L-9756) is added to 10 ml buffer 3 immediately before use.

14. One or two percent normal sheep serum: Reconstitute lyophilized normal sheep serum (Sigma, S-2382) in sterile water and dilute to 1 or 2% (as required in protocol) in buffer 1.

Resolution

The degree of cellular resolution obtained with probes labeled in this manner is far superior to radiolabeled probes. Individual cell profiles were easily defined and multiple cells could be distinguished within deeper layers of the tissue section. Figure 2 is an example of the resolution achieved with a Dig–dUTP-labeled oligonucleotide (24 bases) which we have shown to be

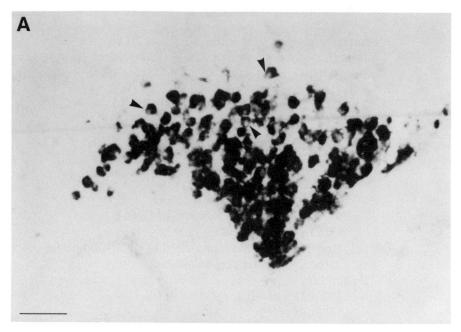

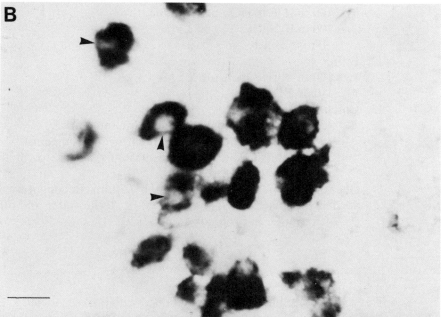

FIG. 2 Bright-field photomicrographs demonstrating *in situ* hybridization histo-chemistry with a 24-base oligonucleotide probe for arginine vasopressin (AVP) labeled on its 3′ end with Dig–dUTP. (A) Low-magnification photomicrograph

highly specific for arginine vasopressin precursor mRNA (2, 20). Hybridization signal was characterized by dense particulate labeling within the cytoplasm and a clear unlabeled nucleus (note arrows in Fig. 2). Little if any hybridization signal extended beyond the soma with this probe. The nonspecific (i.e., background) labeling was also considerably less than that observed with radiolabeled probes. Moreover, hybridization and detection of these probes was obtained within 24 hr compared to the 8–10 weeks required to detect single cell profiles with ^{35}S- or ^{3}H-labeled probes.

Concluding Remarks

High-resolution *in situ* hybridization histochemistry can be readily performed with alkaline phosphatase–Dig–dUTP-labeled oligonucleotide probes. The ease of performance, safety, and rapidity of detection render this methodology a useful alternative to that employing radiolabeled probes for the detection of mRNAs in the CNS or any organ system where cellular resolution is essential.

A further advantage of this particular nonradioactive method is that since several substrates are presently available for alkaline phosphatase, it should be possible to detect multiple mRNAs within a single cell. It should also be possible to detect two different species of mRNA by combining an enzyme-labeled probe with a radiolabeled probe.

One interesting feature inherent to the use of the digoxigenin–dUTP system is the advantage of amplification by the enzymatic addition of multiple digoxigenin–dUTPs, which, when coupled with standard double- or triple-bridging techniques with alternate species antisera, should permit the detection of even the rarest mRNA species.

Acknowledgments

The authors gratefully acknowledge the technical assistance of Elaine Robbins and Kathleen V. Callison (Cephalon, Inc.) and the advice and expertise of Dr. Debra S. Grega and Dr. Rick Martin (Boehringer Mannheim, Inc.). The secretarial skills of Linda W. Morrison are also appreciated. This work was supported in part by Boehringer Mannheim, Inc.

---

showing the cellular distribution of AVP mRNA in the supraoptic nucleus. Bar, 200 μm. (B) High-magnification photomicrograph of magnocellular neurons in the paraventricular nucleus. Arrowheads point to cell nuclei in both photomicrographs. Bar, 50 μm.

References

1. M. Schalling, T. Hökfelt, B. Wallace, M. Goldstein, D. Fier, C. Yamin, and D. H. Schlesinger, *Proc. Natl. Acad. Sci. U.S.A.* **83,** 6208 (1986).
2. F. Baldino, Jr., and L. G. Davis, *in* "*In Situ* Hybridization in Brain" (G. R. Uhl, ed.), pp. 97–116. Plenum, New York, 1986.
3. F. Baldino, Jr., M.-F. Chesselet, and M. E. Lewis, *in* "Methods in Enzymology" (P. M. Conn, ed.), Vol. 168, p. 761. Academic Press, San Diego, California, 1989.
4. M. E. Lewis, R. G. Krause II, and J. M. Roberts-Lewis, *Synapse* **2,** 308 (1988).
5. M. E. Lewis, T. G. Sherman, and S. J. Watson, *Peptides* **6,** 75 (1985).
6. J. P. Card, S. Fitzpatrick-McElligott, I. Gozes, and F. Baldino, Jr., *Cell Tissue Res.* **252,** 307 (1988).
7. A. T. Haase, P. Ventura, C. J. Gibbs, Jr., and W. W. Tourtellotte, *Science* **212,** 672 (1981).
8. M. Mechanic, *Immunochemica* **2,** 12 (1988).
9. M. Wilchek and E. P. Bayer, *Anal. Biochem.* **171,** 1 (1988).
10. A. F. Cook, E. Vuocolo, and C. L. Brakel, *Nucleic Acids Res.* **16,** 4077 (1988).
11. J. C. McInnes, S. Dalton, P. D. Vize, and A. J. Robins, *BioTechnology* **5,** 269 (1987).
12. R. H. Singer and D. C. Ward, *Proc. Natl. Acad. Sci. U.S.A.* **79,** 7331 (1982).
13. D. Myerson, R. C. Hackman, J. A. Nelson, D. C. Ward, and J. K. McDougall, *Hum. Pathol.* **15,** 430 (1984).
14. C. Ruppert, D. Goldowitz, and W. Wille, *EMBO J.* **5,** 1897 (1986).
15. D. Goldowitz, D. Bartels, and W. Wille, *Soc. Neurosci. Abstr.* **13,** 385.11 (1987).
16. H. Arai, P. Emson, S. Agrawal, C. Christodoulou, and M. Gait, *Mol. Brain Res.* **4,** 63 (1988).
17. A. F. Guitteny, B. Fouque, C. Mougin, R. Teoule, and B. Bloch, *J. Histochem. Cytochem.* **36,** 563 (1988).
18. J. L. Ruth, *DNA* **3,** 123 (1984).
19. E. Jablonski, E. W. Moomaw, R. H. Tullis, and J. L. Ruth, *Nucleic Acids Res.* **14,** 6115 (1986).
20. B. Wolfson, R. W. Manning, L. G. Davis, R. Arentzen, and F. Baldino, Jr., *Nature (London)* **315,** 59 (1985).

[17] Quantitation of Nuclear Low-Level Gene Expression in Central Nervous System Using Solution Hybridization and *in Situ* Hybridization

Mariann Blum and James L. Roberts

Introduction

Messenger RNA is transcribed in the nucleus from chromatin by RNA polymerase II, as outlined in Fig. 1. The resulting primary transcript must go through several posttranscriptional modifications before the mature mRNA is transported to the cytoplasm. In addition to the "capping" of the 5′ end of the mRNA with a 7-methylguanosine and the "tailing" of most mRNAs on the 3′ end with a poly(A) tract, there are also internal regions within primary transcripts called intervening sequences or introns which must be spliced out within the nucleus. The remaining segments, which must be precisely religated together, constitute the mature mRNA and are called exons. It is generally believed that the half-life of a primary transcript is only about 10 to 20 min. It is either rapidly degraded or processed into a mature mRNA which is subsequently transported to the cytoplasm. The spliced-out introns are very rapidly degraded and are usually present at a steady-state level of less than 1% of the primary transcript. Each of these steps in the biosynthesis of mRNA is a potential site for regulation of gene expression. The protocols outlined in this chapter are designed to enable one to study possible regulation of neural gene expression in the nucleus at each of these posttranscriptional sites of mRNA biosynthesis. We describe a nuclease protection/solution hybridization assay, which can be used to quantitate the amount of the primary transcript, processing intermediates, or mature mRNA in the nucleus, and intervening sequence *in situ* hybridization histochemistry, which can detect the level of the primary transcript in individual cell nuclei.

Solution Hybridization/Nuclease Protection Assay

Analysis of neural gene expression can be performed with either fresh brain tissue or primary cell or clonal cell line cultures. The basis of the solution

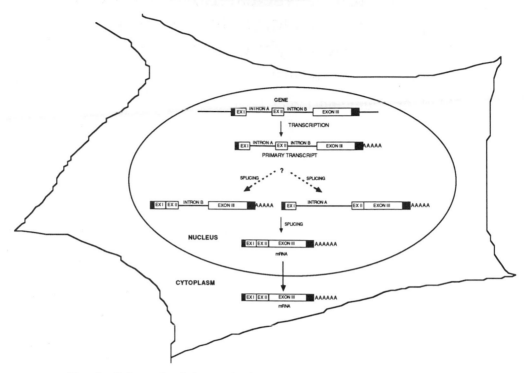

FIG. 1   Schematic of the synthesis and processing of nuclear RNAs in the neuron.

hybridization/nuclease protection assay is to treat either the animal *in vivo* or the culture *in vitro* with the desired hormone, behavioral paradigm, etc., for a specified time and then to isolate the cell nuclei by homogenizing the tissue in a cold buffer containing detergent, which solubilizes the cell membrane and allows for the cell nuclei to be pelleted away from the cytoplasm at low-speed centrifugation. The resulting postnuclear supernatant contains the cytoplasmic RNA and also peptides or proteins of interest and can be saved for further analysis.

The primary transcripts, processing intermediates, and mature mRNA from the pelleted nuclei can be purified so that one can determine if the experimental treatment affects RNA processing. To quantitate the amount of the primary transcript, processing intermediates, and the mature mRNA, a high-specific-activity radioactive (10^9 cpm/μg) RNA probe complementary to an intron/exon junction is synthesized. The RNA samples are then hybridized with the probe in solution. A standard curve is set up with a known amount of coding RNA so that the number of counts per minute protected in the sample hybrids can be converted into picograms of a specific RNA species per microgram of total RNA. After the hybridization reaction goes to completion, any nonhybridized RNA remaining is digested away with either S_1 nuclease or RNase A/RNase T_1 (see Fig. 2). The protected double-stranded RNA is then run on an acrylamide gel so that each of the protected bands can be resolved. The bands are then cut out of the gel and counted in a scintillation counter. The level of radioactivity in the excised bands is then converted into picograms of RNA from the standard curve.

Isolation of Cell Nuclei and Cytoplasm

This protocol was initially developed so that you can rapidly process a large number of samples with little transfer of the sample (1). This is in contrast to several of the published protocols which require an ultracentrifugation step and at least two transfers of the nuclei. To isolate cell nuclei from fresh tissue, homogenize between 25 and 50 mg wet weight ($\sim 3 \times 10^6$ cells) per milliliter of cold RNase-free AT buffer [10 mM Tris-HCl, pH 8, 3 mM $CaCl_2$, 2 mM $MgCl_2$, 0.5 mM dithiothreitol (DTT), 0.3 M sucrose, 0.15% Triton X-100] in a glass/Teflon homogenizer. In general, the primary transcript is present at a level of about 1% of the steady-state mRNA levels. Thus, the amount of tissue that will be required to perform the analysis will depend on the level of gene expression of the gene of interest. For the neuroendocrine peptide genes thus far analyzed from brain tissue, one usually needs to pool together microdissected tissue from several animals to get enough material ($\sim$1,000,000 nuclei), although this will obviously vary with every system. To completely homogenize the tissue, it usually only requires 10 strokes done by hand. Then, carefully layer the homogenate over 400 μl of 0.4 M AT buffer (the same as AT buffer except that it contains 0.4 M sucrose rather than 0.3 M sucrose) in a 1.5-ml microcentrifuge tube. Centrifuge at 2500 g for 10 min at 4°C. The supernatant, leaving behind the 0.4 M AT cushion, is removed and can be used for cytoplasmic RNA and protein analysis. Discard the 0.4 M AT cushion from the nuclei pellet. The cushion serves to protect the nuclear fraction from contamination of any RNase present in the cytosol fraction. Add 1 ml of 0.3 M AT buffer to the nuclear pellet and very gently resuspend the nuclei by flicking the tube with your finger. Do not vortex, as this tends to lyse the nuclei and release DNA, which will make the solution very viscous and interfere with subsequent RNA isolation. Centrifuge once again at 2500 g for 10 min at 4°C. Remove the supernatant and the pellet is the nuclear fraction to be used for RNA isolation.

To isolate nuclei from cells in culture, merely remove the tissue culture media, which you may want to save to quantitate peptide or neurotransmitter release, and add cold AT buffer. For example, with a 100-mm confluent tissue culture dish (~5 × 10^6 cells) add 2 ml of AT buffer, scrape the cells off with a rubber policeman, and split into two tubes each containing 400 μl of 0.4 M AT buffer and proceed as described above.

Quantitation of Nuclear hnRNA and mRNA

This section will describe how to quantitate RNA using a very sensitive solution hybridization S_1 nuclease protection assay [Ref. (2), modified from Durnam and Palmiter (3)]. With the availability of a new generation of vectors which contain promoters for specific bacteriophage RNA polymerases, it is possible to synthesize high-specific-activity antisense RNA probes. In addition, large quantities of sense RNA can also be synthesized with these vectors to make well-characterized standards. Having both of these tools, one can hybridize RNA samples in solution with a high-specific-activity antisense RNA probe and set up a standard curve with synthetic sense strand. By having a standard curve with a known amount of RNA it makes it possible to then express the hybridized radioactivity in the unknown samples as a mass amount rather than a relative density number or equivalents, as done with either Northern or dot-blot analysis. This allows one to compare across experiments or with other laboratories. With the high-specific-activity antisense probe, it is possible to routinely detect less than 0.5 pg of a specific RNA, allowing for analysis of the low levels of the primary transcript, processing intermediates, and the amount of mature mRNA in the nucleus, as well as the low levels of gene expression often seen in the central nervous system (CNS).

To purify the primary transcript, processing intermediates, and mature mRNA in the nucleus, first isolate the nuclear pellet as described above. Resuspend the pellet in 300 μl of DNase buffer (50 mM Tris-HCl, pH 8, 5 mM MgCl$_2$, 1 mM MnCl$_2$, 1 mM DTT), and 1 μl of RNasin (20 U/μl), 2 μl of DNase I (20 μl/μl, Worthington ultrapure and RNase-free) and incubate for 5 min at 37°C. Then add 30 μl of 10× SET (1× SET: 1% SDS, 5 mM EDTA, 10 mM Tris-HCl, pH 8) and 3 μl of proteinase K (10 mg/ml) and incubate for 1 hr at 45°C. Add 175 μl of phenol (saturated with TE), vortex, and then add 175 μl of chloroform. Vortex again and centrifuge (16,000 g) at room temperature for 5 min, remove the aqueous phase and transfer it to a 1.5-ml microcentrifuge tube. Add 40 μl of 3 M ammonium acetate and 1 ml of 100% ethanol and store at −20°C until ready to use.

To quantitate the amount of a specific RNA by the protection assay, first synthesize the sense strand to be used for a standard, so it is possible to express the data in picograms of a specific RNA per amount of total RNA put into the assay. The synthesis is done as outlined by Promega. Briefly, linearize the probe 3' to the insert. If using a vector which has a promoter on either side, linearize such that the coding sequence can be made. Set up the reaction as follows: 28 μl H_2O, 10 μl 5× transcription buffer (200 mM Tris-HCl, pH 7.5, 30 mM $MgCl_2$, 10 mM spermidine, 50 mM NaCl), 0.5 μl of 1 M DTT, 2 μl RNasin, 0.5 μl of 50 mM ATP, 0.5 μl of 50 mM CTP, 0.5 μl of 50 mM GTP, 0.5 μl of 50 mM UTP, 5 μl of linearized DNA template (1 μg/μl), 2 μl (of the appropriate polymerase: SP6, T3, or T7) RNA polymerase (5 U/μl). Incubate for 1 hr at 37°C. Then add 50 μl of H_2O, 5 μl of 1 M Tris-HCl, pH 8, 1 μl of 1 M $MgCl_2$, 1 μl RNasin, 1.5 μl of DNase I (10 ng/μl, Worthington ultrapure) and incubate at 37°C for 30 min. To purify the probe away from any unincorporated nucleotides run the sample on a Sephadex G-100 column (4). Usually around 10 to 20 μg is synthesized in this reaction. To quantitate the amount of RNA synthesized, one can either read the optical density or include in the reaction 0.5 μl of [α-^{32}P]UTP (400 Ci/mmol), calculate the percentage incorporation and thus determine the amount synthesized. The resulting specific activity is only about 1 cpm/pg so it will not interfere with the assay. Once you determine the concentration of the probe, make several 1:10 serial dilutions until you get to the desired working concentration. We have found that the RNA synthesized for standard is stable when stored at −70°C. Several aliquots of the lower dilutions are made and frozen away. For long-term stability, the highest concentration can be then stored precipitated under ethanol at −20°C.

To quantitate the amount of RNA in the 0.250- to 5-pg range, synthesize the antisense strand at a specific activity of ~2 × 10^9 cpm/μg. This is done by drying down 200 μCi of [α-^{32}P]UTP (~800 Ci/mmol), then adding 3.5 μl of H_2O, 2 μl of 5× transcription buffer, 1 μl of 100 mM DTT, 0.5 μl of RNasin, 0.5 μl of 50 mM ATP, 0.5 μl of 50 mM CTP, 0.5 μl of GTP, 1 μl of linearized DNA template (1 μg/μg), and 0.5 μl of the specific RNA polymerase (10 U/μl) and incubating at 37°C for 1 hr. After the incubation, add 92 μl of H_2O and take two 1-μl aliquots to determine the total counts per minute incorporated and the total counts per minute in the reaction. In this way, determine the fraction of incorporation and calculate the amount synthesized. Add 5 μl of 1 M Tris-HCl, pH 8, 1 μl of 1 M $MgCl_2$, 1 μl of yeast RNA (10 μg/μl), 1 μl of RNasin (20 U/μl), and 1 μl of DNase I (10 ng/μl, Worthington ultrapure and RNase free) and incubate at 37°C for 30 min to remove the DNA template. Purify the probe by running on a Sephadex G-100 column. Probes synthesized at this specific activity are not very stable and can only be used to nuclease protection assays for 3 days at most. The reason is that, wherever the ^{32}P decays, the probe breaks into smaller and smaller pieces until finally the probe will only give a smear instead of a protected band. One should verify that the probe synthesized is full length before using it by running it on a Tris/borate/EDTA acrylamide gel (4) as described for the assay below.

To perform a nuclease protection assay, first set up a series of tubes for a standard curve; for example add 0 RNA to tube 1, 0.5 pg of specific coding RNA to tube 2, 1 pg of specific coding RNA to tube 3, etc. Add TE to the standard tubes to bring the final volume up to 5 μl. Add your "unknown" RNA samples to the next set of tubes also in a final volume of 5 μl. Then, to each tube add ~100 pg of the newly synthesized antisense RNA probe (~10^9 cpm/μg) in a volume of 5 μl. One should add at least 10-fold excess probe to the expected sample RNA so that the hybridization will be driven to completion; therefore, when analyzing in the 0.5- to 5-pg range, one should add between 50 and 100 pg of probe. Finally, add 20 μl of the hybridization mix (60% formamide, 0.9 *M* NaCl, 6 m*M* EDTA, 60 m*M* Tris-HCl, pH 7.4, 2.5 mg/ml yeast RNA), mix, and add two drops of mineral oil over each sample to prevent evaporation. Heat denature at 85°C for 5 min and incubate overnight (~16 hr) at 68°C. This hybridization time allows for even very-low-abundance RNAs to hybridize to completion. Transfer the samples to fresh microcentrifuge tubes, leaving behind the oil. Add 300 μl of 1× S$_1$ nuclease buffer (0.3 *M* NaCl, 30 m*M* sodium acetate, pH 4.8, 3 m*M* ZnCl) and add the S$_1$ nuclease, which you will have to titer. For S$_1$ nuclease purchased from Sigma, usually about 1500 to 2500 U is required to completely digest the unprotected material. Some investigators like to use RNase A and RNase T$_1$ rather than S$_1$ nuclease. RNase works well, it is cheaper, and can even give a cleaner signal. However, we prefer in general not to use it because it is harder to control than S$_1$ nuclease, which needs to be at an acidic pH and requires zinc, whereas RNase can work under any condition, i.e., it is hard to get rid of. So when one is working with precious RNA samples we find it safer not to work with large quantities of RNase. However, we have found that some double-stranded sequences are suscepti-ble to S$_1$ nuclease digestion but are resistant to RNase digestion and vice versa. Therefore in some cases RNase protection is the method of choice. When RNase is used it should also be titrated rather than just using the 40 μg/ml of RNase A and 2 μg/ml of RNase T$_1$ as described in the Promega protocol, for you may overdigest your samples. After adding the S$_1$ nuclease to the samples, incubate for 1 hr at 56°C. Add 40 μl of 5 *M* ammonium acetate, pH 4.8, 1 μl of 0.5 *M* EDTA, 1 μl of yeast RNA (10 μg/ml), 150 μl of phenol (saturated with TE), vortex samples, and add 150 μl of chloroform. Vortex samples and centrifuge (16,000 *g*) for 5 min. Extract the samples and transfer to 1.5-ml microcentrifuge tubes and add 600 μl of 2-propanol and store at −20°C for at least 1 hr. Then spin down the samples in a microfuge for 10 min, pour off the supernatant, and add 0.5 ml of 70% ethanol, vortex, and centrifuge for 5 min. Carefully take off the supernatant, for the pellets can be a bit slippery, then dry them. Resuspend the pellets in 4 μl of 1× TE and 1 μl of 5× dye mix. Heat denature at 65°C for 5 min. Load the samples on a Tris/borate/EDTA acrylamide gel (4). After running the gel, dry it and expose to X-ray film with an intensifying screen at −70°C. Then, using the X-ray film as a guide, cut out the protected bands and count them in a scintillation counter. Some investigators (3) merely TCA precipitate the protected material, collect the precipitate onto filters, and count the filters, rather than running the gel. However, we have found that fractionating the protected material on a gel gives much more sensitivity necessary for low-level nuclear RNA detection by spreading the background throughout the gel and gives additional information, such as protected fragment size, making it easier to trouble shoot when something goes wrong with the assay. One other major advantage is that multiple species can be detected in a single assay, as shown in Fig. 2, greatly increasing the information obtained from precious samples. It is possible to quantitate 500 fg and, if you use very fresh probe, it is possible to detect down to 200 fg. We have found the standard curve to be very reproducible; however, the actual amount of radioactivity (counts per minute) protected for each point varies as the probe gets older. Usually we analyze each "unknown" sample two to three times and have found the assay to be very reproducible despite the numerous transfers. Our interassay coefficient of variation from an aliquoted 10 pg standard has been 4.3%.

If a probe is synthesized that is complementary to an intron–exon–intron junction, it is possible to detect the primary transcript which will protect the full-length probe (see Fig. 2). It is also possible to detect processing intermediates with this probe. By synthesizing the probe such that the regions that are complementary to the two different introns are of unequal lengths, it can be determined which of two possible pathways processing takes. And finally, with this same probe, the amount of mature mRNA in the nucleus can be measured. One thing that you need to consider when measuring nuclear RNA compared to cytoplasmic RNA is to make sure that the probe is in 10-fold excess for all protected bands being measured. For example, the amount of primary transcript may be in 10-fold excess of the processing intermediates and the mature mRNA. In addition, one would need the standard curve to span a wider range.

Normally, data from this type of assay are expressed relative to total amount of RNA, which is measured by optical density at 260 nm. However, the excess of DNA relative to RNA in the nucleus (about 5-fold) makes it difficult to perform such analysis, even after extensive DNase digestion. Therefore, we have expressed the data either per amount of DNA or per nuclei since each nuclei should contain the same amount of DNA. To do this, an aliquot of the nuclei is taken before the final centrifugation step and either counted in a hemocytometer or used in a DNA quantitation assay (4).

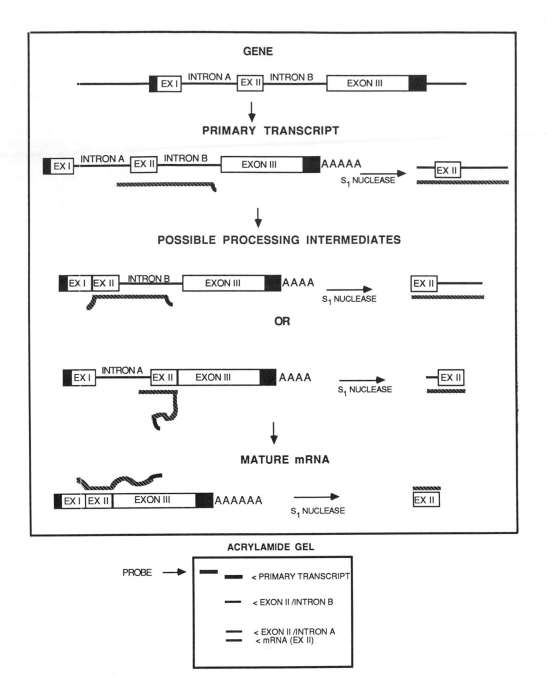

FIG. 2 Schematic of the nuclease protection/solution hybridization outlining the various protected RNA species in the assay. Note that the probe contains a nonhomologous extension on the 5′ end, which is derived from the promoter in the vector. Thus, undigested probe is always different from fully protected RNA.

Intervening Sequence *in Situ* Hybridization

Quite often in the complex and heterogeneous CNS there may be more than one cell type in the region of interest expressing the gene you are studying. In that case, the data on nuclear RNA levels you obtain by the solution hybridization/nuclease protection assay will reflect contributions from all of them, giving you an average, albeit very accurate, value. One way to combine the anatomical resolution of histological procedures with measurements of posttranscriptional nuclear events is to utilize the procedure of *in situ* hybridization with probes that recognize only nuclear species of the RNAs from the gene of interest. As discussed in the first paragraph of this chapter, the intervening sequences are located exclusively in the nucleus (Fig. 1) and are present in significant quantities only in the primary transcript and its processing intermediates. Thus, this assay utilizes intervening sequence-specific probes in an *in situ* hybridization protocol on sections of brain tissue.

Basically the procedure of intervening sequence *in situ* hybridization is similar to that of cytoplasmic RNA *in situ* hybridization in which radioactive nucleic acid probes are used to identify specific sequences of nucleotides in RNAs fixed in the tissue section (5). We have already used this procedure to analyze proopiomelanononocortin (POMC) primary transcripts in the anterior pituitary and verified its value in studying gene expression at the single-cell level (6). More recently, we have extended it to the CNS, which is the basis of the procedure described here (7).

Our initial attempts to perform the brain intervening sequence *in situ* assay were done with hypothalamic sections from cardiac perfused rats [4% (w/v) paraformaldehyde in PBS, 4°C, 20 min, 120–155 mm Hg] as reported previously for our pituitary POMC intervening sequence *in situ* hybridizations (6). While this approach worked for the pituitary (a highly vascularized tissue with fenestrated blood vessels), we failed to obtain a detectable signal from perfusion-fixed hypothalamic neuronal nuclei. We reasoned that possibly it may take too long for the paraformaldehyde to reach the brain neuron nuclei and the primary transcript was being lost due to its extremely short half-life ($t_{1/2} < 15$–30 min). Switching to a rapid postfixing procedure with the same fixer allowed us to detect nuclear primary transcripts from the POMC gene.

After experimental manipulation, rats are decapitated and the brains quickly dissected, placed on ice-cold M-1 embedding medium (Lipshaw Manufacturing Co.) and frozen in liquid ntirogen. Twelve-micrometer crystat sections are cut, thaw-mounted onto gelatin- and poly(lysine)-coated glass microscope slides (5), and stored at −70°C until use. When ready to perform the experiment, tissue sections are postfixed by thawing in ice-cold

4% paraformaldehyde in PBS for 10 min. Following postfixation with paraformaldehyde, the sections are washed for 10 min in 2× SSC. Tissue sections are then covered with prehybridization solutions [50% formamide, 0.6 *M* NaCl, 10 m*M* Tris-HCl, pH 7.5; 0.02% Ficoll, 0.02% poly(vinylpyrolidine), 0.1% bovine serum albumin, 1 m*M* EDTA, pH 8.0; 50 μg/ml salmon sperm DNA, 500 μg/ml yeast total RNA, 50 μg/ml yeast transfer RNA] and prehybridized for 60–120 min at 50°C. Following prehybridization, the buffer is removed, and the tissue sections were covered with hybridization solutions [50% (w/v) formamide, 0.6 *M* NaCl, 10 m*M* Tris-HCl, pH 7.5; 0.02% Ficoll, 0.02% poly(vinylpyrrolidone), 0.1% bovine serum albumin, 1 m*M* EDTA, pH 8.0; 10 μg/ml salmon sperm DNA, 50 μg/ml yeast total RNA, 50 μg/ml yeast transfer RNA, 10 m*M* DTT, 10% dextran sulfate] containing 2.5 to 10 × 10^6 cpm/ml ^{35}S-labeled intervening sequence complementary RNA probe which has been heat denatured for 10–15 min at 65°C. The sections are then hybridized for 16–18 hr at 50°C in boxes humidified with 50% formamide and 4× SSC. Following hybridization, the sections are washed in 3 liters of 2× SSC at 45°C for 30 min and subjected to RNase A digestion (30 μg/ml in 500 m*M* NaCl, 10 m*M* Tris-HCl, pH 7.5) for 60 min at 37°C. The sections are then washed in 3 liters of 2× SSC at 45°C for 60 min followed by a final high-stringency wash in 4 liters of 0.1× SSC, 0.15% sodium pyrophosphate, and 14 m*M* 2-mercaptoethanol for 3 hr at 50°C followed by an overnight wash in the same buffer at room temperature. The sections are dehydrated through graded alcohols containing 0.3 *M* ammonium acetate and dried in a vacuum desiccator. For visualization of the hybrids, the slides are dipped in Kodak NTB2 nuclear track emulsion (Eastman Kodak Co.) and exposed for the indicated time at 4°C in light-tight boxes with desiccant capsules. Development was carried out in Kodak D-19 developer as described by the manufacturer. After fixation, the slides are washed for 30 min in distilled water and stained with hematoxylin and eosin to visualize cytoplasm and nucleus.

Following a 6- to 8-week exposure, silver grains are specifically localized over the nuclei of neurons, paralleling the distribution previously established by immunohistochemistry for the gene of interest. Thus, the autoradiographic signal obtained with the intervening sequence probes appears to result from specific hybridization to primary transcripts of the gene localized in the nuclei of the expressing neurons. Consistent with the observation that there is approximately one to two orders of magnitude less nuclear primary transcript relative to the related cytoplasmic mRNA, considerably longer exposure times (6–8 weeks) are required with intervening sequence probes for a detectable autoradiographic signal compared to the mRNA-specific probes (3–5 days).

The grains over the nuclei can be counted manually or by any one of many commercially available image analysis systems. The grain count per nucleus is relatively proportional to the amount of intervening sequence present in the nucleus. This value should be treated semiquantitatively, however, since the efficiency of hybridization of the probe to the nuclear RNA is unknown. In addition, the possibility that the availability of the RNA in the tissue section to the probe might vary with the experimental treatment further complicates interpretation of the data. However, even with these caveats, we have still been able to use this system to analyze transcription of the POMC gene in a tissue accurately where we could verify the results.

Conclusion

In conclusion, we have described two assays, one biochemical and one histochemical, to study posttranscriptional events in the nucleus. While the solution hybridization/nuclease protection assay is very accurate and yields much information concerning the levels of all the different RNA species derived from a gene, its resolution is defined by the tissue dissection from which the RNA was isolated. The *in situ* hybridization assay gives excellent single-cell anatomical resolution, but fails to resolve the different RNA species. The best study, therefore, is one that combines both assays to give a comprehensive view of nuclear posttranscriptional events in the brain.

References

1. M. Blum, B. S. McEwen, and J. L. Roberts, *J. Biol. Chem.* **262,** 817 (1987).
2. M. Blum, *In* "Methods in Enzymology" (P. M. Conn, ed.), Vol. 168, p. 618. Academic Press, San Diego, California, 1989.
3. D. M. Durnam and R. D. Palmiter, *Anal. Biochem.* **131,** 385 (1983).
4. T. Maniatis, E. F. Fritsch, and J. Sambrook, *in* "Molecular Cloning: A Laboratory Manual." Cold Spring Harbor Laboratory, Cold Spring Harbor, New York, 1982.
5. J. N. Wilcox, C. E. Gee, and J. L. Roberts, *in* "Methods in Enzymology" (P. M. Conn, ed.), Vol. 124, p. 510. Academic Press, Orlando, Florida, 1986.
6. R. T. Fremeau, Jr., J. R. Lundblad, D. B. Pritchett, J. N. Wilcox, and J. L. Roberts, *Science* **234,** 1265 (1986).
7. R. T. Fremeau, D. J. Autelitano, M. Blum, J. N. Wilcox, and J. L. Roberts, *Mol. Brain Res.,* in press, 1989.

Section III

Screening, Sequencing, and Cloning

[18]   Immunoscreening λgt11 cDNA Library

John S. Kizer and Thomas O. Brock

Bacteriophage λgt11 is an extremely useful cloning vector that can cause its bacterial host to express a foreign protein (1). This characteristic of λgt11 makes it possible to recognize a complementary DNA clone (cDNA) if one has the wherewithal to identify the protein. Because of the rarity with which expressed proteins are fully biologically functional, immunological detection of the expressed proteins is usually the most practical.

Theory

λgt11 is a double-stranded DNA bacteriophage whose genome has been modified so as to contain an exon for β-galactosidase. Included near the end of the β-galactosidase gene is an *Eco*RI restriction enzyme site. Because this restriction site is unique, "libraries" of cDNAs can be constructed by ligating cDNA mixtures with attached *Eco*RI termini into the λ genome at this site.

When a suitable *Escherichia coli* host (such as Y1090) that lacks β-galactosidase is infected with the modified phage, the introduction of the β-galactosidase exon (*lac*Z) into the host by the phage permits the cell to synthesize β-galactosidase in the presence of an inducer such as IPTG (isopropylthio-β-galactoside). Thus, phage λgt11 grown on a bacterial lawn will produce blue plaques in the presence of IPTG and the indicator substrate X-gal (5-bromo-4-chloro-3-indolyl-β-D-galactoside). If, however, a cDNA has been inserted into the *Eco*RI restriction site of the β-galactosidase gene of λ, then the plaques will be clear, indicating that the β-galactosidase gene is no longer intact. Furthermore, in place of the β-galactosidase which can no longer be synthesized in its entirety, the host will synthesize a fusion protein comprising the N-terminal fragment of β-galactosidase coupled to the peptide corresponding to the cDNA insert. The phage plaques can then be directly blotted onto a solid support, and the blots screened immunologically for the presence of β-galactosidase–peptide fusion proteins using an antiserum raised against a peptide of interest.

It is important to remember, however, that immunological screening of a λgt11 cDNA library is only one-sixth as likely to detect a clone of interest as is hybridization screening because the cDNA insert must have the proper 5′–3′ orientation and the proper reading frame within the β-galactosidase gene to direct the correct translation of the corresponding peptide.

Methods in Neurosciences, Volume 1

Choice of Antiserum

As a rule, in immunoscreening a λgt11 library, monospecific polyclonal antibodies are likely to be more useful than monoclonal antibodies. There are several reasons for this. (1) Polyclonal antisera are more likely to contain at least one clone that will recognize the antigen in an altered conformation, i.e., blotted onto a solid phase. (2) Polyclonal antisera may contain several clones reacting with different antigenic sites on the peptide of interest, thereby increasing the likelihood of detecting partial cDNAs during screening. (3) Polyclonal antisera are easier to obtain. (4) Polyclonal antisera are more likely to recognize nonglycosylated forms of a glycosylated immunogen, an important consideration since the fusion proteins generated in *E. coli* are not glycosylated.

Before undertaking to screen a cDNA library, it is important to test the usefulness of potential antisera under conditions similar to those that will be used for the screening, i.e., by testing the ability of the antisera to detect proteins blotted onto a solid support such as nitrocellulose. Not all antisera that are useful for radioimmunoassay of a given protein will detect the same protein immobilized on a membrane. Thus, if this step is bypassed, negative results from immunoscreening may indicate only a unsuitable antiserum, not the absence of clones containing the desired fusion protein.

Antisera of high titer are easier to work with than those of low titer because high working dilutions of primary antiserum (usually greater than 1 : 1500) give a very low background by diluting out endogenous antibodies against *E. coli* proteins. This usually obviates the need for preabsorption of the antiserum with *E. coli* lysates (see below).

Finally, in our laboratory, purified IgG has not proved to be superior to diluted, unpurified antisera for immunoscreening.

Preparation of Plates

Plates of 150 mm diameter are filled with 75 ml or 90-mm plates filled with 30 ml of "bottom agar" (1.5% agar) made up according to the following recipe for 1 liter:

LB broth	25 g
(Bacto tryptone 10 g/liter, Bacto yeast extract 5 g/liter, NaCl 10 g/liter)	
Distilled water	1.0 liter

| 10 *M* NaOH | 0.35 ml |
| Bacto agar | 15 g |

Autoclave for 20 min and cool to 52°C (the bottom agar may be kept for extended periods at this temperature). Before pouring the plates, add 4 ml of ampicillin from a stock solution of 25 mg/ml in distilled water (final concentration 100 μg/ml).

Allow the plates to cool and solidify with the tops removed (to prevent contamination, this is best carried out in a laminar flow hood for 30 min or in a UV box for several hours). The purpose of this step is to dry the medium sufficiently so that the top agar will adhere tightly and not peel off as the blotting membranes are removed. If a laminar flow hood is not available for the drying step, the plates should be incubated for 24–48 hr at 37°C to allow for further drying. They may be stored for several weeks at 4°C if tightly wrapped. Before use they should be incubated for several hours at 37°C.

Eighty-millimeter plates are most useful for titering phage, whereas 150-mm plates are most useful for plaque screening and amplification.

Preparation of Top Agar

Top agar (0.8%) may be prepared in small quantities for immediate use or in large batches. When large quantities are prepared, these should be divided into 100- or 200-ml aliquots and stored for later use at room temperature without ampicillin. When needed, aliquots can be rapidly melted in a microwave oven at the defrost setting.

LB broth	25 g
(Bacto tryptone 10 g/liter, Bacto yeast extract 5 g/liter, NaCl 10 g/liter)	
Distilled water	1.0 liter
10 *M* NaOH	0.35 ml
1 *M* MgCl$_2$	20 ml
Agarose*	8 g

Autoclave and cool to 52°C. If the top agar is to be used the same day, add 4 ml of ampicillin (25 mg/ml in distilled water) and maintain at 52°C in a water bath for pouring.

---

* Agarose should be used to prepare "top agar" due to its better tensile strength as compared to agar. This is important when overlaying the plate with a nitrocellulose or other membrane to prevent tearing of the top agar layer as the membrane is removed.

If X-gal is to be included in the top agar, to 100 ml of top agar add 2 ml of a 25 mg/ml of X-gal dissolved in *N,N*-dimethylformamide. (Please note: formamide is not the same chemical and will chemically destroy the X-gal). The final concentration in the agar will be 50 μg/ml.

Selection of Bacterial Host

The most widely used hosts for λgt11 are *E. coli* Y strains (1, 2). All these strains contain an ampicillin resistance plasmid, while some strains contain other important and useful genes that may vary depending on the commercial source. For example, Y1088 is *hsdR*⁻, which means that the strain does not synthesize restriction enzymes that may damage the infecting λ DNA (3). This host is best for amplification of a cDNA library to ensure that no fragments are lost. Usually, Y1090 and Y1089 are not *hsdR*⁻, but these two strains are *hsdR*⁻ when obtained from Promega (Madison, WI) and can be used for amplification also. In addition, Y strains (except Y1088) are also usually protease negative (lon) so that fusion proteins are not rapidly degraded. Y1090 and Y1089 differ in that the latter has the *hflA* mutation, resulting in a very high frequency of λ lysogeny. Thus, Y1090 grows temperately, resulting in lytic as well as lysogenic growth and is the best host for plaque immunoscreening of a cDNA library. Y1089, on the other hand, does not grow lytically and, therefore, is most useful for expressing large amounts of fusion protein.

Preparation and Plating of Phage

SM buffer [Maniatis *et al.* (4)]: This buffer is an all-purpose buffer used for storage, dilution, and manipulation of phage.

NaCl	5.8 g
MgSO₄·7H₂O	2.0 g
1.0 *M* Tris-HCl (pH 7.5)	50 ml
2% gelatin	5 ml

Autoclave for 15 min and store in small aliquots of 50–100 ml.

To grow the phage, it is first necessary to streak out the host Y1090 on LB plates to obtain single colonies. These are grown overnight at 37°C until bacterial growth is clearly visible. Next, a single colony is removed from the plate with a sterile loop and inoculated into 5 ml of LB broth (see above; no agar added) to which has been added 20 μl of ampicillin (25 mg/ml), 50 μl of sterile 1.0 M MgSO$_4$, and 50 μl of sterile 20% maltose. (The plate may now be stored at 4°C for several weeks and single colonies removed as needed.) The broth tube is incubated in an orbital shaker (250–300 rpm) at 37°C for 3–5 hr until visibly turbid. For each plate that is to receive phage, aliquot 0.3 ml (0.5 ml if 150-mm plates are used) of the broth culture into a separate 15-ml culture tube. The λ phage are diluted as necessary with SM buffer and added to the tubes of broth in volumes of 5–20 μl. For titering, serial 100-fold dilutions are most useful. Next the tubes are incubated at 37°C for 15–20 min to allow the phage to adsorb to the bacteria and inject their DNA.

To plate the phage-infected bacteria, 3–4 ml (8–9 ml for 150-mm plates) of the top agar solution is added to the broth tubes and plated on *prewarmed* LB plates. The top agar solution should be added to a single tube, quickly vortexed, and spread as rapidly and evenly as possible over the bottom agar by tilting the plate back and forth. Bubbles should be quickly removed by poking with a sharp, sterile needle. With practice, the top agar can be spread evenly without bubbles, although at first the rapid solidification of the top agar can be frustrating. The plates are inverted and incubated overnight at 37°C. Plaques may first be visible within 6–8 hr and are almost always fully developed within 12–16 hr. The titer of phage particles [plaque-forming units (pfu)/ml] may then be calculated.

Amplification by Plate Lysis

If the cDNA library is already amplified, then it is only necessary to titer the library to determine the number of plaque-forming units per milliliter. If the library has not been amplified, it should be amplified in either *E. coli* Y1088 or Y1090 containing the *hsdR*⁻ mutation.

For amplification of a newly constructed library, a small aliquot of the total ligated and packaged cDNA is plated on X-gal LB media, and the total number of plaque-forming units and the ratio of blue to clear plaques are determined. This provides an index of the total number of recombinants or the degree of "complexity" of the library. Next, the entire remainder of the ligated and packaged cDNA is mixed with host cells and amplified by the plate lysate method (see below). After amplification, a reserve of the library (see below) should be stored in SM buffer with 7% DMSO (dimethyl sulfoxide) at −70°C.

To amplify a single plaque, one first obtains a "plug" from a plate with a sterile pipette or touches the tip of a sterilized toothpick to the center of a plaque. The phage on the tip of the toothpick may be inoculated directly into the broth as outlined in *Preparation of Top Agar*. The agar plug is best placed in a 1.5-ml polypropylene microcentrifuge tube along with 1 ml of SM buffer and 30 μl of chloroform. The tube is vortexed and allowed to sit at room temperature for 1–2 hr. At this point, the phage may be pipetted from the liquid above the agar into the host-containing broth as outlined in *Preparation of Top Agar*.

Amplification of a library is carried out in much the same manner, but one should be very careful not to add so many plaque-forming units or allow growth to continue so long that the plaques touch one another. If the plaques grow together or the plate is allowed to incubate until confluent lysis is obtained, there is the potential for recombination among the phage, with a consequent degeneration of the library.

The phage are "harvested" by adding 5 ml of sterile SM buffer to the plates, replacing the lids, and agitating on an orbital shaker at 60–70 rpm for 2 hr. Alternatively, the plates may be incubated at 4°C overnight, and agitated briefly the next morning with equally good results. The SM buffer is then carefully poured or pipetted into a polypropylene tube and chloroform added to a final concentration of 3.0%. The bacteria will lyse and settle to the bottom, leaving the phage in the aqueous layer. The phage are stable in this solution at 4°C for many months.

Preparation of Membrane Blots of Plaques

Once the library is amplified and titered, then one may begin to immunoscreen the library for positive clones. In deciding how many plaque-forming units to screen, it is necessary to know the original complexity (base number of recombinants) within the library and the titer of the amplified library. As a general rule, one should screen enough plaques to give confidence that, statistically, at least one of each type of recombinant phage derived from the original library has been examined. For example, if the amplified library contains 10^9 pfu/ml, and the original library contained 0.5×10^6 pfu with 75% recombinants, then at a minimum one would need to screen 0.67×10^6 pfu (0.67 μl) from the amplified library. In practice, it is useful to screen a 20–30% excess to provide for a statistical margin of error. When the volume to be removed from the library is determined, this volume should be removed all at the same time and either screened or placed in another tube since withdrawing portions of the library at different times destroys the selection statistics of a single removal.

In our laboratory, we have found that screening is best carried out on 150-mm plates carrying about 30,000 plaques per plate. The phage are grown and plated as described *Preparation and Plating of Phage*. Instead of incubating the plated phage at 37°C, however, the plates are incubated at 42°C for 3.5 hr. While the plates are incubating, prepare a solution of IPTG (10 mM in distilled water; sterilized by filtration) and soak the required number of 137-mm-diameter nitrocellulose membranes thoroughly in this solution. (The most economical means to do this is to fill a sterile petri dish with 50 ml of the IPTG solution and individually layer the membranes into the dish, carefully wetting both sides before inserting the next membrane.) After soaking, the filters should be laid out to dry *thoroughly*. In our laboratory, a laminar flow hood is the best way to accomplish this, not only drying the membranes but keeping them as sterile as possible. (The membranes should be handled with forceps and gloves at all times.) If the membranes are dry before applying to the plates, there is better adhesion of the plaque proteins to the membrane. Before the membranes are applied to the plates, they should be marked at the edge with a No. 2 pencil for identification.

After the 3.5 hr, 42°C incubation, the plates are carefully covered with the dry IPTG membranes without trapping air bubbles between the membrane and the agar. (The easiest method for applying the filters is to grasp them at 9 o'clock and 3 o'clock and fold the membranes together. Next place the long axis of the fold into the center of the plate and allow the moisture in the agar to pull the membrane down onto the surface of the plate. Once the membranes have touched the agar, they should not be repositioned.) The tops of the petri dishes are replaced and the plates incubated for a further 3.5 hr at 37°C.

At the end of the second 3.5-hr incubation, the plates are ready for removal of the membranes. (If a duplicate membrane is desired, a second IPTG-saturated membrane may be applied after removal of the first and the plates incubated for a further 3.5 hr. In our laboratory, this second blot is not of as high a quality as is the original.)

Before removing a blotted membrane from a plate, its position on the agar should be marked by inserting a sterile needle through the membrane in at least two different sites. This is necessary so that the position of the membrane relative to the agar can be determined after screening. After the membrane is removed, the plate is covered and stored at 4°C until the screening is completed.

(The screening of the membrane should be completed as soon as possible so that the plates will not suffer overgrowth or excessive phage diffusion. If the plates develop white granular growth or other fungus growth within 2–3 days, this is due to contamination of the plates during set up. In our laboratory, because all these steps are carried out in a laminar flow hood we have had few problems with contamination of the cultures.)

Immunoscreening of the Blotted Membrane

After the membranes are lifted from the plates, they are allowed to completely dry, *plaque side up,* in a laminar flow hood.

[NOTE: In almost all instruction manuals, one is cautioned not to let the membranes dry. This is not only not necessary, but counterproductive since the proteins will adhere more tightly to the membrane if allowed to dry thoroughly. Sometimes one may find that the immobilized antigen is more readily recognized by the screening antiserum if the dry membrane is first heated to 50–60°C in an oven for 15 min or treated with 1% KOH for 5 min, rinsed, and redried. Conditions such as these, however, should be developed before screening (see *Choice of Antiserum*).]

Once the membranes are dry, they are ready for immunoscreening. There are many protocols and commercial kits and reagents available for immunoblotting, and there is not one particular method or source that is better than another, all work well. Any method that works well for standard protein blotting will also work well for screening an expression library. The only important choice with respect to method concerns the manner of detection of the immobilized immune complexes. Second antibody–peroxidase conjugates are nearly 5- to 10-fold less sensitive than those composed of alkaline phosphatase. Newer polyconjugates of alkaline phosphatase can increase the sensitivity to almost another order of magnitude, but this degree of sensitivity is not necessary for plaque screening. Other methods of detection such as radiolabeled protein A can be used, but this requires autoradiography, and orientation of the position of the membrane with respect to the original plate is more complicated. Thus, for ease of use, quick results, and sensitivity, we recommend alkaline phosphatase as the reporter. [See Bers and Garfin for a readable summary of considerations in immunoblotting with an excellent bibliography (5). The following protocol is adapted from many of their suggestions.]

Solutions

> TBS (Tris-buffered saline)
>   400 mM NaCl, 20 mM Tris-HCl, pH 7.5
> Tween TBS
>   TBS containing 0.05% Tween 20
> Blocking TBS
>   TBS containing 3.0% gelatin
> Antibody TBS
>   Tween TBS containing 1.0% gelatin
> Color development solution

0.1 *M* NaHCO$_3$, 1.0 m*M* MgCl$_2$, pH 9.8. Containing 1 ml each of
BCIP and NBT stocks

BCIP (5-bromo-4-chloro-3-indoylphosphate *p*-toluidine salt). Made as a
stock solution (0.035 *M* in dimethylformamide). May be stored at 4°C
for many months if shielded from light

NBT (nitroblue tetrazolium). Made as a stock solution (0.035 *M* in 70%
dimethylformamide/water). Store similarly to BCIP

Gelatin is used for blocking in our laboratory, although we have determined that nonfat dry milk and high concentrations of albumin work equally
well.

Second antibody–alkaline phosphatase conjugates may be purchased from
several different commercial sources. Most are affinity purified and reason-
ably priced. One should follow the manufacturer's directions for the
recommended dilutions of these conjugates which can be made in antibody
TBS buffer. In addition, the manufacturer's recommendations for the
incubation conditions necessary for the enzymatic hydrolysis of the BCIP–
NBT substrate by the antibody alkaline phosphatase conjugate should also
be followed. Usually, either a sodium bicarbonate or borate buffer,
pH 9.6–9.8, containing 1.0 m*M* MgCl$_2$ is advised. The borate buffer is more
stable, but seems to give slightly poorer color development. The sodium
bicarbonate buffer should be made freshly every other month.

Protocol

For immunoscreening, the 137-mm membranes are transferred *plaque-side
up* to clean 150-mm petri dishes. All steps may be carried out in the same
dish, and the spent reagents removed by vacuum aspiration. Furthermore,
we have not found that incubation in the cold improves the results;
therefore, all steps in the screening are carried out at room temperature.
Continuous shaking of the dishes to ensure adequate flow of reagents is
necessary throughout.

1. Thoroughly wet the dried membranes in TBS (usually 5–10 min).
2. Wash twice for 5 min with Tween-TBS.
3. Wash for 1–2 hr with Blocking TBS
4. Wash twice for 5 min with Tween-TBS.
5. Incubate for 2 hr in primary antiserum diluted in Tween-TBS.
6. Wash twice for 5 min with Tween-TBS.
7. Incubate for 1–2 hr in second antibody. (Species-specific IgG–alkaline
   phosphatase conjugate.)
8. Wash twice for 5 min with Tween-TBS.
9. Wash once for 5 min with TBS.

10. Incubate for 0.5–5 hr in NBT/BCIP color development solution. Cover the dish to shield from light.
11. Wash membrane with distilled water for 5 min.

It is often suggested that the sensitivity of the immunooverlay can be improved by overnight incubations in the primary antiserum. In plaque screening, however, the amount of fusion protein on the blotted membrane is usually substantial, rendering prolonged incubations of only occasional help.

The optimal time of incubation for color development is variable and should be optimized for each lot of alkaline phosphatase–IgG conjugate. Usually, development for 90 min provides the best contrast between background and signal.

If the background is quite dark and there is concern lest the signal be difficult to discern, there are two possible approaches. First, use the antiserum at the highest possible dilution (see *Choice of Antiserum*). Second, add an *E. coli* lysate to the immune serum at a concentration of 10 mg/ml, or soak several membranes in an *E. coli* lysate, dry them, and incubate the serum with them for several hours. (*Escherichia coli* lysate affinity columns can be obtained commercially, but we have not found them to be useful.) It is important to remember not to discard the primary antibody solution after screening, especially if initially a high background is a problem, because the performance of the antiserum will improve with repeated use.

What Is a Positive Result?

One of the more frequent questions from those just beginning plaque immunoscreening concerns the identification of a positive clone. To help illustrate the identification of positive clones, we have photographed a membrane taken from a plate containing plaques derived from a single λ clone. Before immunoscreening, the membrane was cut in half, and the left half was screened with immune serum, while the right half was screened with immune serum in the presence of 10 μg/ml of the peptide used to generate the antiserum (Fig. 1). It is not difficult to distinguish positives from the background, which is usually a soft, light purple compared to the deep, dark blackish-purple of the positives. In addition, the morphology of the reaction product is helpful in identifying positive clones. Although not obvious in the photograph in Fig. 1 due to the intense deposition of reaction product, true positive staining appears as a small "doughnut" with a clear center due to the heavier synthesis of fusion protein at the margins of the

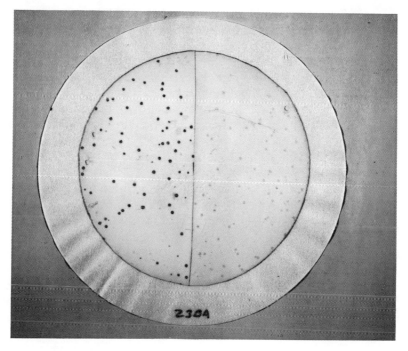

FIG. 1   Nitrocellulose membrane (0.45 μm) blotted onto a lawn of *E. coli* Y1089 infected with a pure clone of λgt11 and immunoscreened using an alkaline phosphatase–second antibody conjugate. See *What Is a Positive Result?* for discussion.

plaque—small solid specks are not positives. Background also has the doughnut configuration, however, making it necessary to use both color and morphology for identification.

The frequency of positive clones on initial screening is also helpful in deciding whether a clone is a true positive. For example, a modestly abundant cDNA will produce about 1–2 positive clones for every 30,000–60,000 clones screened. Screening for very abundant cDNAs, such as that for actin, may produce 10 times this frequency of positives.

Plaque Purification

Once a clone is identified by immunoscreening, the next step is to extract it from among all the other plaques on the plate and by repeated plating to purify it to a single homogeneous λ clone. To do this, one must be able to determine the location of the positive clone on the original plate. In our laboratory, we have found the following method to be simple and accurate.

1. Turn the membrane plaque side up and draw a 5-mm circle around the positive plaque with a felt-tip marker so that the color seeps through the membrane to the other side.
2. Where the needle holes penetrated the membrane (see *Preparation of Membrane Blots of Plaques*), dot the felt-tip marker so that the color also seeps through the membrane.
3. Turn the membrane plaque side down, place the corresponding plate on top of it, and align the needle marks in the agar with the corresponding marks on the membrane.
4. Cut the tip from a 1-ml plastic pipette tip so that the internal diameter is about 0.75 cm.
5. The inked circles marked on the membrane will show through the agar. Directly above each circle, "plug" the plaque(s) from the agar and blow them into a 1.5-ml microcentrifuge tube.
6. Add 1 ml of SM buffer and 30 μl of chloroform and follow the procedures outlined in *Preparation and Plating of Phage* to regrow the phage.
7. Repeat the steps of growth, screening, and plugging until it is certain that the clone is pure. Then plaque purify one further time.
8. The clone is pure and ready for further use. Remember to store an aliquot for back up as outlined in *Amplification by Plate Lysis*.

Acknowledgments

We thank Ms. Debbie Lowery for preparation of the manuscript. J. S. Kizer is a recipient of a NIMH Research Scientist Career Development Award (#K02-MH00114). Other grant support was provided by NIMH (RO1-MH41461) and NICHD (T32-HD07201).

References

1. R. A. Young and R. W. Davis, *Proc. Natl. Acad. Sci. U.S.A.* **80,** 1194 (1983).
2. R. A. Young and R. W. Davis, *Science* **222,** 778 (1983).
3. T. V. Huynh, R. A. Young, and R. W. Davis, *in* "DNA Cloning: A Practical Approach" (D. M. Glover, ed.), Vol. 1, p. 49. IRL Press, Oxford, 1985.
4. T. Maniatis, E. F. Fritsch, and J. Sambrook, "Molecular Cloning: A Laboratory Manual," p. 443. Cold Spring Harbor Laboratory, Cold Spring Harbor, New York, 1982.
5. G. Bers and D. Garfin, *BioTechniques* **3,** 276 (1985).

[19]   Rapid Identification of DNA Clones: Utilization of Same Degenerate Oligonucleotides for Both Screening and Sequencing

R. Nichols and Jack E. Dixon

Introduction

The efficient isolation of specific DNA sequences depends, to a great extent, on an effective assay to allow for the identification of the clone of interest. Knowledge of the correct DNA sequence makes it possible to virtually eliminate mismatches or false positives by the choice of appropriate hybridization conditions. The difference in the thermal stability makes it possible to eliminate formation of mismatched duplexes without affecting the formation of perfectly matched ones (1).

When amino acid sequence information is available for a given gene, it may be possible to predict the nucleotide sequence and then synthesize an oligonucleotide that can be used to identify clones containing the desired sequence. However, due to redundancy in the genetic code it is not usually possible to predict a unique nucleotide sequence from the amino acid sequence and so a mixture of oligonucleotides is synthesized. In addition, when the amino acid sequence of the desired gene is not known, an oligonucleotide mixture may be designed based on the sequence of the same gene product from another species or a closely related gene product. The potential ambiguities or mismatches present in the sequences of a highly redundant oligonucleotide mixture or oligonucleotides based on cross-species or closely related sequences may result in the identification of positively hybridizing colonies containing incorrect sequences or false positives, as well as colonies containing the clone of interest. The presence of false positives greatly increases the difficulty of identifying the correct clone and is often very time-consuming.

Mixtures of oligonucleotides are frequently used in the identification of specific clones in a cDNA or genomic library (2–4). Therefore, it is important to distinguish accurately and efficiently between the colonies containing correct sequences and the colonies containing incorrect, false positives.

DNA sequencing is perhaps the single, most important method to distinguish between positive-hybridization signals and false positives. The Sanger dideoxynucleotide chain-termination sequencing procedure is a widely used method for determining the nucleotide sequence of a single-stranded cloned fragment of DNA (5). The chain-termination sequencing procedure is based on the enzymatic synthesis of a radioactive complementary strand from the single-stranded template DNA utilizing a universal sequencing primer to initiate synthesis and dideoxynucleotides to randomly terminate synthesis. The universal primer is annealed to the region of the M13 vector directly adjacent to the cloned DNA and extended enzymatically to synthesize the complementary strand of the cloned DNA adjacent to the primer site. The resulting products are subsequently separated electrophoretically to obtain the sequence information.

Although the dideoxynucleotide sequencing method has been applied successfully to single-stranded DNA and can generate readable DNA sequences of 400–600 nucleotides in length, it remains both a time-consuming and labor-intensive task when it is necessary to sequence a large number of potentially positive clones to ultimately identify the specific DNA of interest. Several strategies have been used to enhance the efficiency of DNA sequencing methods. The random-cloning or partial-nuclease-digestion methods currently employed require generation and sequencing of numerous subclone constructions (6–9). An alternative method is to synthesize sequence-specific oligonucleotide primers (10, 11). This method can reduce the time required for the analysis of an individual DNA sequence. However, it is costly and remains a time-consuming method for screening numerous colonies.

The isolation of a specific DNA sequence depends on the ability to distinguish between a clone that contains the correct sequence and a false hybridization positive or background signal. A simple and rapid strategy for the analysis of positive colony hybridization signals is described. This procedure utilizes the same oligonucleotide mixture both as a screening probe and as a sequencing primer. The mixture of oligonucleotides is used as a primer to obtain sequence information directly from the plasmid DNA. Conditions for sequencing with oligonucleotides having up to 64-fold degeneracy are described. In addition, the effect on sequencing efficiency of the location of mismatches within a homologous series of oligonucleotides was examined. The main advantage of the degenerate oligonucleotide sequencing method is the rapid, reliable identification of authentic versus false hybridization positives without subclining into single-stranded M13 phage, without sequencing large regions of DNA, or without synthesizing sequence-specific primers.

A rapid, simple method is described for distinguishing between authentic and false positives utilizing the oligonucleotide screening probe as a sequence-specific primer for double-stranded plasmid sequencing. This method of degenerate oligonucleotide sequencing (DOS) provides an approach to identify authentic positives by utilizing the oligonucleotide mixture both to screen the library for positively hybridizing colonies and also as a primer to initiate sequencing reactions. This method is rapid since the sequence data obtained are adjacent to the site of oligonucleotide hybridization to the cloned DNA and can be compared to a minimal length of the known DNA or amino acid sequence to determine the authenticity of the isolated clone. Also, the double-stranded plasmid dideoxynucleotide sequencing method is reliable and the protocol is straightforward and rapid, since it avoids additional subcloning steps (12).

Materials and Methods

Oligonucleotides

Oligonucleotide mixtures were synthesized with an Applied Biosystems 380A DNA synthesizer using β-cyanoethylphosphoramidite chemistry. Oligonucleotides were purified on denaturing 20% acrylamide gels in 100 mM Tris, 65 mM borate, and 2 mM EDTA, pH 8.3–8.5. Approximately one-third or 0.030 μmol of the total oligonucleotide synthesis was loaded onto the gel and electrophoresed. The oligonucleotides were visualized by placing the gel directly onto an intensifying screen and illuminating with a short-wavelength (254 nm) ultraviolet light. The full-length oligonucleotides and shorter truncated synthesis products were easily visualized. The band corresponding to the full-length oligonucleotides was excised and eluted for ≥3 hr at 37°C in 1–3 ml of 0.5 M ammonium acetate and 1 mM EDTA. The acrylamide was removed by centrifugation through a glass wool plug. The oligonucleotide mixture was desalted by gel filtration through a Sephadex G-25 (fine) column equilibrated with 50 mM tetraethylammonium carbonate, pH 8. One-half milliliter fractions were collected and the fractions containing oligonucleotides identified by absorbance at 260 nm. These fractions were dried in a Speed-Vac Concentrator (Savant, Farmingdale, NY) and the pellet was resuspended in water to a final concentration of 100 ng/μl.

Preparation of Template DNA for Sequencing

The alkaline lysis method of Birnboim and Doly (13) was used to isolate plasmid DNA from overnight bacterial cultures. Plasmid DNA was further purified on a cesium chloride gradient (14). The supercoiled plasmid DNA band was well separated from the RNA, the chromosomal DNA, and linear plasmid DNA after a short ultracentrifugation, e.g., 4 hr at 60,000 rpm. The final DNA pellet was resuspended in 10 mM Tris, 1 mM EDTA, pH 8, at a concentration of 1 μg per microliter.

To accommodate the analysis of numerous colonies, the procedure for plasmid preparation can be simplified. Supercoiled plasmid DNA can be prepared from small bacterial cultures by the alkaline lysis method (12, 15, 16). This template DNA is suitable for dideoxy double-stranded sequencing.

DNA Sequencing Reactions

The DNA sequencing protocol described by Chen and Seeburg (12) was used with a few modifications. The dideoxy sequencing reactions were done using [^{32}P]dATP and 1 μg of the denatured plasmid. The primer-to-plasmid ratio was dependent on the redundancy of the specific oligonucleotide mixture being used (see *Results*). The annealing reaction was at 55°C for 10–15 min. The annealing mixture was allowed to cool to 42°C. One microliter of avian myeloblastosis virus (AMV) reverse transcriptase (Seika-gaku America, Inc., St. Petersburg, FL) and 2 μl [^{32}P]dATP (PB 10164, Amersham, Arlington Heights, IL) were added to the annealed mixture and 4-μl aliquots dispensed to each of the four reaction tubes containing the appropriate dideoxy- and deoxynucleotide mixtures (5). The reaction tubes were mixed quickly and incubated at 42°C for 15–20 min. One microliter of chase solution (0.5 mM dNTPs) was then added to each reaction tube and the reactions incubated at 42°C for an additional 5–10 min. The reactions were stopped by adding 5 μl of stop solution (5) (formamide–dye mix). The samples were heated for 3–5 min at 95–100°C, chilled on ice, and then applied to a sequencing gel.

Gel Electrophoresis

Electrophoresis of the sequencing samples was in 8% (w/v) acrylamide–7 M urea gels, 40 cm × 20 cm × 0.4 mm. Samples (2–3 μl) were loaded and electrophoresed at 1500 V until the xylene cyanole (XC) reached the bottom of the gel. At that time, a second loading was made and electrophoresis continued until the bromphenol blue (BPB) migrated to the bottom of the gel. After electrophoresis, the gel was transferred to a support, e.g., an old film, and exposed 12–20 hr at −20°C with no intensifying screen.

Results

To determine the feasibility of utilizing the DOS strategy to identify positive clones rapidly among a series of potential false positives, we applied the technique to a genomic clone which had been isolated using an oligonucleotide mixture and sequenced with sequence-specific primers (17).

The *Drosophila* genomic library was screened for sequences which hybridized to a peptide which had been previously isolated from the cockroach (18). The amino acid sequence of the cockroach peptide leucosulfakinin (LSK) is shown in Fig. 1A. No amino acid sequence is available for a corresponding *Drosophila* peptide since the *Drosophila* peptide has neither been identified nor isolated.

The screening-sequencing probes were designed based on the amino acid sequence for the cockroach peptide. Several positively hybridizing phages were isolated. The positively hybridizing DNA fragments were identified by Southern blot (19) and were subsequently subcloned into pUC18. The design of an oligonuceotide mixture (shown in Fig. 1B) hybridizes to the *Drosophila* clone. It consists of 14 bases with 16-fold degeneracy. If a DNA fragment isolated from a library indeed corresponds to the *Drosophila* LSK-like peptide, one would anticipate that the sequence information would correspond to an amino acid sequence of -Tyr-Gly-His-Met-Arg-Phe- or a peptide which is highly homologous to this peptide sequence (refer to Fig. 1). Reactions were performed as described under *Materials and Methods*. The data shown in Fig. 2 indicate that the DNA sequence contains codons which exist adjacent to the sequencing primer that correspond to the deduced amino acid sequence -Gly-His-Met-Arg-Phe-Gly-. Although the sequence data in Fig. 2 are easy to analyze, close scrutiny of the film suggests that a background or secondary sequence exists. The source of this sequence was of concern since it could represent anomalous priming. However, the source of this background sequence was understood when a complete sequence of the cloned DNA was determined. A second, distinct

A Glu – Gln – Phe – Glu – Asp – Tyr – Gly – His – Met – Arg – Phe – NH_2

B $GA_G^A \ CA_G^A \ TT_T^C \ GA_T^C \ GA$

FIG. 1 (A) Sequence of leucosulfakinin (LSK) from cockroach head extracts (18). (B) Nucleotide sequence of the degenerate oligonucleotide screening/sequencing probe mixture. The 14-base sequences were predicted from *Drosophila* codon usage tables. [Reproduced with permission from R. Nichols and J. E. Dixon, *Anal. Biochem.* **170,** 110 (1988).]

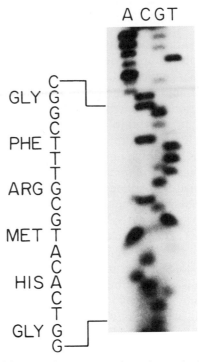

FIG. 2   Dideoxy double-stranded sequencing data obtained from a positively hybridizing clone utilizing the 14-base, 16-fold degenerate screening/sequencing primer as the sequencing primer. (Refer to Fig. 1 for information regarding the design of the 14-base oligonucleotide mixture.) [Reproduced with permission from R. Nichols and J. E. Dixon, *Anal. Biochem.* **170,** 110 (1988).]

but related sequence is present in the same DNA insert. The extent of this background sequence was lessened when the sequencing reactions conditions were increased in stringency by raising the annealing reaction temperature.

It should be pointed out that an oligonucleotide mixture complementary to the sequence shown in Fig. 1 could be synthesized to obtain sequence information in the opposite direction. Using a complementary oligonucleotide mixture as a primer, DNA data can be obtained from which the amino acid sequence corresponding to the amino terminal extension of the peptide could be predicted.

To further explore the feasibility of using the DOS strategy, we undertook a systematic investigation of oligonucleotide mixtures with increasing degeneracies that could be used directly as primers for double-stranded DNA sequencing. The same *Drosophila* LSK-like DNA fragment was used for these model studies. Oligonucleotide primers of 14 bases in length and increasing degeneracy were examined. Initial experiments utilized a constant molar ratio of probe to template DNA. The intensity of the sequencing bands suggested that the effective concentration of the correct sequence within the mixture was an important determinant in using degenerate oligonucleotide mixtures as primers (data not shown). To further test the ratio of primer to DNA template, a purified nondengerate 14-base primer was used in various amounts with 1 μg of denatured plasmid template. The quality of the sequence data was comparable for reactions of 5–100 ng primer to 1 μg plasmid (data not shown). (An unpurified, nondegenerate 14-base primer synthesized with high stepwise yields, e.g., >98%, gave the best sequence data at the higher primer-to-plasmid ratio of 100 ng to 1 μg.)

The oligonucleotide mixtures listed in Table I which have up to 32-fold degeneracy were used in sequencing reactions at ratios of 200 ng primer to 1 μg plasmid. The oligonucleotide mixture of 64-fold degeneracy was used at a ratio of 300 ng primer to 1 μg plasmid. The sequence data were compared to a nondengerate primer used at 10 ng to 1 μg plasmid (Fig. 3). The quality of the sequence data obtained from the degenerate oligonucleotide mixtures was indistinguishable from the specific, nondegenerate sequencing primer.

The effect, if any, of the location of degeneracies within the oligonucleotide on sequence data was investigated by designing oligonucleotides with redundancy at various positions (refer to Table I). The design of the oligonucleotides includes redundancy at positions along the 14-base sequence and at the initiation site of the sequence reaction, the 3' end. As can be observed in Fig. 3, the location of the redundancy has no apparent effect on the sequencing data.

Collectively, these results suggest that oligonucleotides as short as 14

TABLE I Oligonucleotide Mixtures

Degenerate sequencing primer (DSP)	Sequences[a]	Degeneracy
DSP1	5'AA TCA GAA AACA AT3'	1
DSP2	AA TCA (A/G) AA (A/G) ACN AT	16
DSP3	AA (C/T) CA (A/G) AA (A/G) ACN AT	32
DSP4	AA TCA (A/G) AA (A/G) AC (A/G) A (C/T)	16
DSP5	AA NCA (A/G) AA (A/G) ACN AT	64

[a] N is equivalent to A, C, G, and T.

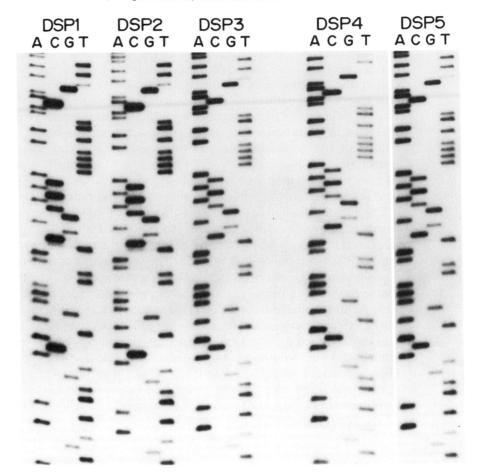

FIG. 3   Dideoxy double-stranded sequencing data utilizing degenerate sequencing primers DSP1–DSP5. (Information regarding the primer sequence design is illustrated in Table I.) [Reproduced with permission from R. Nichols and J. E. Dixon, *Anal. Biochem.* **170,** 110 (1988).]

bases in length and 64-fold degenerate can be used for both screening and rapidly identifying authentic clones among false positives. It is necessary to alter the effective primer concentration-to-plasmid ratio in order to obtain high-quality sequence data.

While using this procedure, occasional problems were encountered that were always traced back to oligonucleotide synthesis problems, the improper primer-to-plasmid ratio, or the suitability of the template DNA for sequencing. Oligonucleotide synthesis problems or improper primer-to-plasmid ratio will often result in poor sequencing data with high background. The suitability of template DNA for sequencing is well documented (12, 15).

Discussion

A method for rapidly and unambiguously verifying the authenticity of colony hybridization positives based on the use of the synthetic oligonucleotide screening probes as sequencing probes has been described. The utilization of the oligonucleotide mixtures as both screening probes and sequencing primers for dideoxy double-stranded plasmid sequencing provides a rapid, reliable method of analysis.

The degenerate oligonucleotide sequencing (DOS) procedure has major advantages over the random-cloning and partial-nuclease-digestion procedures (6–9) as well as the specific oligonucleotide primer-directed sequencing procedures (10, 11). This technique requires no subclone construction and does not require the sequencing of large stretches of DNA. One sequencing reaction per clone will yield the necessary data to determine the authenticity of the hybridization positive.

An important factor in utilizing oligonucleotide mixtures as sequencing primers is the effective concentration of the correct sequence. The degree of redundancy in those oligonucleotide mixtures studied (16- to 64-fold), as well as the position of the redundancy, did not affect the quality of sequence data.

The use of the oligonucleotide mixture as both screening probes and sequencing primers greatly simplifies the identification of colony positives as authentic clones. Although the application of this methodology to bacteriophage λ was not studied, several articles suggest that this method may be applicable to directly sequencing large double-stranded DNA (20, 21).

References

1. W. I. Wood, J. Gitschier, L. A. Lasky, and R. M. Lawn, *Proc. Natl. Acad. Sci. U.S.A.* **82,** 1585 (1985).
2. R. B. Wallace, J. Schaffer, R. P. Murphy, J. Bonner, T. Hirose, and K. Itakura, *Nucleic Acids Res.* **6,** 3543 (1979).
3. R. B. Wallace, M. J. Johnson, T. Hirose, T. Miyake, E. H. Kawashima, and K. Itakura, *Nucleic Acids Res.* **9,** 879 (1981).
4. D. E. Woods, A. E. Markham, A. T. Richer, G. Goldberger, and H. R. Colten, *Proc. Natl. Acad. Sci. U.S.A.* **79,** 5661 (1982).

5. F. Sanger, S. Nicklen, and A. Coulson, *Proc. Natl. Acad. Sci. U.S.A.* **74,** 5463 (1977).
6. S. Anderson, *Nucleic Acids Res.* **9,** 3015 (1981).
7. G. F. Hong, *Biosci. Rep.* **2,** 907 (1982).
8. G. F. Hong, *J. Mol. Biol.* **158,** 539 (1982).
9. A. Frischauf, H. Garoff, and H. Lebrach, *Nucleic Acids Res.* **8,** 5541 (1980).
10. R. Sanchez-Pescador and M. S. Urdea, *DNA* **3,** 339 (1984).
11. E. C. Strauss, J. A. Kobori, G. Sin, and L. E. Hood, *Anal. Biochem.* **154,** 353 (1986).
12. E. Y. Chen and P. H. Seeburg, *DNA* **4,** 165 (1985).
13. H. C. Birnboim and J. Doly, *Nucleic Acids Res.* **7,** 1513 (1979).
14. D. B. Clewell and D. R. Helinski, *Proc. Natl. Acad. Sci. U.S.A.* **62,** 1159 (1969).
15. R. G. Korneluk, F. Quan, and R. A. Gravel, *Gene* **40,** 317 (1985).
16. M. Hattori and Y. Sakaki, *Anal. Biochem.* **152,** 232 (1986).
17. R. Nichols, S. A. Schneuwly, and J. E. Dixon, *J. Biol. Chem.* **263,** 12167 (1988).
18. R. J. Nachman, G. M. Holman, W. F. Haddon, and N. Ling, *Science* **234,** 71 (1986).
19. E. Southern, *Nucleic Acids Res.* **9,** 3015 (1981).
20. X.-Y. Liu, S. Maeda, K. Collier, and S. Pestka, *Gene Anal. Tech.* **2,** 83 (1985).
21. R. J. Zagursky, K. Baumeister, N. Lomax, and M. L. Berman, *Gene Anal. Tech.* **2,** 89 (1985).

[20]   Molecular Cloning of Nicotinic Acetylcholine Receptor Genes

Jim Boulter and Paul D. Gardner

Introduction

The purpose of this chapter is to present and discuss methods for the molecular cloning of members of the nicotinic acetylcholine receptor (nAChR) gene family. The emphasis will be on those techniques and strategies that are most frequently used in our laboratory; however, in cases where an alternate or more complete discourse on theory or practical

Methods in Neurosciences, Volume 1

aspects of given techniques is required, specific literature references will be cited. The chapter will be divided into a consideration of the following topics and relevant methods: (1) the cloning and characterization of complementary DNAs (cDNAs) for vertebrate muscle and neuronal nAChR genes and (2) the genomic cloning of members of the nAChR gene family.

Cloning of cDNAs for Muscle and Neuronal Nicotinic Acetylcholine Receptors

A project to construct and screen a cDNA library can be organized into a few basic steps: isolation of poly(A)$^+$ RNA, synthesis of first-strand cDNA, synthesis of the second DNA strand to yield double-stranded cDNA (dscDNA), modifying the ends of the dscDNA to facilitate ligation to bacterial or viral vectors, ligations to an appropriate vector, plating and screening the library, and, finally, characterizing individual cDNA clones. At each phase of the project there are procedural and tactical choices to be made which will affect the overall quality of the library and its suitability for a given purpose.

Detailed protocols for all methods utilized in the construction of cDNA libraries have been published. They represent a valuable but complex resource for the molecular neurobiologist. In the following pages we will present an integrated strategy for cloning nAChR genes from cDNA libraries built from poly(A)$^+$ RNA obtained from either muscle or neuronal tissue. The actual synthesis of dscDNA, ready for ligation into selected cloning vectors, will be discussed in detail; adjunct methodologies will, of necessity, be treated less completely.

Isolation of RNA

General Considerations

The overall quality of a cDNA library is determined by the integrity of the poly(A)$^+$ RNA used for the first-strand cDNA synthesis. The size of the RNA and its suitability as template for reverse transcriptase are the major determinants in generating a representative and useful cDNA library. The major concern during this phase of the project, then, is to isolate undegraded poly(A)$^+$ RNA from a tissue or cellular source rich in nicotinic acetylcholine receptors.

We used the mouse BC3H-1 muscle cell line as a source of RNA for the cloning of muscle-type nAChR subunit genes. This cell line is easy to maintain in culture and synthesizes high levels of a muscle type nAChR (1).

RNA isolated from either the pheochromocytoma cell line PC12 (2) or portions of adult rat brain was used to clone neuronal nAChR subunit genes.

It is essential that ribonuclease activity be minimized when isolating RNA. Specific suggestions for creating a ribonuclease-free working environment are discussed in detail elsewhere and *must be followed* (3). Endogenous tissue ribonucleases are best rendered tractable by isolating total cellular RNA using procedures which employ guanidine salts as strong protein denaturing reagents (4). Early RNA isolation protocols using guanidine hydrochloride (5) or guanidine thiocyanate (6) have proved quite successful. In the following procedural section, a modification of the guanidine thiocyanate extraction protocol (7) is presented which has several advantages over previous methods: (1) it is rapid, (2) it does not require ultracentrifugation, (3) it can be scaled to accommodate small (100 mg) or large (several grams) amounts of starting material as well as the processing of large numbers of samples, and (4) it yields high-quality total cellular RNA with excellent recoveries.

Procedure

The following volumes are prescribed for 1 g starting material or, in the case of cultured cells, for each 100-cm tissue culture dish. Have ready the following solutions and reagents.

> Diethyl pyrocarbonate (0.1%, v/v)-treated H_2O (DEPC-H_2O)
> 0.5% (w/v) sodium dodecyl sulfate in DEPC-H_2O
> 2-Propanol
> Chloroform–isoamyl alcohol (24 : 1, v/v)
> Redistilled phenol saturated with DEPC–H_2O
> 2 M sodium acetate adjusted to pH 4.0
> Guanidine thiocyanate solution (GTC solution): 4 M guanidine thiocyanate, 25 mM sodium citrate, pH 7.0, 0.5% (w/v) N-lauroylsarcosine (sodium salt), 100 mM 2-mercaptoethanol

To dissolve the GTC solution completely, heat at 50–60°C (minus the 2-mercaptoethanol). Pass the solution through a 0.45-μm filter and store at room temperature. Add the 2-mercaptoethanol just before use. With 2-mercaptoethanol, the GTC solution is reported to be stable for 1 month at room temperature.

1. Homogenize the tissue in 10 ml GTC solution in a 50-ml sterile, disposable screw-capped plastic (polypropylene) centrifuge tube. Use a polytron homogenizer (Brinkmann Instruments, Westbury, NY) at maximum setting. Use three 10-sec pulses. For cultured cells, use 600 μl GTC solution per 100-cm tissue culture dish or 100 μl per 1×10^6 cells.

2. Add in the following order: 1.0 ml 2 M sodium acetate, pH 4.0, 10 ml H_2O-saturated phenol, 2.0 ml chloroform–isoamyl alcohol. Mix well after each addition and place on ice for 15 min. For cultured cells the volumes are 60, 600, and 120 μl, respectively.

3. Transfer the homogenate to an acid-washed, baked 30-ml Corex glass centrifuge tube and spin at 10,000 g for 20 min at 4°C. For cultured cells, use a 1.5-ml autoclaved microfuge tube.

4. Transfer the upper, aqueous phase to a 50-ml polypropylene centrifuge tube. Discard the lower, organic phase. Add an equal volume (approximately 11 ml) of 2-propranol to the aqueous phase. Place at −20°C for 60 min.

5. Transfer to a 30-ml Corex tube and centrifuge at 10,000 g for 20 min at 4°C.

6. Aspirate supernatant and discard. Resuspend pellet in 3.0 ml of GTC solution. Vortex to ensure pellet is completely dissolved. For cells use 225 μl.

7. Add 3.0 ml 2-propanol and place at −20°C for 60 min. Centrifuge as above.

8. Wash pellet once with 75% (v/v) ethanol. Centrifuge at 10,000 g for 5 min at 4°C. Dry pellet under stream of nitrogen or under vacuum.

9. Resuspend pellet in 500 μl of 0.5% sodium dodecyl sulfate. Heat to 65°C for 5–10 min to completely dissolve RNA. For cells, resuspend pellet in 20 μl.

10. Measure absorbance of RNA at 260 and 280 nm. The ratio of A_{260} to A_{280} should be approximately 1.8.

The yield of total cellular RNA will depend on the cell type or tissue. For cultured cells, yields are on the order of 40–80 μg per 100-cm culture dish while, for whole organ or tissue, RNA yields are typically 2–5 mg/g of tissue. At this point the total RNA should be poly(A)$^+$ selected using oligo(dT)-cellulose (8) or poly(U)-Sepharose (9) affinity chromatography. The poly(A)$^+$ RNA should be analyzed on a denaturing agarose gel to assess its size (see Ref. 10 for electrophoresis conditions).

Synthesis of Size-Fractionated, EcoRI Linkered dscDNA

General Considerations

The following protocol can generate size-fractionated, dscDNA ready for ligation into an appropriate vector in 2 days. The first day ends with the ligation of the phosphorylated *Eco*RI linkers to the blunt-ended dscDNA and the second day ends with the precipitation of the fractions from the agarose

A 50-m column. A less hectic pace is obtained by stopping the procedure at the ethanol precipitation step after the S_1 nuclease digestion and starting the *Eco*RI methylase reaction on the morning of the second day. Ligation of the *Eco*RI linkers to the dscDNA ends the second day. The procedure was designed to minimize handling steps (e.g., multiple phenol extractions and ethanol precipitations, changes in reaction tubes). Starting from 10 μg poly(A)$^+$ RNA, one can expect to generate a cDNA library with an unamplified base of between several hundred thousand and several million elements. This rather broad range may reflect differences in the quality of the individual poly(A)$^+$ RNA used for first-strand template as well as variations in the efficacies of individual steps in the procedure. The notes presented in the following section are designed, in part, to help minimize the latter.

Procedure

The following reaction conditions are for 10 μg poly(A)$^+$ RNA. You will need the following reagents.

> 10× avian myeloblastosis virus reverse transcription buffer (10× AM-VRT buffer, 500 mM Tris, pH 8.5, at room temperature, 400 mM KCl, 80 mM MgCl$_2$). Autoclave and store in aliquots at $-20°$C. Add 1 μl 1.0 M DTT to 49 μl 10× AMVRT buffer immediately before use
> Oligo(dT)$_{12-18}$ at 1 mg/ml DEPC-H$_2$O
> Deoxyribonucleotide triphosphates (stock dATP, dCTP, dGTP, dTTP at 10.0 mM each, pH 7.5, in DEPC-H$_2$O)
> 10× second-strand buffer (10× SS buffer, 200 mM Tris, pH 7.4, 100 mM (NH$_4$)$_2$SO$_4$, 50 mM MgCl$_2$)
> MgCl$_2$, 100 mM
> KCl, 1 M
> Ammonium acetate, 10 M
> β-NAD, 10 mM stock
> EDTA, 500 mM, pH 8
> Ether
> Ethanol (absolute)
> Bovine serum albumin, nuclease free, 1 mg/ml stock
> Avian myeloblastosis virus reverse transcriptase (10–20,000 U/ml)
> DNA polymerase I (5,000 U/ml)
> *Eco*RI methylase (20,000 U/ml)
> RNase H (3,000 U/ml)
> T4 DNA ligase (1–3,000 U/ml)
> *Escherichia coli* DNA ligase (1 mg/ml stock)
> *Eco*RI (100–130,000 U/ml)

2× S$_1$ nuclease buffer [56 mM NaCl, 100 mM sodium acetate, pH 4.6, 15 mM ZnSO$_4$, 10 μg/ml denatured calf thymus DNA, 10% (v/v) glycerol]

5× EcoRI methylase buffer (250 mM Tris, pH 8.0, 5 mM EDTA)

Phenol : CHCl$_3$: isoamyl alcohol (50 : 48 : 2, v/v/v)

TE buffer (10 mM Tris, pH 8.0, 1 mM EDTA)

SM buffer (10 mM NaCl, 50 mM Tris, pH 7.5, 10 mM MgSO$_4$, 0.01% gelatin)

Phosphorylated EcoRI linkers (10-mer, 5′-pd[CCGAATTCGG]-3′, 500 μg/ml)

10× T4 DNA ligase buffer (500 mM Tris, pH 7.8, 100 mM MgCl$_2$, 2 mM spermidine-HCl, 100 mM DTT, 100 mM ATP)

2× EcoRI buffer (50 mM Tris, pH 7.4, 10 mM MgSO$_4$, 200 mM NaCl)

BioGel agarose A-50m dye mix (50% glycerol, 0.25% bromphenol blue)

BioGel agarose A-50m (100-200 mesh) chromatography resin

1. The first-strand cDNA synthesis reaction mixture contains the following components: 5 μl 10× AMVRT buffer, 2 μl RNase inhibitor, 4 μl each stock dNTPs, 10 μg poly(A)$^+$ RNA, 2 μl stock oligo(dT)$_{12-18}$, 60 units of AMVRT in a total volume of 50 μl. Mix the RNA and H$_2$O in a 1.5-ml microfuge tube and heat to 68°C for 2 min. Quickly cool on ice and add the remaining ingredients. Add the AMVRT and incubate at 42°C for 60 min. Stop the reaction by placing the tube on ice.

2. The second-strand DNA synthesis reaction is performed using the RNase H procedure of Okayama and Berg (11) as modified by Gubler and Hoffman (12) and contains 50 μl first-strand synthesis, 10 μl 10× SS buffer, 10 μl stock KCl, 5 μl stock BSA solution, 1 μl each of 10.0 mM dNTPs, 5 μl β-NAD stock, 2.5 μl E. coli DNA ligase, 2 μl RNase H, 5 μl [^{32}P]dCTP (1 mCi/ml, 800 Ci/mmol), 5 μl DNA polymerase I, and H$_2$O to 100 μl. Keep all reagents ice cold. After addition of DNA polymerase I, place reaction mixture in a 12°C H$_2$O bath for 60 min then transfer to a 22°C H$_2$O bath for an additional 60 min.

3. Remove second-strand reaction from H$_2$O bath and immediately place on ice. Add 100 μl 2× S$_1$ nuclease buffer followed by S$_1$ nuclease to a final concentration of 750 U/ml. Incubate at 37°C for 30 min. Stop the reaction with 4 μl 500 mM EDTA. Remove 2 μl of the reaction mixture to 18 μl TE buffer and freeze at −20°C. This sample should be used to determine the amount of second-strand synthesis using the DE-81 filter paper binding assay (13) as well as to ascertain the size of the dscDNA (neutral agarose gel electrophoresis) or the average size of the second-strand DNA itself (alkaline agarose gel electrophoresis). Yields of dscDNA at this point range from 0.5 to 4 μg.

4. Extract S_1 nuclease-treated dscDNA once with phenol:CHCl$_3$: isoamyl alcohol. Transfer upper, aqueous phase to a clean 1.5-ml microfuge tube. Reextract organic phase with 36 μl TE buffer. Combine aqueous phases and extract three times with ether. Remove ether from final aqueous phase by heating at 45°C for 5–10 min. Add 60 μl 10 M ammonium acetate and 600 μl ethanol. Place on dry ice for 5 min followed by 25 min at 4°C. Warm to room temperature and spin in a microcentrifuge at maximum speed for 30 min. Aspirate supernatant and discard. Do not dry pellet. Add 40 μl TE buffer and resuspend pellet with vortexing. If necessary, warm to 40°C for 5 min. Add 10 μl 10 M ammonium acetate and 10 μl ethanol. Repeat precipitation as above. Aspirate supernatant and dry pellet under vacuum.

5. Add 13 μl TE buffer to dried pellet. Warm to 37°C and vortex to resuspend. Add 4 μl 5× EcoRI methylase buffer, 2 μl stock BSA solution, and 1 μl EcoRI methylase. The final volume is 20 μl. Incubate at 37°C for 30 min. Stop reaction by placing on ice.

6. The ends of the dscDNA are rendered flush using DNA polymerase I as follows. To the EcoRI methylase-treated dscDNA, add 2.5 μl stock MgCl$_2$, 2.5 μl of a mixture of the four dNTPs at 250 μM each, and 2.5 U DNA polymerase I (0.5 μl of stock DNA polymerase at 5,000 U/ml). The final volume is 25.5 μl. Incubate at room temperature for 15 min. Stop the reaction by addition of 2 μl 500 mM EDTA and 12.5 μl TE buffer. Extract once with phenol:CHCl$_3$:isoamyl alcohol. Remove and save aqueous phase. Reextract organic phase with 15 μl TE buffer and pool aqueous phases. Extract with ether three times. Warm aqueous phase to 45°C for 10–15 min to remove excess ether. Add 10 μl 10 M ammonium acetate and 100 μl ethanol. Place on dry ice for 5 min then transfer to 4°C for 25 min. Warm to room temperature and spin in a microcentrifuge for 15 min. Aspirate supernatant and discard. Do not dry pellet. Resuspend in 20 μl TE buffer, add 5 μl 10 M ammonium acetate, 50 μl ethanol, and repeat precipitation. Dry pellet under vacuum.

7. Ligation of phosphorylated EcoRI 10-mer linkers (5'-pdCCGAATTCGG-3') to the ends of the dscDNA is accomplished as follows: the dried pellet from step 6 is resuspended in 9 μl TE buffer with brief heating to 40–45°C and vortexing. Place dscDNA on ice and add 1.5 μl 10× T4 DNA ligase buffer, 3 μl phosphorylated EcoRI linkers (at 500 μg/ml) followed by 1.5 μl T4 DNA ligase. Final volume is 15 μl. Incubate reaction in a 12°C H$_2$O bath overnight.

8. To remove excess EcoRI linkers, the ligation mixture is treated as follows. Add 15 μl of 2× EcoRI buffer and heat to 68°C for 10 min to inactivate the T4 DNA ligase. Cool on ice and add 1 μl EcoRI (100–120,000 U/ml). Final volume is 31 μl. Incubate at 37°C for 2 hr. Stop reaction with 1.5 μl 500 mM EDTA. Place EcoRI linkered, dscDNA on ice.

At this point, it is necessary to separate the digested linkers from the dscDNA. This is best achieved by passing the dscDNA over a sizing column since, in addition to effectively removing excess EcoRI linkers, it also allows one to enrich for large, full-length dscDNA. In the following paragraphs, we describe a simple procedure for size-fractionating the dscDNA using agarose BioGel A-50m.

1. Prepare agarose BioGel A-50m as follows. Place 25 ml (packed bed volume) A-50m into a 1-liter graduated cylinder. Add sterile H_2O containing 0.5 mM EDTA to about 800 ml. Seal the top with parafilm and place cylinder on its side. Slowly rock for 24–36 hr at 4°C. Change H_2O–EDTA washing solution every 8 hr by letting the A-50m settle out and decanting the supernatant. After last wash, resuspend resin in A-50m running buffer (150 mM NaCl, 10 mM Tris, pH 7.4, 1 mM EDTA). This washing procedure is reported to remove compounds which inhibit ligation.

2. Siliconize and bake a 0.2 × 35 cm glass column (3 mm OD, Corning Glassworks). Place a small plug of siliconized glass wool in one end. Attach a 25-gauge, $\frac{5}{8}$-in. syringe needle to the bottom of the column. Fill the column with A-50m buffer from the *bottom up* using a syringe filled with buffer and attached to the 25-gauge needle. Pack the column by allowing the degassed resin to flow down from the top (a 10-ml plastic syringe barrel attached to the top of the column with a Tygon tubing collar is a good way to get a small reservoir for packing and running the column). Equilibrate and run the column at a flow rate of 0.5 to 1 ml/hr.

3. Add 3 μl of A-50m dye mix to the EcoRI digested dscDNA (final volume 34 μl). Load the sample using a Hamilton syringe by underlaying the dscDNA on top of the A-50m. Collect four-drop (approximately 30 μl) fractions. The excluded volume is about 300–350 μl (fractions 10–11), and it is here that the first radioactivity appears. If you collect fractions in microfuge tubes (with tops cut off), you can place them in scintillation vials and count directly using Cerenkov radiation.

4. The dscDNA elutes over about 15 fractions. To determine which samples to pool, take a small aliquot (2–5 μl) of every other fraction and electrophorese on a 1% agarose gel along with radiolabeled DNA molecular weight standards. Store remainder of fractions at 4°C. The results of such an analysis are presented in Fig. 1. Pool the desired fractions, adjust to 2 M ammonium acetate, and ethanol precipitate as usual. Resuspend the dried pellet in 20 μl TE buffer. The dscDNA can be stored in TE buffer at −20°C.

The dscDNA should be characterized with respect to (1) size, (2) yield, and (3) "ligatability." The size of the dscDNA can be estimated from the autoradiograph of the agarose gel using radiolabeled DNA fragments as

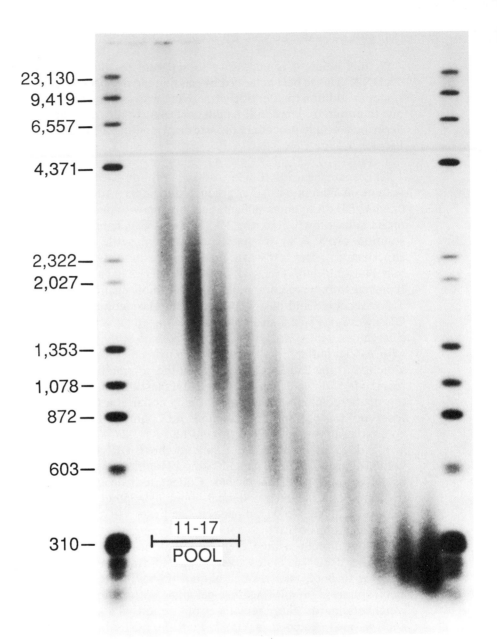

FRACTION NUMBER

FIG. 1   Autoradiogram of fractions taken from a BioGel A-50m chromatography column loaded with ^{32}P-labeled, *Eco*RI-linkered dscDNA prepared from PC12 cell poly(A)+ RNA (see the text for details of sample preparation and chromatography conditions). Aliquots of the indicated fractions were electrophoresed on a 1% neutral agarose gel at 17 mA constant current for 16 hr. The gel was dried and exposed to Kodak XAR-5 X-ray film for 15 hr at −70°C. DNA molecular weight standards are in base pairs. Pool volume was 210 μl.

molecular weight standards. The yield of dscDNA can be estimated from the results of the DE-81 cellulose binding assay performed after the S_1 nuclease digestion step. This assay gives you the total number of [^{32}P]dCTP counts per minute (cpm) in the reaction mixture as well as the cpm incorporated into dscDNA. Dividing the bound cpm by the total cpm and multiplying by the number of cpm per picomole dNTP in the second-strand synthesis yields the number of picomoles cDNA made. Using an average of 330 pg/pmol DNA, one can calculate the weight of dscDNA in the final A-50m pool.

One significant indicator of success can be determined by performing a ''self-ligation'' of the dscDNA obtained from the A-50m column. It is a direct demonstration of whether the dscDNAs have cohesive *Eco*RI linkers on *both* ends. Even if the yield of dscDNA is good and the size acceptable, the ligation of the *Eco*RI linkers may have been incomplete because all the dscDNA ends were not flush. Without linkers on both termini, and the cohesive ends generated by *Eco*RI cleavage, subsequent ligation to *Eco*RI cut cloning vectors will not work. Perform a self-ligation as follows.

1. To each of two 0.5-ml microfuge tubes add 2 μl of the A-50m pooled dscDNA and 1 μl 5× T4 DNA ligase buffer. To one of the tubes add 1 μl T4 DNA ligase. Adjust final volumes to 5 μl with H_2O and incubate tubes in a 12°C H_2O bath overnight.

2. Load samples, including radiolabeled DNA molecular weight standards, on an 0.8% agarose gel. Run the gel, dry, and expose to X-ray film. If the dscDNA has *Eco*RI linkers on both ends, the sample treated with T4 DNA ligase will form high-molecular-weight concatamers and the distribution of radioactivity will shift toward the top of the gel. If this doesn't happen, or there is just a modest increase in the average size distribution, it is likely that only a fraction of the dscDNA has been properly linkered.

cDNA Cloning Vectors, Ligation, and Packaging

General Considerations

Once made, the *Eco*RI-linkered dscDNA must be enzymatically ligated to a suitable cloning vector. Vectors are key elements in the construction of cDNA libraries and are of two general types: plasmid and viral. Plasmid vectors are small extrachromosomal, circular DNA molecules which are replicated in appropriate bacterial hosts. Such vectors are capable of harboring up to several kilobase pairs of foreign DNA. Viral vectors are derivatives of naturally occurring bacterial, plant, insect, and animal cell viruses which have been engineered to accommodate moderate-sized fragments (0–20 kilobase pairs) of cloned DNA.

In recent years, recombinant DNA methodologies have been applied to many of the original general-purpose cloning vectors in an effort to increase their usefulness for specific applications. The evolution of these second-generation, multipurpose vectors has been extremely rapid. A choice must first be made between plasmid and bacteriophage vectors and, second, among the diverse vectors of each type. A variety of factors bear on the choice of a particular vector over another, but a detailed discussion of these considerations is beyond the scope of this chapter; however, the reader is enjoined to give this aspect of the project serious thought. In the present context, we will discuss only the use of bacteriophage λ vectors (e.g., λgt10 (14)]; however, a more complete listing of currently available cloning vectors and their applications is shown in Table I.

Procedure

The final stages of cDNA library construction involve the ligation of the *Eco*RI-linkered, dscDNA to a λgt10 vector having *Eco*RI-compatible termini. The ligation is followed by the *in vitro* assembly of recombinant λgt10 phage particles via a packaging reaction and subsequent infection of a susceptible bacterial host. Optimal ligation conditions are achieved at high DNA concentrations (vector plus dscDNA, 100–200 μg/ml) and at approximately a 2:1 molar ratio of dscDNA to vector. In practice, however, it is difficult to determine the molar concentration of dscDNA since a knowledge of both the weight and average length of the dscDNA is required to make such a calculation. It is better to take an empirical approach and set up several small-scale, trial ligations and packagings.

1. To each of five siliconized, autoclaved 0.5 ml microfuge tubes add 1 μl *Eco*RI cut λgt10 vector DNA diluted to 500 ng/μl. Place tubes on ice and add 1 μl 6× T4 DNA ligase buffer. To reaction tubes 2–3 add 2 μl and 1 μl of undiluted *Eco*RI-linkered dscDNA from the A-50m column pool, respectively. Make a 1:5 and 1:10 dilution of the dscDNA. Place 2 μl of the 1:5 dilution and 2 μl of the 1:10 dilution to reaction tubes 4–5, respectively. To all tubes add 1 μl T4 DNA ligase, adjust volume to 6 μl final with DEPC-H$_2$O and incubate in a 12°C H$_2$O bath overnight. As an approximation, assume a yield of 1 μg size-fractionated dscDNA from the A-50m column pool and 50 ng dscDNA/μl TE final concentration. If the average length of the dscDNA is 2 kilobase pairs, the estimated molar ratio of insert:vector in the trial ligations will span the range of 4:1 through 0.4:1.

2. Ligated λgt10 DNA is then assembled into intact phage particles using commercially available packaging reagents (e.g., Gigapak Plus, Stratagene, Inc.) following the manufacturer's instructions. Packaging reactions are terminated by addition of 500 μl SM phage dilution buffer and phage are

TABLE I   Characteristics of Some Frequently Used cDNA and Genomic Cloning Vectors[a]

Library type	Vector	Vector size (kb)	Insert size (kb)	MCS	Directional cloning	Amp selection	Biological selection	lacZ selection	Promoter T3	T7	SP6	Reference[b]
cDNA												
Plasmid												
	pBR322	4.4	0–8	No	No	Yes	No	No	−	−	−	1
	pUC	2.7	0–8	Yes	Yes	Yes	No	Yes	±	±	−	2
	pBluescript	3.0	0–8	Yes	Yes	Yes	No	Yes	+	+	−	3
	Okayama–Berg	3.1	0–8	No	Yes	Yes	No	No	−	−	±	4
Viral												
	λgt10	43.3	0–7.6	No	No	No	Yes	No	−	−	−	5
	λgt11	43.7	0–7.6	No	No	No	No	Yes	−	−	−	6
	λZAP	40.8	0–10	Yes	Yes	Yes	No	Yes	+	+	+	7
	λGEM-2	NA	0–7.1	Yes	Yes	No	No	No	−	+	+	8
	λGEM-4	NA	0–4.7	Yes	Yes	Yes	No	No	−	+	+	8
	λLONG C	39.6	0–10	Yes	Yes	No	No	No	−	−	−	9
Genomic												
Viral												
	λCharon4a	45.5	0–7.1	Yes	NA	No	No	No	−	−	−	10
	λEMBL3	42.4	9–23	Yes	NA	No	Yes	No	−	−	−	11
	λFIX	41.9	9–23	Yes	NA	No	Yes	No	+	+	−	9
	λDASH	41.9	9–23	Yes	NA	No	Yes	No	+	+	−	9
	λGEM-11	41.5	9–23	Yes	NA	No	Yes	No	−	+	+	8

[a] MCS, Multiple cloning site; kb, kilobase pairs; NA, not available. Directional cloning pertains to any strategy that allows one to construct a cDNA library in which all the inserted dscDNAs have been ligated in a single orientation. In principle, any cloning vector with more than one cloning site can be used for constructing directional libraries using appropriate primer/adapters and linkers. In this context, biological selection refers to the ability to distinguish between recombinant phage particles and the nonrecombinant, parental phage. For λgt10 vectors, the selection is obtained by plating the library on *E. coli* C600 *Hfl*. For genomic libraries constructed with λ replacement vectors, one can plate the library on strains of *E. coli* lysogenic for the phage P2. Only recombinant phage missing the *red* and *gam* genes (deleted with the central "stuffer" fragment) can form plaques. T3, T7, and SP6 promoter refer to the presence of specific RNA polymerase promoters for the bacterial viruses T3, T7, and SP6.

[b] References: (1) F. Bolivar, R. L. Rodriguez, P. J. Greene, M. C. Betlach, H. L. Heynecker, H. W. Boyer, J. H. Crosa, and S. Falkow, *Gene* **2**, 95 (1977); (2) J. Vieira and J. Messing, *Gene* **19**, 259 (1982); (4) H. Okayama and P. Berg, *Mol. Cell. Biol.* **3**, 280 (1983); (5) R. D. Young and R. W. Davis, *Science* **222**, 778 (1983); (6) T. V. Huynh, R. A. Young, and R. W. Davis, *in* "DNA Cloning Techniques: A Practical Approach" (D. Glover, ed.), Vol. 1, p. 49. IRL Press, Oxford, 1984; (7) J. M. Short, J. M. Fernandez, J. A. Sorge, and W. D. Huse, *Nucleic Acid Res.* **16**, 7583 (1988); (8) Promega, Madison, WI; (9) Stratagene, La Jolla, CA; (10) F. R. Blattner, B. G. Williams, A. E. Blechl, K. Denniston-Thompson, H. E. Faber, L.-A. Furlong, D. J. Grunwald, D. O. Kiefer, D. D. Moore, J. W. Schumm, E. O. Sheldon, and O. Smithies, *Science* **196**, 161 (1977); (11) A. M. Frischauf, H. Lehrach, A. Poustka, and N. Murray, *J. Mol. Biol.* **170**, 827 (1983).

titered on *E. coli* strains C600 and C600 *Hfl*. The titer on strain C600 represents both wild-type λgt10 as well as recombinant phage particles, while the titer on the C600 *Hfl* strain reflects the number of packaged phage which harbor dscDNA inserts in the *Eco*RI cloning site. (For a complete discussion of the basis for the difference in plating efficiencies of recombinant versus nonrecombinant phage on the two strains, see Ref. 15.)

The phage titer of the control ligation tube (ligation tube 1 above, λgt10 vector DNA alone) should be about 1×10^6 pfu/μg vector on C600 and less than 1×10^4 pfu/μg vector on C600 *Hfl*. Titer the packaged phage stocks from each of the experimental ligations (tubes 2–5) on C600 *Hfl* and determine the ratio of insert : vector which yields the highest number of recombinant phage particles per microgram vector using the smallest amount of dscDNA. These conditions can be used as guidelines for scaling up the number of ligations required to obtain the desired unamplified library base. The phage titers of ligation tubes 2–5 using C600 *Hfl* as host can often be as high as 1×10^6/μg vector; however, titers as low as 1×10^5/μg are acceptable and represent, on average, a 10-fold stimulation over the background of nonrecombinant λgt10 vector. Newly packaged, unamplified phage stocks should be stored at 4°C over a few drops of $CHCl_3$.

Library Plating, Screening, and Isolation of cDNA Clones

Procedure

Have available the following reagents and media (amounts indicated in the text are those suggested for screening 1×10^6 plaques).

> NZY medium (per liter, 5 g NaCl, 5 g yeast extract, 10 g tryptone, 2 g $MgSO_4 \cdot 7H_2O$. Adjust to pH 7.4 with NaOH)
> NZY agar plates (as above but with 15 g agar per liter)
> NZY soft agarose (as above but with 7.5 g agarose per liter)
> 20% (w/v) maltose (sterilize by filtration through a 0.22-μm filter)
> Sterile plastic petri dishes (150 × 15 mm; 100 × 15 mm)
> Sterile polystyrene/polypropylene tubes (17 × 100 mm)
> Nylon membrane filters for plaque transfers (137 mm diameter)
> Nitrocellulose membrane filters (Schleicher and Schuell, BA85, 0.45 μm, 82 mm diameter)
> Hybridization buffer [1 *M* NaCl, 1% (w/v) sodium dodecyl sulfate, 100 μg/ml denatured salmon sperm DNA, 5× Denhardt's solution, 0.1% sodium pyrophosphate, 50 m*M* Tris, pH 8.5 (at 22°C)]

1. The library can be plated on 150 × 15 mm NZY agar plates. At a

plating density of 4×10^4 plaques/plate and a library base of 1×10^6 phage, you will need 25 plates. Pour plates 2–3 days before scheduled plating and use between 100 and 120 ml NZY agar per plate (8–10 plates per liter of media). Plates should be poured on a level surface. Do not stack the plates after agar has hardened. On the day of the library plating, the surfaces of the plates should be dried by placing them in a sterile hood with the tops *completely* removed for 1 hr. Slight ripples will appear on the agar surface when dry. Replace covers and place the NZY plates in the 37°C incubator for *no less than* 3 hr prior to plating. This ensures that the plates are 37°C when used and permits the molten NZY soft agarose to flow completely over the surface of the plate before hardening.

2. The highest plating efficiency is achieved when the *E. coli* C600 *Hfl* cells are in mid-log phase when used. Streak a fresh NZY agar plate with a stock of *E. coli* C600 *Hfl* to obtain single, well-isolated colonies. The morning of the library plating, pick a single colony to 50 ml NZY liquid media containing 0.2% (w/v) maltose. Grow cells at 37°C with vigorous aeration in a 500-ml flask. Monitor the growth of the cells and harvest cells at an OD_{600} of 0.3 by centrifugation in a 50-ml sterile polypropylene centrifuge tube at 1500 g for 10 min. Resuspend cells in 50 ml of sterile 10 mM Tris, pH 7.4, 5 mM MgSO$_4$, by gentle swirling.

3. In a sterile 50-ml polypropylene tube add 20 ml of the suspension of *E. coli* C600 *Hfl* host cells and 1×10^6 phage from the library stock. Mix gently and allow phage to adsorb to bacteria by placing in a 37°C H$_2$O bath for 30 min. Distribute 800 μl of the adsorbed phage–bacteria mixture to each of 25 17 × 100 mm sterile polystyrene tubes. Each aliquot contains 4×10^4 phage particles and approximately $1–2 \times 10^8$ bacteria.

4. Prepare fresh NZY soft agarose (200 ml) and place in a H$_2$O bath adjusted to 46–48°C. Allow adequate time for the top agarose to equilibrate.

5. Remove five NZY agar plates from the 37°C incubator at a time and stack to maintain temperature. Add 6.5 ml NZY soft agarose to a single aliquot of the phage–bacteria mix and vortex gently for 5–7 sec. Pour entire contents onto agar plate and gently but quickly tilt and roll the plate so molten agarose covers entire surface before hardening. Immediately place plate on a level surface. Proceed to next plate and repeat.

6. Allow 10–15 min for the soft agarose to harden. Return plates to 37°C and incubate for 8–10 hr.

Prior to lifting the plaques onto membrane filters, the plates should be placed at 4°C for at least 2 hr to prevent the soft agarose from adhering to the filter. A variety of filter types are available for lifting the plaques prior to screening the library. We have had the best results (signal-to-noise) with nylon-based membranes (e.g., Amersham's Hybond-N, DuPont's Colony/

Plaque Screen, or ICN's Biotrans, all 137 mm diameter circles). Detailed protocols for the transfer of plaques, denaturation of DNA, and neutralization of filters are supplied by the manufacturer. After plaque transfer, the plates are stored at 4°C.

We used the following basic protocol for high-stringency screening of cDNA libraries for mouse muscle and for rat neuronal nAChR subunit clones. The membrane filters were prehybridized for 4–6 hr in 500 ml hybridization buffer at 65°C using plastic dishes with air-tight lids. This prehybridization solution was discarded and replaced with 250 ml fresh, prewarmed hybridization buffer containing [^{32}P]CTP radiolabeled DNA as probe. Probe DNAs were labeled by nick translation or random primed with mixtures of hexanucleotides to specific activities of $5\text{--}10 \times 10^8$ cpm/μg and were used at final isotopic concentrations of $2\text{--}4 \times 10^5$ cpm/ml hybridization buffer. A description of the specific DNA probes used to isolate each of the muscle and neuronal AChR subunit cDNAs is presented in Table II. Filters were hybridized for 12–18 hr. They were washed twice in 500-ml volumes of 2× SSPE containing 0.5% sodium dodecyl sulfate at 65°C for 30 min, each followed by 0.2× SSPE plus 0.5% sodium dodecyl sulfate at 65°C for 60 min. For low-stringency hybridization screening, the hybridization temperature was adjusted to 50°C. After hybridization, the filters were washed extensively in 2× SSPE plus 0.5% sodium dodecyl sulfate at room temperature. Filters were exposed to Kodak XAR-5 film with Cronex Quanta II/III intensifying screens at −70°C for 18–36 hr prior to development. Positively hybridizing plaques were purified as follows.

1. The plates were aligned on the X-ray film and the region corresponding to a positively hybridizing plaque was removed by taking a core of the agar using the large end of a Pasteur pipette. The agar plug was placed in 1 ml of SM buffer containing 50 μl of CHCl$_3$, vortexed briefly, and stored at 4°C overnight to allow the phage particles to leach out of the soft agarose.

2. The primary plug phage stocks were diluted 10^{-4} and 20-, 50-, and 100-μl aliquots mixed with 200 μl log phase *E. coli* C600 *Hfl,* 4 ml melted NZY soft agarose and plated on 100×15 mm NZY agar plates. Plates were incubated at 37°C for approximately 8–10 hr.

3. Secondary plaque lifts were made using nitrocellulose membrane filters following established protocols. The filters were prehybridized and hybridized as in the primary screening with the exception that the hybridization buffer contained 0.1% sodium dodecyl sulfate.

4. Single plaques that rescreened positive were picked with the small end of a Pasteur pipette and expelled into 1 ml SM buffer containing 50 μl CHCl$_3$. Purified plaques can be stored in this manner for several months with minimal loss of titer. For long-term storage, however, it is recommended that high-titer lysates be prepared for each λ clone (see below).

TABLE II   Probes and Hybridization Conditions Used for Isolation of
Muscle and Neuronal Nicotinic Acetylcholine
Receptor Subunit cDNAs[a]

Acetylcholine receptor subunit	Clone designation	Probe	Stringency	Reference[b]
Mouse				
Muscle α	λBMA407	Chicken muscle α	High	1
Muscle β	λBMB49	Mouse muscle γ	Low	1
Muscle γ	λBMG419	Human muscle γ	High	2
Muscle δ	λBMD451	Mouse muscle γ	Low	1
Rat				
Neuronal $\alpha2$	λHYP16	Neuronal $\alpha3$	Low	3
Neuronal $\alpha3$	λPCA48	Mouse muscle α	Low	4
Neuronal $\alpha4$	λHYA23-1	Neuronal $\alpha3$	Low	5
Neuronal $\alpha5$	λHIP6E	Neuronal $\beta3$	Low	6
Neuronal $\beta2$	λPCX49	Neuronal $\alpha3$	Low	7
Neuronal $\beta3$	λESD-7	Neuronal $\alpha3$	Low	8
Neuronal $\beta4$	λPC852	Neuronal $\beta4$	High	9

[a] Mouse muscle cDNA clones were isolated from BC3H-1 cell line poly(A)⁺ RNA. Rat neuronal cDNA clones were isolated from libraries constructed from either brain or PC12 cell line poly(A)⁺ RNA. High- and low-stringency hybridization and washing conditions are described in the text.

[b] References: (1) J. Patrick, J. Boulter, D. Goldman, P. Gardner, and S. Heinemann, *Ann. N.Y. Acad. Sci.* **505,** 194 (1987); (2) J. Boulter, K. Evans, G. Martin, P. Mason, S. Stengelin, D. Goldman, S. Heinemann, and J. Patrick, *J. Neurosci. Res.* **16,** 37 (1986); (3) K. Wada, M. Ballivet, J. Boulter, J. Connolly, E. Wada, E. S. Deneris, L. W. Swanson, S. Heinemann, and J. Patrick, *Science* **240,** 330 (1988); (4) J. Boulter, K. Evans, D. Goldman, G. Martin, D. Treco, S. Heinemann, and J. Patrick, *Nature (London)* **319,** 368 (1986); (5) D. Goldman, E. Deneris, W. Luyten, A. Kochhar, J. Patrick, and S. Heinemann, *Cell* **48,** 965 (1987); (6) unpublished observations; (7) E. S. Deneris, J. Connolly, J. Boulter, E. Wada, K. Wada, L. W. Swanson, J. Patrick, and S. Heinemann, *Neuron* **1,** 45 (1988); (8) E. S. Deneris, J. Boulter, L. W. Swanson, J. Patrick, and S. Heinemann, *J. Biol. Chem.* in press; (9) unpublished observations.

Characterization of λ cDNA Clones

General Considerations

Hybridization of λ clones to radiolabeled probes made from existing nAChR subunit DNAs, even at elevated stringencies, was not an adequate criterion for determining that the cloned dscDNA were derived from nAChR subunit genes. The nucleotide sequence and a demonstration of function were the best criteria that the cloned dscDNA encoded nAChR subunits. In the case of the mouse muscle nAChR subunit cDNAs, the sequence of the cloned DNA was sufficient data to confirm the identity of the cloned gene since published reports containing the nucleotide sequences of the *Torpedo* electric organ, calf and chicken skeletal muscle nAChR were available. Sufficient interspecies nucleotide and deduced amino acid sequence identity allowed for the unambiguous assignment of the cloned mouse nAChR genes as either the α, β, γ, or δ subunit cDNAs. However, when a novel nAChR subunit cDNA (e.g., the ε subunit of calf muscle) or putative neuronal nAChR cDNAs were isolated, it became necessary to demonstrate that the protein encoded by the cloned gene actually functioned as part of a bonafide nAChR. A list of muscle- and neuronal-type acetylcholine receptors and related genes cloned from a variety of species is presented in Table III.

Procedure

The first step in sequencing or expressing the cloned cDNA is to isolate sufficient amounts of the insert fragment for subcloning into bacteriophage M13 and a suitable expression vector. The following protocol yields approximately 10–20 μg of phage λ DNA. You will need the following reagents:

Tris, 1 M, pH 7.5
NaCl, 5 M
Polyethylene glycol 6000 (PEG 6000)
10× *Eco*RI buffer (250 mM Tris, pH 7.4, 50 mM MgCl$_2$, 1 M NaCl)
10× Tris-acetate electrophoresis buffer (500 mM Tris-acetate, pH 8.3)
*Eco*RI (100–120,000 U/ml)
Pancreatic RNase (20 mg/ml in 50 mM Tris, pH 7.5, 100 mM NaCl)
DNase I (10 mg/ml in 50 mM Tris, pH 7.5, 5 mM MgCl$_2$, 100 mM NaCl, 50% glycerol)
EDTA (500 μM, pH 8.0)
Ammonium acetate, 10 M
Low-melting-point agarose
Phenol : CHCl$_3$: isoamyl alcohol (50 : 48 : 2, v/v/v)
Ether
Ethanol (absolute)

1. To 10 ml of NZY medium add 500 μl log phase *E. coli* C600 *Hfl* plus 10 μl of purified λ phage stock. Grow phage at 37°C with vigorous shaking in a 250-ml flask.
2. When turbidity of culture decreases (in about 4–5 hr) add 500 μl CHCl$_3$ and continue shaking for 10 min.
3. Transfer phage lysate to a 15-ml polypropylene tube and centrifuge at 3000 g for 15 min. Carefully remove 8 ml of the supernatant to a fresh tube.
4. Add 160 μl of 1 M Tris, pH 7.5, and RNase and DNase to final concentrations of 2 μg and 1 μg/ml, respectively. Vortex and incubate in a 37°C H$_2$O bath for 30 min.

5. Filter lysate through a 0.45-μm filter and add 0.88 g of PEG 6000 and 500 μl of 5 M NaCl. Mix well and place on ice for 30 min.
6. Transfer PEG-treated lysate to a 15-ml Corex tube and centrifuge at 10,000 g for 30 min at 4°C. Decant and discard supernatant. Allow tube to drain in an inverted position for 10–15 min. Wipe sides of tube with a paper towel to remove excess PEG solution.
7. Resuspend pellet in 500 μl 20 mM Tris, pH 7.5, and transfer to a 1.5-ml microfuge tube. Extract with 2 vol of CHCl$_3$. Centrifuge to separate phases. Be careful not to disturb PEG pellicle at interface. Repeat for a total of three extractions.
8. Add 20 μl 500 mM EDTA, pH 8.0, followed immediately by 500 μl phenol : CHCl$_3$: isoamyl alcohol. Vortex for 1 min at maximum speed. Centrifuge for 5 min in a microfuge. Remove top, aqueous phase to a fresh microfuge tube. Extract two times with 1-ml aliquots of ether. Spin briefly to separate phases and discard top ether layer each time.
9. Place the opened tube in a 45°C H$_2$O bath for 5–10 min to evaporate residual ether. Measure volume, add 0.1 vol 10 M ammonium acetate and 2 vol ethanol. Place at −20°C for 10 min and on ice for 20 min. Spin in microfuge for 30 min.
10. Dry pellet under vacuum. Resuspend pellet in 50 μl TE buffer.

At this point, the λ DNA containing the cloned gene should be cleaved with *Eco*RI and electrophoresed on an agarose gel to determine both the size as well as the number of cloned *Eco*RI fragments present. Since it is often the case that multiple *Eco*RI fragments derived from different genes may have been ligated to a single vector, an aliquot of the λ DNA should also be used for a Southern blot and probed with the radiolabeled DNA used to isolate the primary clone. The remainder of the digest can be electrophoresed on a low-melting-point agarose gel and the desired fragment excised and subcloned into *Eco*RI cleaved M13 and plasmid vectors. Set up the following.

1. To 45 μl of the resuspended DNA add 5 μl 10× *Eco*RI buffer and 1 μl *Eco*RI. Incubate at 37°C for 2 hr.
2. Add RNase to a final concentration of 40 μg/ml and continue incubation for an additional 15 min.
3. Remove 10 μl and load directly onto a 0.8% (w/v) standard agarose gel. Load the remainder in two lanes of a low-melting-point agarose gel. For improved resolution, run gels at 4°C.

If the *Eco*RI digest shows a single insert fragment, it can be excised from the low-melting-point agarose gel and subcloned into bacteriophage M13 for

TABLE III cDNA Clones for Muscle and Neuronal Type Acetylcholine Receptors and Related Genes[a]

Acetylcholine receptor type	Species	RNA source	Designation	Type	Function	Reference[b]
Muscle	Torpedo californica	Electric organ	pSPα	α	Yes	1
			2D8	α	No	2
			pSS-2-α	α	Yes	3
			pSPβ	β	Yes	1
			pSS-2-β	β	Yes	3
			4D8	γ	Yes	4
			pSPγ	γ	Yes	1
			pSS-2-γ	γ	Yes	3
			pSPδ	δ	Yes	1
			pSS-2-δ	δ	Yes	3
	Torpedo marmorata	Electric organ	pα1	α	No	5
			NA	α	No	6
	Mouse	BC3H-1 cell line	pMARα15	α	No	7
			pBMA407	α	Yes	8
			NA	α	nt	9
			β7gt11	β	Yes	10
			pBMB49	β	Yes	8
			M169	γ	Yes	11
			pBMG419	γ	Yes	12
			λ58	δ	Yes	13
			pBMD451	δ	Yes	8
	Calf	Fetal skeletal muscle	pSPcα	α	Yes	14
			pSPcβ	β	Yes	14
			pSPcγ	γ	Yes	14
			pSPcδ	δ	Yes	14
			pSPcε	ε	Yes	14
	Rat	Skeletal muscle	NA	ε	nt	14a
	Xenopus laevis	Embryos	NA	α	nt	15
			NA	γ	nt	15
			NA	δ	nt	15
	Human	TE671 cell line	TE 1.1	α	nt	16

			Clone	Subunit	Expressed	Reference
Neuronal	*Drosophila melanogaster*	Head	ARD1	Non-α	nt	17
		Instar larvae	ALS	α	nt	18
	Rat	Brain	pHYP16	α2	Yes	19
			pHYA23-1	α4-1	Yes	20
			pHIP3C	α4-2	nt	21
			pPC989	α5	No	21
			rESD76	β3	No	22
		Superior cervical ganglion	SCG3	Non-α2	nt	22a
		PC12 cell line	pPCX49	β2	Yes	23
			pPCA48	α3	Yes	24
	Chicken	Brain	NA	α4	Yes	25
			NA	Non-α	Yes	25
			pCh23.1	Non-α	nt	26

[a] In cases where overlapping cDNA clones have been isolated for a single nAChR gene, only one of the clones has been entered. The function of the clones was, in most cases, determined by using electrophysiological techniques. The cloned DNAs were used as templates for *in vitro* synthesis of RNA followed by microinjection of the transcripts into *X. laevis* oocytes. The *T. californica* electric organ cDNA clones engineered in the pSS-2 vector have also been expressed in stably transfected mammalian cell lines. NA, Specific clone designation not available; nt, not tested.

[b] References: (1) M. Mishina, T. Tobimatsu, K. Imoto, K. Tanaka, Y. Fujita, K. Fukuda, M. Kurasaki, H. Takahashi, Y. Morimoto, T. Hirose, S. Inayama, T. Takahashi, M. Kuno, and S. Numa, *Nature (London)* **313**, 364 (1985); (2) *Cold Spring Harbor Symp. Quant. Biol.* **83**, 71 (1983); (3) T. Claudio, *Proc. Natl. Acad. Sci. U.S.A.* **84**, 5967 (1987); (4) M. Ballivet, J. Patrick, J. Lee, and S. Heinemann, *Proc. Natl. Acad. Sci. U.S.A.* **79**, 4466 (1982); (5) A. Devillers-Thiery, J. Giraudat, M. Bentaboulet, and J. Chargeux, *Proc. Natl. Acad. Sci. U.S.A.* **80**, 2067 (1983); (6) K. Sumikawa, M. Houghton, J. C. Smith, L. Bell, B. M. Richards, and E. A. Barnard, *Nucleic Acids Res.* **10**, 5809 (1982); (7) J. Boulter, W. Luyten, K. Evans, P. Mason, M. Ballivet, D. Goldman, S. Stengelin, G. Martin, S. Heinemann, and J. Patrick, *J. Neurosci.* **5**, 2545 (1985); (8) J. Patrick, J. Boulter, D. Goldman, P. Gardner, and S. Heinemann, *Ann. N.Y. Acad. Sci.* **505**, 194 (1987); (9) K. E. Isenberg, J. Mudd, V. Shah, and J. P. Merlie, *Nucleic Acids Res.* **14**, 5111 (1986); (10) A. Buonanno, J. Mudd, V. Shah, and J. P. Merlie, *J. Biol. Chem.* **261**, 16451 (1986); (11) L. Yu, R. J. LaPolla, and N. Davidson, *Nucleic Acids Res.* **14**, 3539 (1986); (12) J. Boulter, K. Evans, P. Mason, S. Stengelin, D. Goldman, S. Heinemann, and J. Patrick, *J. Neurosci. Res.* **16**, 37 (1986); (13) R. J. LaPolla, K. Mixter Mayne, and N. Davidson, *Proc. Natl. Acad. Sci. U.S.A.* **81**, 7970 (1984); (14) T. Takai, M. Noda, M. Mishina, S. Shimizu, Y. Furutani, T. Kayano, T. Ikeda, T. Kubo, H. Takahasi, T. Takahashi, M. Kuno, and S. Numa, *Nature (London)* **315**, 761 (1985); (14a) M. Criado, V. Witzemann, M. Koenen, and B. Sakmann, *Nucleic Acids Res.* **16**, 10920 (1988); (15) T. Baldwin, C. M. Yoshihara, K. Blackmer, C. R. Kintner, and S. J. Burden, *J. Cell Biol.* **106**, 469 (1988); (16) R. Schoepfer, M. Luther, and J. Lindstrom, *FEBS Lett.* **226**, 235 (1988); (17) I. Hermans-Borgmeyer, D. Zopf, R. Ryseck, B. Hovemann, H. Betz, and E. D. Gundelfinger, *EMBO J.* **5**, 1503 (1986); (18) B. Bossy, M. Ballivet, and P. Spierer, *EMBO J.* **7**, 611 (1988); (19) K. Wada, M. Ballivet, J. Boulter, J. Connolly, E. Wada, E. S. Deneris, L. W. Swanson, S. Heinemann, and J. Patrick, *Science* **240**, 330 (1988); (20) D. Goldman, E. Deneris, W. Luyten, A. Kochhar, J. Patrick, and S. Heinemann, *Cell* **48**, 965 (1987); (21) unpublished observations; (22) E. S. Deneris, J. Boulter, L. W. Swanson, J. Patrick, and S. Heinemann, *J. Biol. Chem.* **264**, 6268 (1989); (22a) K. E. Isenberg and G. E. Meyer, *J. Neurochem.* **52**, 988 (1989); (23) E. S. Deneris, J. Connolly, J. Boulter, E. Wada, K. Wada, L. W. Swanson, J. Patrick, and S. Heinemann, *Neuron* **1**, 45 (1988); (24) J. Boulter, K. Evans, D. Goldman, G. Martin, D. Treco, S. Heinemann, and J. Patrick, *Nature (London)* **319**, 368 (1986); (25) P. Nef, C. Oneyser, C. Alliod, S. Couturier, and M. Ballivet, *EMBO J.* **7**, 595 (1988); (26) R. Schoepfer, P. Whiting, F. Esch, R. Blacher, S. Shimasaki, and J. Lindstrom, *Neuron* **1**, 241 (1988).

sequencing. If more than one insert fragment is present, excise each fragment from the low-melting-point agarose and store at 4°C. To identify the fragment(s) of interest, perform a Southern blot on the standard agarose gel and hybridize to the probe used in the initial library screening. Protocols for ligations using low-melting-point agarose (16) and for DNA sequencing (17) are detailed elsewhere.

Genomic Cloning of Nicotinic Acetylcholine Receptors

The key to a successful genomic DNA library screening is to construct a library that contains as complete a representation of genomic sequences as possible. There are, of course, a number of practical aspects which must be considered in constructing such a library, the most important being the ability to achieve full genomic representation with as few clones as possible, thus simplifying the screening process. In the discussion that follows, we will present our approach to this problem and describe in detail the strategy we employed to generate a genomic DNA library from rat liver DNA and the screening procedure we used to isolate genomic DNA clones coding for several members of the neuronal nAChR gene family. Furthermore, we will illustrate how recently developed bactriophage λ vector technology was used to identify a cluster of receptor-related genes.

Construction of a genomic DNA library proceeds in three phases: (1) isolation of high-molecular-weight genomic DNA, (2) generation of randomly cleaved DNA, and (3) cloning of the cleaved DNA into a suitable vector.

Isolation of High-Molecular-Weight Genomic DNA

General Considerations

It is critical that the genomic DNA used to generate the recombinant library be of high molecular weight (>100 kb). A number of precautions should be taken to ensure that this is the case. First, the activity of endogenous nucleases can be minimized by processing tissue rapidly and at low temperatures. Second, genomic DNA is susceptible to shearing forces when being extracted and thus mixing should be gentle. Finally, prior to size fractionation of the DNA, organic solvents and salts should be removed by dialysis rather than ethanol precipitation.

Procedure

The volumes indicated are recommended for 2–3 g of starting material. The following solutions are needed.

0.15 M NaCl, 10 mM Tris, pH 7.5

Buffer A: 0.32 M sucrose, 3 mM CaCl$_2$, 2 mM magnesium acetate, 0.1 mM EDTA, 0.1% Triton X-100, 1 mM dithiothreitol, 0.1 mM phenylmethylsulfonyl fluoride, 10 mM Tris, pH 8.0

Buffer B: 2 M sucrose, 5 mM magnesium acetate, 0.1 mM EDTA, 1 mM DTT, 10 mM Tris, pH 8.0

Buffer C: 25% glycerol, 5 mM magnesium acetate, 0.1 mM EDTA, 5 mM DTT, 50 mM Tris, pH 8.0

Buffer D: 0.625% SDS, 0.625 mM NaCl, 12.5 mM EDTA, 62.5 mM Tris, pH 8.0

Redistilled phenol

Phenol : chloroform : isoamyl alcohol (50 : 48 : 2, v/v/v)

Ether

Proteinase K

TE buffer (10 mM Tris, pH 8.0, 1 mM EDTA)

DNase-free RNase

Note: Unless otherwise indicated, steps 1–6 are done at 4°C.

1. Immediately after dissection, wash and mince neonatal rat livers (day 1) in ice-cold 0.15 M NaCl, 10 mM Tris, pH 7.5.
2. Gently homogenize (6–8 strokes) the tissue with a Teflon dounce homogenizer in 8 ml buffer A.
3. Pass homogenate through cheesecloth to remove large tissue fragments and gently homogenize again with ~15 strokes.
4. Dilute homogenate with 2 vol of buffer B.
5. Overlay 8 ml of diluted homogenate onto a 3-ml cushion of buffer B in a Beckman SW41 polyallomer tube. A total of four tubes will be necessary. Centrifuge the tubes in a Beckman SW41 rotor at 30,000 rpm for 50 min at 2°C.
6. Discard supernatant and resuspend pelleted nuclei in 2 ml buffer C. The nuclei can be stored at −100°C or processed further.
7. Adjust volume to 10 ml with buffer D then add proteinase K to a final concentration of 50 μg/ml. Incubate at 37°C for 30 min.
8. Extract the DNA with an equal volume of redistilled phenol.
9. Extract the DNA two times with an equal volume of phenol : CHCl$_3$: isoamyl alcohol.
10. Extract the DNA two times with an equal volume of ether.
11. Dialyze the DNA extensively against TE at 4°C.
12. Add DNase-free RNase to a final concentration of 50 μg/ml and incubate at 37°C for 2 hr.
13. Repeat steps 8–11.

14. Determine concentration and purity of DNA. Highly purified DNA will have an A_{260} to A_{280} ratio of about 1.8.

Approximately 4–5 mg of DNA can be expected from 2–3 g of tissue. Agarose gel electrophoresis should be done to assess the size and integrity of the genomic DNA.

Partial Digestion and Size Fractionation of Genomic DNA

General Considerations

As mentioned earlier, the critical step for a successful genomic DNA library screening is the construction of a recombinant library that is as complete as possible. This can be accomplished by cloning large (~15–20 kb) DNA fragments generated by random cleavage of genomic DNA. Under such conditions, the number of clones, N, that must be screened to identify a particular sequence with a probability, P, can be estimated by

$$N = \ln(1 - P)/\ln(1 - f)$$

where f is the size of the fragment expressed as a fraction of the genome (18). For example, to achieve a 99% probability of isolating a given DNA sequence in a library consisting of 15-kb fragments from a typical mammalian genome (3×10^9 bp):

$$N = \ln(1 - 0.99)/\ln[1 - (1.5 \times 10^4/3 \times 10^9)] = 9.2 \times 10^5 \text{ clones}$$

It is important to realize that this statistical analysis is based on the assumption that the genomic sequences are randomly represented in the cloned DNA fragments. Mechanical shearing is the only technique which can approach totally random cleavage of genomic DNA. Unfortunately, randomly sheared DNA must be subjected to a number of additional manipulations prior to cloning, which renders this procedure a relatively inconvenient way of constructing a genomic DNA library. The method of choice which, while reducing the number of subsequent manipulations, still yields sufficiently random cleavage of genomic DNA, is partial digestion of DNA with restriction enzymes. A detailed discussion of genomic sequence representation in a library constructed in this fashion is beyond the scope of this chapter; however, the reader is referred to Seed *et al.* (19) for an excellent treatment of the subject.

The enzymes most commonly used for partial digestion of genomic DNA, *Mbo*I and *Sau*3A, are advantageous for two reasons. (1) They recognize a tetranucleotide sequence which results in a more random collection of DNA fragments than enzymes which recognize hexanucleotide sequences and (2) they produce fragments that can be directly ligated into *Bam*HI-cut vectors. Because of our choice of cloning vectors (see below), we used *Mbo*I to partially restrict the genomic DNA. Before carrying out a large-scale partial restriction, it is necessary to perform an analytical experiment to determine the optimal conditions for the partial digestion.

Procedure

The following reagents are needed.

> High-quality *Mbo*I ($\sim$10,000 U/ml)
> 10× *Mbo*I buffer (1 M NaCl, 100 mM Tris, pH 7.4, 100 mM MgCl$_2$, 10 mM DTT)
> 0.5 M EDTA
> 10× agarose gel loading dye (150 mg/ml Ficoll-400, 2.5 mg/ml bromphenol blue, 2.5 mg/ml xylene cyanole)
> Phenol : CHCl$_3$: isoamyl alcohol (50 : 48 : 2, v/v/v)
> 10 M ammonium acetate
> Ether
> TE buffer
> Ethanol (absolute)

1. In a 1.5-ml microfuge tube, mix 10 μg genomic DNA and 15 μl 10× *Mbo*I buffer. Adjust the volume to 150 μl with H$_2$O.
2. Label nine microfuge tubes 1–9 and place on ice.
3. Add 30 μl of the DNA mix to tube 1 and 15 μl to tubes 2–9.
4. Add 2 units of *Mbo*I to tube 1 and mix well. This gives a final enzyme concentration of 1 U/μg of DNA. Transfer 15 μl of this reaction mixture to tube 2, thus diluting the enzyme 2-fold and giving a final concentration of 0.5 U/μg of DNA. Continue serially diluting the enzyme 2-fold in this manner through to tube 8 (final *Mbo*I concentration in tube 8 = 0.0075 U/μg DNA). Add no enzyme to tube 9.
5. Incubate all the tubes at 37°C for 1 hr.
6. Stop the reactions by adding 1 μl of 0.5 M EDTA.
7. Add 2 μl of gel loading dye to each sample and electrophorese through a 0.4% agarose gel. Be sure to run size markers on the outside lanes of the gel. The electrophoresis is done slowly (1–2 V/cm) until the bromphenol blue has just migrated off the gel.
8. Photograph the gel and determine the amount of enzyme required to produce the maximum ethidium bromide staining in the 15- to 20-kb region of the gel (Fig. 2). The staining intensity is related to the mass

AMOUNT OF <u>Mbo</u>I (units/μg)

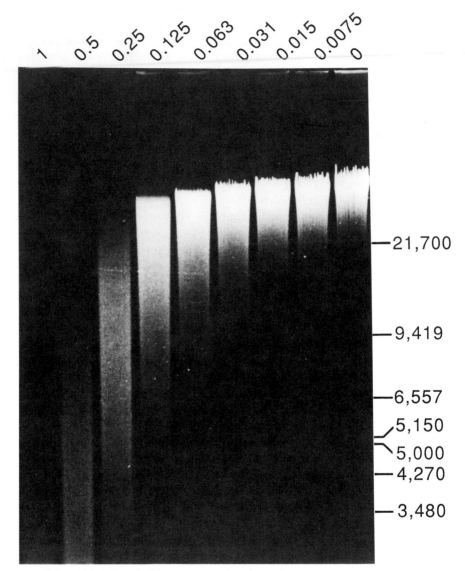

FIG. 2 Ethidium bromide-stained agarose gel showing digestion patterns of high-molecular-weight genomic DNA cut with varying concentrations of *Mbo*I. DNA molecular weight standards are in base pairs. *Mbo*I partial digestion and agarose gel electrophoresis conditions are described in the text.

distribution of the DNA. In order to generate the maximum number of DNA molecules in the 15- to 20-kb range, use half of the amount of *Mbo*I that produces the most intense staining (see Ref. 19 for a complete discussion of partial digestion of genomic DNA). In the experiment shown in Fig. 2, 0.125 U of *Mbo*I/μg of DNA was found to give the most intense staining in the 15- to 20-kb range. Therefore, we used 0.0625 U/μg of DNA for the preparative procedure.

9. Based on the analytical experiment, partially digest 200 μg of high-molecular-weight genomic DNA with the appropriate concentration of *Mbo*I using identical reaction conditions.
10. Run 1 μg of the restricted DNA through a 0.4% agarose gel to check that the size distribution is as expected.
11. Extract the DNA with an equal volume of phenol : $CHCl_3$: isoamyl alcohol.
12. Extract the DNA with ether.
13. Precipitate the DNA using 10 M ammonium acetate and 100% ethanol. Resuspend the DNA in 200 μl of TE.

At this point, the partially digested genomic DNA is usually size-fractionated. However, the cloning system we used, λGEM-11, requires that the *Mbo*I ends of the genomic DNA be partially filled-in prior to ligation to the vector (see below). Therefore, we carried out a partial fill-in reaction before size-fractionating the DNA.

Procedure

The following reagents are needed.

> *Mbo*I partially digested genomic DNA
> Klenow fragment of *E. coli* DNA polymerase I (5,000 U/ml)
> 10× Klenow buffer (0.5 M Tris, pH 7.2, 0.1 M MgSO$_4$, 1 mM DTT)
> 5 mM dGTP
> 5 mM dATP
> 0.5 M EDTA

1. Add in order 200 μl *Mbo*I partially restricted genomic DNA, 30 μl 10× Klenow buffer, 10 μl 5 mM dGTP, 10 μl 5 mM dATP, 45 μl H$_2$O, 5 U of Klenow fragment.
2. Incubate at room temperature for 45 min.
3. Stop the reaction by adding 15 μl 0.5 M EDTA and heating at 68°C for 10 min.

The partially digested, partially filled-in genomic DNA is now ready to be size-fractionated.

Procedure

The following solutions are needed.

> 5% NaCl in 10 mM Tris, pH 8.0, 5 mM EDTA
> 25% NaCl in 10 mM Tris, pH 8.0, 5 mM EDTA
> 10× agarose gel loading dye
> TE buffer
> Ethanol (absolute)

1. Prepare a 5–25% linear NaCl gradient in a Beckman SW41 polyallomer tube.
2. Carefully layer the partially digested, partially filled-in, genomic DNA onto the salt gradient.
3. Centrifuge the gradient in a Beckman SW41 rotor at 35,000 rpm for 4.5 hr at 20°C.
4. Puncture the bottom of the tube and collect 0.33-ml fractions.
5. Mix 5 μl of every other fraction with 15 μl H_2O and 2 μl 10× agarose gel loading dye. Electrophorese the samples through a 0.4% agarose gel with appropriate molecular weight size markers.
6. Photograph the gel (Fig. 3). Pool the gradient fractions containing DNA migrating in the 15- to 20-kb range. In the experiment shown in Fig. 3, fractions 19 and 20 were pooled.
7. Ethanol precipitate the pooled DNA and resuspend in TE to a final concentration of ~500 ng/μl.

Genomic DNA Library Construction

General Considerations

The last phase of genomic DNA library construction involves the ligation of the size-fractionated genomic DNA to an appropriate cloning vector. The two primary classes of genomic cloning vectors are bacteriophage λ vectors and hybrid plasmid vectors called cosmids. Bacteriophage λ vectors are most commonly used because of their relatively high cloning efficiency and ease of manipulation. While cosmids can accommodate genomic DNA inserts approximately twice as large as λ vectors (e.g., 30 to 40 kb), they are technically difficult to handle.

As is the case with cDNA cloning vectors, the application of recombinant DNA techniques to genomic cloning vectors has led to a second generation of λ vectors. These multipurpose vectors have been designed to satisfy a number of cloning requirements (e.g., large DNA insert size, multiple cloning sites). A representative sample of these vectors and their character-

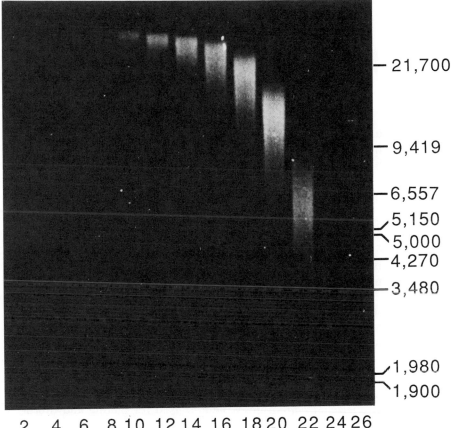

FIG. 3   Size fractionation of *Mbo*I partially digested genomic DNA. The DNA was fractionated by centrifugation through a 5–25% NaCl gradient. Aliquots of every other fraction were analyzed by agarose gel electrophoresis as described in the text. Fractions 19 and 20 were pooled and used to construct a genomic DNA library in λGEM-11.

istics is presented in Table II. Below, we describe the use of one of these vectors, λGEM-11 (Fig. 4) to construct a rat genomic DNA library.

λGEM-11 affords several advantages for genomic cloning. (1) It can harbor genomic DNA inserts of 9–23 kb. (2) λGEM-11 has a multiple cloning region with several unique restriction sites permitting versatility in the choice of enzymes used for cloning. In addition, the multiple cloning region

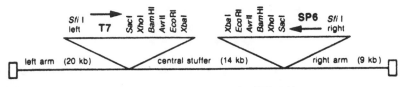

FIG. 4   Structural map of λGEM-11.

allows more efficient restriction endonuclease mapping strategies to be used in characterizing the cloned genes. (3) The multiple cloning region is flanked by the SP6 and T7 RNA polymerase promoters. These promoters can be used for making radiolabeled end-specific probes that permit rapid gene mapping and chromosome walking.

Procedure

λGEM-11 has been engineered in such a way that the efficiency of insertion is higher than other λ-based vectors, the background of nonrecombinant phage is minimized, and the possibility of multiple inserts is eliminated. The cloning strategy is diagrammed in Fig. 5. λGEM-11 is digested with *Xho*I and then partially filled-in with dTTP and dCTP. This leaves the vector with 5'-TC extensions that cannot self-ligate but can ligate with genomic DNA partially digested with *Mbo*I and partially filled-in with dGTP and dATP (prepared as described above). Genomic DNA fragments prepared in this way cannot self-ligate themselves. The ligated λGEM-11 is assembled into intact phage particles as described for the construction of a cDNA library. *Escherichia coli* strain MB406 is used for plating and titering the genomic library.

Plating and Screening the Genomic DNA Library

Procedure

The procedures used for plating and screening genomic and cDNA libraries are essentially the same. The major difference is the *E. coli* host used for plating: *E. coli* C600 *Hfl* is used for a λgt10 cDNA library while *E. coli* MB406 is used for the λGEM-11 library. Plaque purification of positively hybridizing genomic DNA clones is also done as described for cDNA clones (although the dilutions for plating may differ, depending on the titer of the phage stocks).

Our initial strategy for screening the λGEM-11 library was straightforward (Fig. 6). The genomic DNA library was screened at high stringency with a nick-translated probe derived from a cDNA clone encoding the neuronal

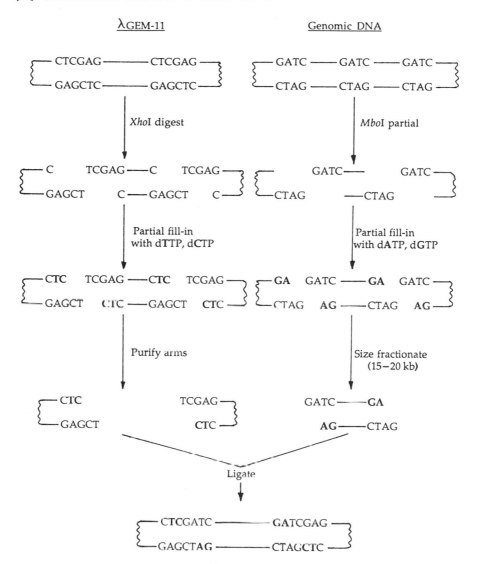

FIG. 5 Strategy used to construct a genomic DNA library in λGEM-11.

nAChR α3 gene (20). The screening was done exactly as described for the high-stringency screening of a cDNA library. This initial screening yielded a genomic clone, λRG518B (Fig. 6A), that was characterized as described below.

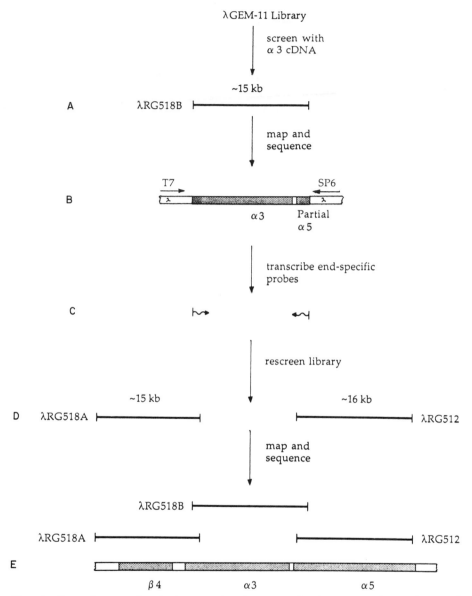

FIG. 6   Procedure used to isolate overlapping genomic clones spanning a cluster of three members of the rat neuronal nicotinic acetylcholine receptor-related gene family.

Characterization of Genomic Clones

Significant amounts of the cloned genomic DNA are required for mapping and subcloning and can be isolated as follows.

Procedure

    NZY agar plates
    λ genomic clone stock
    Escherichia coli strain MB406
    10 mM Tris, pH 7.4, 5 mM MgSO$_4$
    NZY soft agarose
    SM saturated with CHCl$_3$ (without gelatin)
    CsCl dissolved in SM (without gelatin) at the following concentrations:
        1.7 g CsCl/ml of SM
        1.5 g CsCl/ml of SM
        1.3 g CsCl/ml of SM
    20% sucrose in SM (without gelatin)
    50% formamide, 200 mM Tris, pH 8.5, 20 mM EDTA
    TE buffer

Steps 1–5 are described in detail above for the plating of a cDNA library.

1. Pour 10 150 × 15 mm NZY agar plates 2–3 days before plating.
2. On the day of plating, grow *E. coli* MB406 to mid-log phase. Harvest cells by centrifugation and resuspend in an equal volume of 10 mM Tris, pH 7.4, 5 mM MgSO$_4$.
3. In a sterile tube mix 2.5 ml MB406 with 5×10^5 phage from the genomic DNA clone stock. Incubate at 37°C for 30 min. Aliquot 250 μl of the adsorbed phage–bacteria mixture to each of 10 17 × 100 mm sterile polystyrene tubes.
4. Add 15 ml molten NZY soft agarose (at 48°C) to each tube. Vortex gently for 3–4 sec, then pour the contents onto an NZY agar plate. Be sure the molten agarose covers the entire surface of the plate.
5. Let the soft agarose harden for 10 min, then incubate the plates at 37°C for 8–12 hr.
6. Harvest the phage by scraping the surface of the plates with a rubber spatula. The soft agarose layer (containing the phage) will come off very easily. Transfer the soft agarose to a beaker.
7. Break up the soft agarose and then add 100 ml SM saturated with CHCl$_3$. Incubate at 4°C overnight.
8. Transfer the soft agarose mixture to a 250-ml centrifuge bottle and centrifuge at 4°C for 20 min at 6000 rpm in order to spin out the agarose.

9. Prepare CsCl block gradients in Beckman SW27 tubes as follows. Place 3 ml of a 1.7 g CsCl/ml SM solution at the bottom of the tube. Carefully layer 4 ml of a 1.5 g/ml solution on top of the 1.7 g/ml solution. Carefully layer 3 ml of a 1.3 g/ml solution on top of the 1.5 g/ml solution. Carefully layer 4 ml of 20% sucrose on top of the 1.3 g/ml solution.

10. Carefully layer ~24 ml of the phage solution on top of the gradient. You will need about four gradients for the entire preparation.

11. Centrifuge at 22,000 rpm for 90 min at 4°C.

12. The phage will appear as a faint blue band at the interface of the 1.3 g/ml and 1.5 g/ml solutions. Remove the phage with a 22-gauge needle and syringe.

13. Dialyze the phage against 50% formamide, 200 mM Tris, pH 8.5, 20 mM EDTA overnight at 4°C with one change of buffer. This step ruptures the phage coat, resulting in the release of the phage DNA.

14. Dialyze extensively against TE at 4°C.

Phage DNA isolated in this manner is suitable for mapping, subcloning and generating chromosome walking probes (see below).

We used the above procedure to isolate phage DNA from one of the genomic clones that hybridized with the α3 cDNA probe. The genomic clone, λRG518B, was mapped with restriction endonucleases and found to contain an insert of ~15 kb (Fig. 6A). Detailed restriction mapping and Southern blot analysis (21) identified a number of genomic DNA fragments that hybridized with various regions of the α3 cDNA. These genomic fragments were subcloned into M13mp19 and sequenced. The sequence analysis indicated that λRG518B contained the majority of the coding region of the α3 gene, lacking only the extreme 5' end of the gene. In addition, a portion of another neuronal nAChR subunit-related gene, α5 (unpublished observation), was found to be located to the right of the α3 gene in λRG518B (Fig. 6B).

In order to isolate the entire α5 gene, we took advantage of the chromosome walking system engineered into λGEM-11. The walking is done by using RNA probes synthesized from the extreme 5' and 3' ends of the cloned insert which are used to rescreen the λGEM-11 library. The RNA probes are made using the SP6 and T7 RNA polymerase promoters located on each side of the multiple cloning region. However, before synthesizing the RNA probes, the genomic clone is digested completely with a frequent cutter such as *Rsa*I to restrict the size of the RNA probes. This system enabled us to make an end-specific RNA probe corresponding to the portion of the α5 gene present in λRG518B using the SP6 RNA polymerase promoter (Fig. 6C). The RNA probe was synthesized as follows.

Procedure

The following reagents and solutions are needed.

> *Rsa*I (~20,000 U/ml)
> 10× *Rsa*I digestion buffer (100 mM Tris, pH 7.9, 500 mM NaCl, 100 mM MgCl$_2$, 60 mM 2-mercaptoethanol)
> Ethanol (absolute)
> 10 M ammonium acetate
> TE buffer
> 5× transcription buffer (200 mM Tris, pH 8, 40 mM MgCl$_2$, 10 mM spermidine, 250 mM NaCl)
> 2.5 mM rATP
> 2.5 mM rGTP
> 2.5 mM rCTP
> 400–800 Ci/mmol, 10 mCi/ml [α-^{32}P]UTP
> 750 mM DTT
> SP6 RNA polymerase (20,000 U/ml)
> RQ1 DNase (Promega, 1,000 U/ml)

1. Digest 2 μg of the genomic clone with 50 U of *Rsa*I in 1× *Rsa*I digestion buffer at 37°C for 2 hr.
2. Ethanol precipitate the digested DNA.
3. Resuspend in 10 μl of TE.
4. Add in order 10 μl restricted genomic clone, 5 μl 5× transcription buffer, 1 μl of each nonradioactive rNTP, 5 μl [^{32}P]UTP, 1 μl DTT, 1 μl SP6 RNA polymerase. Incubate at 40°C for 30 min.
5. Add RQ1 DNase to a final concentration of 1 U/μg of template. Incubate for 10 min at 37°C.
6. Ethanol precipitate as usual and resuspend in 50 μl of TE.

The RNA probe was used to rescreen the λGEM-11 library. Because the probe used was an RNA probe, hybridization conditions were somewhat different from those used for a cDNA probe. The hybridization buffer was 1 M NaCl, 50 mM Tris, pH 8.3, 50% (v/v) formamide, 10% PEG 6000, 5× Denhardt's, 100 mg/ml salmon sperm DNA. The hybridization was done at 42°C.

This screening yielded a genomic clone, λRG512 (Fig. 6D), that by restriction mapping was shown to overlap λRG518B. In addition, sequence analysis indicated that λRG512 contained the entire α5 gene (Fig. 6E). Thus, in one walking step we were able to identify two contiguous genomic clones spanning ~31 kb of DNA and containing two neuronal nAChR genes.

We then used this technology to walk in the opposite direction using the T7 RNA polymerase promoter and the left end of λRG518B as template (Fig.

6C). Using this end-specific probe to rescreen the λGEM-11 library, we isolated another clone, λRG518A (Fig. 6D), which by mapping, overlaps λRG518B (Fig. 6E). Sequence analysis of λRG518A showed that this clone contained the extreme 5' end of the α3 gene and at least a portion of yet another neuronal nAChR subunit-related gene, β4 (unpublished observation, Fig. 6E).

In summary, using the λGEM-11 genomic cloning system, we were able to isolate three contiguous genomic clones spanning approximately 45 kb of DNA. Within this span of DNA, we identified a cluster of three members of the nicotinic acetylcholine receptor-related gene family.

Acknowledgments

We thank Anne O'Shea-Greenfield for her able assistance in preparing the tables and manuscript. The unpublished work presented in this chapter was carried out in the laboratory of Dr. James Patrick at The Salk Institute and was supported by grants from the Amoco Foundation, the National Institutes of Health, the Muscular Dystrophy Association, and a contract with the Department of Defense.

References

1. D. Schubert, A. J. Harris, C. E. Devine, and S. Heinemann, *J. Cell Biol.* **61,** 398 (1974).
2. L. A. Greene and A. S. Tischler, *Proc. Natl. Acad. Sci. U.S.A.* **73,** 2424 (1976).
3. D. D. Blumberg, *in* "Methods in Enzymology" (S. L. Berger and A. R. Kimmel, eds.), Vol. 152, p. 20. Academic Press, Orlando, Florida, 1987.
4. J. A. Gordon, *Biochemistry* **11,** 1862 (1972).
5. R. A. Cox, *in* "Methods in Enzymology" (L. Grossman and K. Moldave, eds.), Vol. 12, p. 120. Academic Press, New York, 1968.
6. J. M. Chirgwin, A. E. Przybyla, R. J. MacDonald, and W. J. Rutter, *Biochemistry* **18,** 5294 (1979).
7. P. Chomczynski and N. Sacchi, *Anal. Biochem.* **162,** 156 (1987).
8. H. Aviv and P. Leder, *Proc. Natl. Acad. Sci. U.S.A.* **69,** 1408 (1972).
9. U. Lindberg and T. Persson, *in* "Methods in Enzymology" (W. B. Jakoby and M. Wilchek, eds.), Vol. 34, p. 496. Academic Press, New York, 1973.
10. R. C. Ogden and D. A. Adams, *in* "Methods in Enzymology" (S. L. Berger and A. R. Kimmel, eds.), Vol. 152, p. 61. Academic Press, Orlando, Florida, 1987.
11. H. Okayama and P. Berg, *Mol. Cell. Biol.* **2,** 161 (1982).
12. U. Gubler and B. J. Hoffman, *Gene* **25,** 263 (1983).
13. T. Maniatis, E. F. Fritsch, and J. Sambrook, "Molecular Cloning: A Laboratory Manual," p. 473. Cold Spring Harbor Laboratory, Cold Spring Harbor, New York, 1982.

14. R. D. Young and R. W. Davis, *Science* **222,** 778 (1983).
15. T. V. Huynh, R. A. Young, and R. W. Davis, *in* "DNA Cloning: A Practical Approach" (D. M. Glover, ed.), Vol. 1. IRL Press, Oxford, 1985.
16. K. Struhl, *BioTechniques* **3,** 452 (1985).
17. R. M. K. Dale, B. A. McClure, and J. P. Houchins, *Plasmid* **13,** 31 (1985).
18. L. Clark and J. Carbon, *Cell* **9,** 91 (1976).
19. B. Seed, R. C. Parker, and N. Davidson, *Gene* **19,** 201 (1982).
20. J. Boulter, K. Evans, D. Goldman, G. Martin, D. Treco, S. Heinemann, and J. Patrick, *Nature (London)* **319,** 368 (1986).
21. E. M. Southern, *J. Mol. Biol.* **98,** 503 (1975).

Section IV

Lineage Analysis

[21] Lineage Analysis in the Vertebrate Nervous System by Retrovirus-Mediated Gene Transfer

Connie Cepko

Introduction

Many applications of interest to neurobiologists require the marking of a cell and its progeny. Cell marking can be used to investigate lineage, identify transplanted cells, or follow cells that have undergone some experimental perturbation, such as injection of a drug or introduction of a foreign gene. Several criteria for an ideal marking method are as follows: (1) stability and the capacity to self-renew in order to endure many rounds of cell division throughout the life of the animal, (2) a straightforward and relatively easy method for introduction and tracing of the marker, and (3) no effect of the marker on the system that is under study. A variety of markers and techniques have been employed and each has its advantages and disadvantages. Classical techniques rely on introduction of nonrenewable markers, such as an enzyme (1) or dye (2). These methods have primarily been limited to use in large, accessible cells, but improvements in injection proficiency and the availability of nondiffusible, stable dyes have allowed an expansion of this technique to smaller cells and complex systems. Reliable labeling of only one cell at a time may provide an advantage for lineage analysis in systems where a great deal of cell migration and mixing occur. Accessibility, long-term stability (i.e., months to years), and dilution effects remain as limits to this type of marking protocol.

Retrovirus vectors provide an alternative to intracellular injections. They deliver a stable, genetic marker of one's choice to cells that are not accessible for intracellular injection. The genetic tag remains with infected cells and their progeny throughout the life of an animal. They also provide an alternative to the transgenic mouse technology as they allow introduction of genes and transcriptional elements (e.g., cell type-specific promoters) for evaluation *in vivo* (and *in vitro*). Potential disadvantages for some applications are that expression of a transduced gene does not occur 100% of the time and lineage mapping in tissues that undergo extensive cell mixing requires tedious statistical analysis for establishment of clonal boundaries. The application of this technique to the analysis of lineage in rat retina (3), mouse epithelium (4), and chick tectum (5) has been quite successful and suggests the utility of this approach. A comparison of lineage data obtained by intracellular injections of nondiffusible tags and retrovirus marking was recently made possible as two different groups used intracellular injections to investigate lineage in *Xenopus* retina (6, 7). Both groups obtained the same lineage patterns that were observed from retroviral marking of the rat retina.

The parameters and protocols of the retroviral marking technique will be discussed below. For a review of retroviruses and their use as vectors, see Weiss *et al.* (8), Brown and Scott (9), Price (10), Cepko (11–13), and Hughes *et al.* (14).

Overall Strategy

A retrovirus vector that is replication-incompetent, infectious, and encodes a histochemical marker gene provides the basis for genetically marking virtually any mitotic cell in certain species. Over the past 7 years, efficient vector systems have been made and are generally available. One can now obtain a histochemical marker virus or appropriate bacterial plasmids for construction of one's own vector. If one obtains vector stocks (i.e., infectious virus particles) then the only other necessity is an infectable cell line for quantitation of vector concentration (i.e., titration). If a vector is obtained as a DNA plasmid, then a packaging cell line should also be acquired for production of virus. After a vector stock is produced or obtained, it is titered, usually concentrated, and used to infect cells *in vivo* or *in vitro*. Assay of the marker gene product can be carried out at any desirable time.

Vector Designs

General Considerations

Retroviruses encapsidate RNA as their genomic material. As RNA is difficult to manipulate, a DNA copy of the genome is used for production of vectors. Retroviruses produce a DNA copy of their genome immediately after infection via reverse transcriptase, a protein encoded by the viral *pol* gene and included in the viral particle ("virion"). The DNA copy is integrated into the host cell genome and is thereafter referred to as a "provirus." Most vectors begin as proviruses that are cloned from cells infected with a naturally occurring retrovirus. Proviruses have been manipulated with standard recombinant DNA techniques to yield a variety of vectors. All vectors contain the cis-acting viral sequences necessary for the viral life cycle. These include the ψ packaging sequence (necessary for recognition of the viral RNA for encapsidation into the viral particle), reverse transcription signals, integration signals, viral promoter, enhancer, and polyadenylation sequences. A cDNA can thus be expressed in a vector using the transcription regulatory sequences provided by the virus. Alternative constructs which lack the viral promoter and/or enhancer have also been made. These constructs are used for certain applications where one wishes to study regulation of an alternative promoter and/or avoid activities which may depress gene expression due to repression of the viral LTR. In addition, crippled vectors can be employed to reduce problems due to helper virus (described later). As vector designs are continually evolving, it is best to obtain vectors from a laboratory which has experience with several different designs and which will advise on their use.

Histochemical Marker

The choice of a gene for use in cell marking is based on several criteria. It is quite useful to have a gene product that enables one to use a known, enzymatic, histochemical stain for easy identification of infected cells. Enzymatic histochemical staining is not an absolute requirement, as immunohistochemical procedures are quite standard, but enzymatic reactions can be easier to perform and more sensitive. They also provide flexibility for secondary characterization of marked cells with antibodies that serve to identify cell types. For example, if one encounters a clone of cells that are labeled with the histochemical marker protein (an enzymatic stain), one can then use a rabbit antineurofilament and a mouse antiglial filament antibody stain (coupled with rhodamine and fluorescein conjugated second antibodies) to identify the nature of the infected cells. A second set of criteria concerns the gene itself. It is helpful if it is already cloned and characterized with respect to its molecular structure. It should also be innocuous, have no effect on development, and not be tissue specific. One must be able to detect it in tissues that already contain many enzymatic activities. Either overexpression of the introduced gene product, relative to the endogenous activity, or a unique gene product or specific assay method is required. Finally, the gene must be transmissible in a retrovirus vector. Although it is possible to transmit more than one (possibly up to three) gene in a retrovirus vector, a single gene is less problematic than multiple genes. In general, genes from any source can be used. Several vector and gene combinations are usually tested in order to obtain high titer transmission and a high level of protein expression.

The *Escherichia coli lacZ* gene, encoding β-galactosidase (β-Gal), has been used in tissue culture cells *in vitro* (15–17); *Drosophila in vivo* (18, 19); in transgenic mice (20, 21); and in many bacterial strains. Hydrolysis of X-Gal (5-bromo-3-chloro-indolyl-β-D-galactopyranoside) by β-Gal results in production of indigo, an intensely blue compound, which enables identification of individual infected cells (22–24). We have found that β-Gal is expressed at high levels in infected cells after infection with the BAG retrovirus (3, 23). Sanes *et al.* (4) similarly found good expression from the SV40 early promoter in their LZ1 retrovirus. Other genes that have been used to mark cells include luciferase [a firefly gene used to mark plants (26)] and *E. coli* β-glucuronidase (27). Alternative markers would be quite useful, particularly due to a technical problem in the use of β-Gal, as detected with X-Gal. The indigo precipitate produced by hydrolysis of X-Gal is so dark that it obscures staining with horseradish peroxidase-coupled secondary antibodies, and it absorbs such a broad spectrum of light that fluorescent secondary antibodies cannot be used. Alternative detection systems for β-Gal, such as anti-β-Gal antibodies, may alleviate this problem.

Expression of Histochemical Marker Gene

The viral promoter LTR has been used in many vector designs to express a wide variety of genes taken from many sources. Genes from bacteria, yeast, (other) viruses, birds, and mammals have been successfully transduced and expressed. Genomic DNAs as well as cDNAs have been used. Basically, any gene is likely to be transducible, but the level at which any given gene will allow viral transmission and expression is unpredictable. Some LTR-promoted genes result in high levels of expression at the RNA level, but give low levels of protein expression. The reason(s) for this is unclear. The LTR promoter appears to be fairly nonspecific in terms of expression in a wide variety of cell types. However, there is evidence that it is inactive in preimplantation mouse embryos and early stem cell lines (28–30). There have also been problems in expression in bone marrow cells, the target for the first gene therapy experiments in humans (29, 30). Current efforts at alleviating the expression problems in this system may provide useful insights into expression in the nervous system, should similar problems arise.

Promoters other than the LTR have been used successfully in several types of vector designs. Internal promoters which direct transcription in the same direction as the LTR have been quite popular (for example, see DO-L in Ref. 33). These internal promoters can be non-tissue specific, or can be used to direct transcription in a specified tissue [e.g., the β-globin promoter

(34)]. Promoters can also be placed in the transcriptional orientation opposite to that of the LTR. In this case, a polyadenylation site and perhaps splicing signals should be included. Some of the internal promoter vectors include LTR activity, while others do not. Deletion of the viral promoter and/or enhancer activity may be desirable if one wants to eliminate any potential activation or suppression of an internal promoter via the enhancer or promoter of the LTR.

For the application of these vectors to the problem of lineage mapping, a promoter that does not exhibit cell type specificity is required. If a promoter were used that only expressed in a few cell types, it would select the spectrum of lineages that could be mapped and could even limit the results to the most obvious or trivial of findings. However, the choice of a constitutive promoter is not a simple one. Promoters for housekeeping functions seem an obvious starting point. However, when one is hoping to map lineages of cells that are postmitotic, and as specialized as neurons, not all housekeeping proteins would be expected to be expressed as fully as they might be in mitotic cells, which are typically used in transfection assays to characterize promoter specificity. Furthermore, the specificity of a promoter when it is inserted into the context of a retrovirus must be established for each promoter and vector. Experiments aimed at demonstrating cell type specificity must be performed with all of the proper controls to establish the efficacy and specificity of the internal, non-LTR promoter, as the retrovirus can influence the specificity of internal promoters. The best cases for the retention of specificity of internal promoters in retrovirus vectors are the human β-globin (34–36) and the light-chain immunoglobulin (37) promoters.

Expression in brain tissue from the wild-type Moloney murine leukemia virus (MMLV) LTR was demonstrated by infection of postimplantation mouse embryos (38). As no histochemistry was performed in these studies, the identity of the neural cells that were expressing the viral RNA was not resolved. Several groups have demonstrated the ability of the LTR promoter, as well as the SV40 early promoter transduced by a retrovirus vector, to express in neural tissue. Neuroblastoma and glioma cell lines are infectable and can express from the LTR, as are all neural cell lines that have been tested. In addition, primary cultures of cerebral cortex, olfactory bulb, retina, cerebellum, neural crest (rat and mouse), and dorsal root ganglion are infectable. Thus we constructed the BAG virus using the MMLV LTR for our first test virus for the lineage mapping protocol (25). Sanes *et al.* (4) used the SV40 early promoter, and Calof and Jessell (39) also used the LTR. It remains to be documented whether these promoters will function in all cell types *in vivo*. Caution is extended here as expression *in vitro* does not necessarily imply that it will occur *in vivo* as well.

Packaging Lines and Virus Production

Rationale

Retrovirus vectors usually do not encode any of the structural genes whose products comprise the viral particle [there are, of course, exceptions (for example, see Ref. 14)]. In order to produce infectious viral particles from a retrovirus plasmid, the viral structural proteins, *gag, pol,* and *env* are supplied by packaging cell lines. These lines are usually stable mouse fibroblast lines that contain the *gag, pol,* and *env* genes as a result of the introduction of these genes by transfection. However, these lines do not contain the packaging sequence, ψ, on the viral RNA that encodes the structural proteins. Thus, the packaging lines make viral particles that do not contain the genes or mRNAs for *gag, pol,* or *env.* Prior to the introduction of vector DNA into these lines, cellular RNAs are randomly encapsidated and budded as "normal" viral particles. When one wants to produce viral particles that contain the vector genome, the vector DNA is introduced via transfection or infection, as described below.

Retrovirus vector particles are essentially identical to naturally occurring retrovirus particles. They enter the host cell via interaction of a viral envelope glycoprotein (a product of the viral *env* gene) with a host cell receptor. The murine viruses have several classes of envelope glycoproteins which interact with different host cell receptors. The most commonly used class of viral glycoprotein is the ecotropic class. These viral glycoproteins allow entry only into rat and mouse cells via the ecotropic receptor on these species. They do not allow infection of humans, and thus are considered relatively safe for gene transfer experiments. Until 1988, the packaging line most commonly in use was the $\psi2$ line of Mann *et al.* (40). It encodes the ecotropic *env* gene and it makes the highest titers of vectors, relative to other packaging lines, for unknown reasons. However, it can also lead to the production of helper virus (discussed below). Helper virus can lead to the spread of marker viruses horizontally and is undesirable for many applications. Two new ecotropic packaging lines, CRE, produced by Danos and Mulligan (41), and GP+E−86, produced by Markowitz *et al.* (42), have not allowed production of helper virus to date and are thus the ecotropic lines of choice. The *env* gene of the amphotropic class endows the virus with a very broad host range, including mouse, human, chicken, dog, cat, and mink. There are several packaging lines for the production of vectors with this coat: ψam (43), PA12 (44), and PA317 (45). As all of these lines can apparently lead to helper virus production, Danos and Mulligan (41) also made a new version of an amphotropic packaging line, named CRIP, and this is currently the amphotropic line of choice as it should not yield helper virus.

Recently, an avian leukemia virus packaging line, Q2bn, was made using the same strategy as was employed in making $\psi 2$ (46). This line is currently being tested and it is not yet clear if it will prove as useful as the murine lines.

Isolation of Specific Producer Line

Introduction of a vector plasmid into a packaging line can be accomplished by transfection or by using virus produced by one line to infect a different packaging line ("cross-infection"). Transfection is a nonspecific entry technique that allows one to introduce any DNA into some types of cells (see protocol below). Transfected DNA can be transcribed transiently in about 10% of the packaging cells, within the period of a few hours to a few days after transfection. However, only about 1 in 5000 cells will stably integrate the DNA. Although the transfected DNA bears the retroviral sequences that are necessary for the precise integration that is the hallmark of the retroviral lifecycle, transfected retroviral DNA does not undergo precise or efficient integration. Transfected retroviral DNA integrates as nonspecifically and with as poor an efficiency as any other plasmid DNA. Apparently, key features of the viral structure and/or enzymatic activities are present only following infection and are absent from transfected plasmid DNA.

Transiently or stably produced vector RNA (which contains ψ) is efficiently packaged and budded from the surface of packaging cells. Thus, the infectious retrovirus vector can simply be harvested by removal of the supernatant of the packaging line. A given line which has stably integrated the virus may produce high amounts of virus indefinitely. Cells which have stably integrated the viral genome are usually selected by application of a drug which selects for a gene encoded by the virus. If no such dominant, selectable gene is encoded by the virus, the transfected cells can be cotransfected with a nonviral plasmid which does encode such a gene. By using a molar ratio of viral : nonviral plasmid of 10 : 1, cells can be selected that have integrated both plasmids. If a producer is generated by cross-infection, a very small amount of virus should be used for the infection. If a high multiplicity of infection (moi) were used, there is a risk of transferring defective genomes, or wild-type helper recombinants (discussed in the next section). In some instances, with some vectors, it appears that cross-infection results in producer clones that have a high probability of producing the maximal titer for a given vector. Producer clones isolated following transfection produce quite variable titers, presumably because transfection results in varied configurations of the transfected DNA. Infection reliably results in a single copy provirus.

Infection of a packaging line by virus produced by the same packaging line is very low in efficiency (although it is not blocked entirely). The viral glycoprotein produced by a packaging line apparently binds the host cell receptor for that env glycoprotein class. A virion bearing that same env class thus cannot easily enter. However, since the different classes of viral glycoproteins use different cellular receptors, virions produced by transfections of one class of packaging line can be used to "cross-infect" another (e.g., CRE-produced virus can infect CRIP quite effectively). There is also an alternative method that allows infection of a packaging line with virions produced by that packaging line class (47). One can use an inhibitor of glycosylation, such as tunicamycin, to transiently block the production of the env glycoprotein. During the application of this drug block, the cells can be infected with virions bearing the same class of env glycoprotein. The drug is then washed out. This method requires careful titration of the drug parameters (time, dose), as these drugs can be toxic to the cells. As it is quite easy to introduce viral genomes using standard transfection methods, these will be outlined here.

The transfection protocol most commonly used, and which is quite reliable and easy to perform, is from Parker and Stark (48) and is a modification of the $CaPO_4$ transfection protocol of Graham and van der Erb (49). Filter sterilize the solutions and work in a sterile hood. Plate packaging cells to about 10–20% the density of confluent cells (referred to hereafter as a 1→10 or a 1→5 split) the day before transfection on a 10-cm dish. (A 10-cm dish is usually used, but a 6-cm dish can be used and all the volumes given here can be scaled down by a factor of 3.) Place 10 μg of the retrovirus vector plasmid DNA into 0.5 ml HEPES-buffered saline (HBS) (137 mM NaCl, 5 mM KCl, 0.7 mM Na_2HPO_4, 6 mM dextrose, 21 mM HEPES, pH 7.05; check the pH, as it is a critical parameter). The DNA need not be sterile. Falcon tubes, #2054, provide for good visibility of the precipitate. If cotransfection is being performed, use a molar ratio of viral to nonviral (or drug marker) plasmid of 10 : 1 and mix them together in the HBS. Add 32 μl of 2 M $CaCl_2$ while gently shaking the tube. Mix in the added $CaCl_2$ by tapping the tube for about 30 sec. Incubate at room temperature for 45 min. A fine, hazy blue precipitate should develop. Large, clumpy precipitates do not work well. Remove medium from packaging cells and gently pipette the HBS–DNA onto the center of the dish. Leave the dish in the hood and gently redistribute the solution from the edges of the dish to the entire surface of the dish after about 10 min. After a total of 20-min exposure to the DNA, add back the medium, and return the cells to the incubator. After 4 hr, remove the medium (aspirate well) and gently add 2.5 ml of HBS containing 15% glycerol (at room temperature). Return the dish to the incubator for 3.5 min. Do not leave in too long. Quickly remove glycerol–HBS and rinse (gently) with 10 ml medium. Repeat medium rinse and add back 5 ml of medium plus serum (use medium and serum recommended for the particular packaging line). In order to harvest the transiently produced virus, 18–24 hr after the glycerol shock, remove the medium and filter through a 0.45-μm filter (the type that easily fits onto a syringe). This "transient" harvest can be stored at $-80°C$ or used immediately for an infection.

In order to make "stable" producers of the virus, the rare cells that stably integrate the transfected plasmid (frequency of 10^{-3} to 10^{-4}) must be identified through drug selection. After harvesting the transiently produced virus, add 10 ml medium back to the transfected cells. If cross-infection is the desired method for transferring the viral genome into the packaging line, the transiently produced virus (1 ml) can be used to infect a packaging line with a different envelope type. (Transiently produced virus is usually low in titer, $10–10^4$ cfu/ml.) Infections are carried out as described in the next section. Split the transfected or infected cells $1\rightarrow10$ or $1\rightarrow20$ 2 days after transfection or infection and plate in selection medium. After 3 days, change the medium to fresh selective medium. After a total of 7 to 10 days, colonies should be visible. Well-isolated colonies can be picked using cloning cylinders and transferred into two wells for each clone in 24-well or 6-well tissue culture dishes. The next stage is to identify those colonies that make a high titer of the correct virus structure. When a good producer clone is identified, many vials of these cells should be stored in liquid nitrogen. Freeze cells in 10–15% DMSO. This is to guard against the typical cell culture hazards, as well as the problem of recombination to generate helper virus and loss of titer (some clones reduce their virus output over time, for unknown reasons).

Determination of Viral Titer and Genome Structure

The concentration (titer, expressed as colony forming units per milliliter cfu/ml) of virus varies widely and depends on a combination of factors. The vector, the insert(s), the packaging line, and the method of harvesting all contribute to the final titer. Although titers from stable producers can be as high as 10^8 cfu/ml, 10^6 cfu/ml is considered to be a good titer for an ecotropic producer. Transient titers are generally low, from $10–10^4$ cfu/ml. In order to identify a stable producer clone that makes a maximal titer, two methods can be employed. One is to analyze quantitatively the producer cells for the presence of viral RNA or protein. In our experience, the amount of β-Gal protein present in a producer line that carries a lacZ vector is directly correlated with the amount of virus in the supernatant. Thus, we screen each clone by X-Gal staining (as described below). Since X-Gal or RNA analysis methods are invasive and lethal, duplicate wells containing the colonies picked from the drug-selection dishes (described above) are made so that a dish of live cells is available after the analysis. One can use RNA dot blots to assess the amount of viral RNA quickly, and this has also been correlated with titer (50). Direct titration of the culture supernatants is the more typical method to screen producer clones, but requires a longer period of time and thus more subcultivations of the producers while awaiting the results.

Producer clone supernatants can be collected from the cells at any time after the clones are picked. For $\psi2$ producers, the best titers are obtained when cells are confluent. For other producers, the optimum cell density and harvest method may need to be determined. A method for $\psi2$ is as follows. The medium above the cells is removed the day they become confluent and is discarded. Half the usual volume of fresh medium is then added and harvested 1 to 3 days later. This is the virus stock and it can be stored at −80°C indefinitely, or used fresh. NIH 3T3 cells are mouse fibroblasts that are frequently used for murine retrovirus infections. Split NIH 3T3 cells at 1→10 to 1→20 onto 60- or 100-mm dishes the day before infection. On the day of infection, remove medium from the NIH 3T3 cells and add virus stock. Use 1–2 ml virus stock (or 1–2 ml of medium containing from 0.01 μl to 0.1 ml of virus stock, depending on the titer) to infect a 60-mm dish of cells (or 3–5 ml for a 100-mm dish). Include Polybrene [Sigma (St. Louis, MO) or Aldrich (Milwaukee, WI)] at a final concentration of 8 μg/ml. Polybrene stock is made up to 800 μg/ml in dH$_2$O, filter sterilized, and stored at −20°C. Leave the cells at 37°C for 1–3 hr. (Some cells can stay overnight in the high Polybrene; other cells are bothered by this. Since the virus only has a half-life of 4 hr, longer incubations do not usually result in significantly more infection. Virus absorption takes place fairly rapidly.) Add medium back to dilute the Polybrene to 2 μg/ml. Incubate for at least 2 or 3 times the length of a cell cycle, to allow for integration and expression of viral genes (1–2 days for NIH 3T3 cells). Split infected cells into selection conditions. If the resistance gene is *neo,* split the cells 1→10 to 1→20 into two dishes (10 cm) containing 1 mg/ml G418 in DME + 10% calf serum. (We calculate 1 mg/ml of G418 based on the weight of the material in the bottle. We do not correct for the percentage of active G418, as our cells are not sensitive to small fluctuations in the percentage of active G418.) After 3 days change the medium. Include drug(s). After 7–10 days (for NIH 3T3 under G418 selection), colonies should be obvious. Count them or pick them or both before they spread (usually before 12 days under selection).

The calculation of titer is made differently in different laboratories, partly because it is difficult to account for the number of cell divisions that occurred after viral integration and before plating the cells into selective media. For example, if there are two cell divisions after viral integration and before G418 selection, a single infectious viral particle could result in four G418 resistant colonies. Recently, with the advent of screenable markers such as *lacZ*, it is possible to titer the colony forming units using a direct measure of the number of X-Gal⁺ colonies present 2 days after inoculation of NIH 3T3 cells. A direct method such as this does not require a subcultivation after infection and before assessment of the number of colonies. There is thus no ambiguity due to the number of cell divisions as each colony is scored as 1 regardless of the number of cells in the colony. Since the BAG virus encodes the *neo* gene as well as *lacZ*, we have been able to compare the G418 resistance titer to the X-Gal titer on cells infected with the same stock at the same time in parallel dishes. We can correct the number of G418 resistance (R) cfu/ml for the number of cell divisions by determining the average number of cells per X-Gal⁺ colony and using that factor as the replication factor in the calculation of G418-R titer (as shown below). When such corrections have been made, the observed X-Gal cfu/ml and the observed G418-R cfu/ml are in agreement to within a factor of 2. When the vector under titration does not have a histochemical marker gene, then a guess should be made for the replication factor. Usually, 2 or 4 is a reasonable guess for the replication factor if 2–3 cell cycle times were allowed prior to selection. A formula for calculation of a G418-R and X-Gal titer is as follows:

$$\frac{\text{Average number of X-Gal}^+\text{ colonies}}{\text{Virus volume (ml)}} = \text{X-Gal cfu/ml}$$

$$\frac{\text{Average number of G418-R colonies}}{\begin{array}{c}\text{Virus volume (ml)} \times \text{replication factor}\\ \times \text{ percentage of infected cells plated}\end{array}} = \text{G418-R cfu/ml}$$

Example: 1 µl virus was diluted into 3 ml medium and inoculated onto a 10-cm dish of NIH 3T3 cells. Two days later, the infected cells were split 1–20 onto 10-cm selection dishes (i.e., the percentage of infected cells plated = 0.05 in the calculation). After 10 days of selection, an average of 20 G418 resistant colonies were observed on each dish. In a parallel set of dishes, also infected with 1 µl of virus, *lacZ* expression was assessed by staining the infected cells with X-Gal 48 hr after infection (i.e., the same time that the selection with G418 was initiated in the parallel cultures). The average number of cells per colony after X-Gal staining was 4 (i.e., replication factor is 4) and the average number of X-Gal colonies per dish was 200. The X-Gal titer would be 2×10^5 cfu/ml and the G418 R titer would be 10^5 cfu/ml.

After a virus producer clone is chosen because it gives high titered stocks, the structure of the viral genome should be investigated. A Southern blot analysis (50) is usually performed on cells infected with virus from the producer clone. Alternatively, or additionally, the proviral genome can be cloned directly from infected cells into bacteria using one of several rescue schemes (51). The cloned provirus can then be examined in great detail. It is often important to analyze RNA structure as well [using a Northern blot or RNase protection assays (52)] especially when the mRNA for the gene of interest is a subgenomic RNA.

Virus Stock Production and Concentration

In order to prepare a stock of virus for multiple experiments, several hundred milliliters to a few liters of producer cell supernatant can be prepared, titered, concentrated, and tested for helper virus contamination. A producer clone that is identified as a high-level producer is usually expanded by subcultivations of 1→10 to 1→40. For a large preparation, split cells 1→10 or 1→20 from newly confluent dishes. Set up 10–50 10-cm dishes or 10–20 15-cm dishes. As soon as the cells become confluent, discard the medium and add half the normal volume (e.g., add 5 ml for a 10-cm dish). After 2 to 3 days, harvest this medium. The cells will be extremely densely packed, but this is normal (for ψ2) and results in higher titer. The stock can be stored at −80°C indefinitely. It is customary to titer before concentration. If the titer is sufficiently high, it can be aliquoted and used without concentration (after a helper assay, see below). Stocks can be concentrated before titration, although sometimes this is wasted effort as the stock may be too low in titer. Two methods for concentration, centrifugation and polyethylene glycol precipitation, are fairly easy to perform. They seem to work best on ecotropic viruses, where they result in 10- to 100-fold concentration. For the centrifugation protocol, spin the virus stock at 14,000 rpm for 20 min at 4°C (e.g., J14 rotor in a Beckman centrifuge in 250-ml bottles that have been sterilized by autoclaving, or in an SW27 rotor for smaller volumes). This step is to pellet cells and debris. Pour the supernatant directly into fresh sterile bottles and put back into same rotor and spin for 5 to 16 hr at 4°C in the same centrifuge at the same speed. (Shorter times yield flaky pellets, which sometimes break up when decanting, while longer spins yield pellets that are harder to resuspend. The type of pellet is also dependent on the producer and the method used to prepare the stock.) Discard supernatant (save a small volume to determine whether all virus has been pelleted), while carefully avoiding discarding the pellet, which some-times dislodges. The pellet is *gently* resuspended in 1% of the original volume. Use DME + 10% calf serum or buffer of your choice (we have not tested different buffers). The resuspension may take 2 hr as the pellet is fairly sticky. It is convenient to leave the centrifuge bottle in an ice bucket in the hood and pipette it every 15 min or so. Store the virus at −80°C in small aliquots. It can be frozen and thawed several times with no loss of titer. Sanes *et al.* (4) resuspend it in 50% serum and store for a short period of time at 4°C.

An alternative method is polyethylene glycol precipitation, with an optional step of chromatography on Sepharose CL-4B (53). Add NaCl to the virus stock while stirring at 4°C, to a final concentration of 0.4 M. Slowly add polyethylene glycol 6000 to a final concentration of 8.5% (w/v) and continue stirring for 1 to 1.5 hr at 4°C. Collect the precipitate by centrifugation at 7000 g for 10 min. Dissolve the pellet in NTE (100 mM NaCl, 10 mM Tris-HCl, pH 7.4, 1 mM EDTA) in 1% of the original volume. The stock can be used directly after this step, or stored at −80°C. It can also be further purified on a Sepharose CL-4B column to remove PEG. Prepare a column of Sepharose CL-4B (Pharmacia Fine Chemicals, Uppsala, Sweden) equilibrated in NTE. Apply the virus to the top and chromatograph at a rate of 1 ml/min. Collect 0.3-ml fractions. Fractions can be assayed for virus by measuring absorbance at 280 or 260 nm. Pooled fractions can then be titered. The PEG protocol does not always work for us, for reasons that are not clear, but this protocol is easy to perform and can result in excellent stocks.

For small volume concentrations, there is an additional method that can be used. Supernatants can be centrifuged through filters, either the Centricon-30 microconcentrators from Amicon or the CentriCell 60 from Polysciences, Inc. (Warrington, PA).

Helper Virus Contamination

The production of wild-type helper virus by the packaging lines is an issue of concern when using replication-incompetent vectors. The genome that supplies the *gag, pol,* and *env* genes in ψ2, ψam, and PA12 and PA317 does not encode the ψ sequence, but can still become packaged, although at a low frequency. If it is coencapsidated with a vector genome, recombination in the next cycle of reverse transcription can occur. If the recombination allows the helper genome to acquire the ψ sequence from the vector genome, a recombinant that is capable of autonomous replication is the result. This recombinant can spread through the entire culture (although slowly due to envelope interference). Once this occurs, it is best to discard the producer clone as there is no convenient way to eliminate the wild type. As would be expected, this happens with a greater frequency in stocks with high titer. The PA317 packaging line has a safer design than ψ2, ψam, and PA12, while the new CRE and CRIP probably have the best design for not producing helper virus. Recombination in CRE and CRIP has not yet been observed, but one must retain caution and assay stocks produced by these lines as well.

There are a variety of assays to test for helper virus. A very sensitive assay that is easy to perform for a variety of vectors is to examine the culture supernatant for the ability to promote horizontal spread of the genome carrying a marker (i.e., spread of the vector genome from an infected cell to neighboring, nonsibling cells). This assay also allows for a test of the host range of the helper. Split NIH 3T3 cells 1→50 onto a 6-cm dish the day before the assay is initiated. Set up one dish for a positive control, two dishes for negative controls, and one dish for each stock to be tested. Infect the NIH 3T3 cells with 1 ml of the virus stock using 8 μg/ml Polybrene. If this is a fresh stock that has not been filtered, make sure to filter it through a 0.45-μm filter before doing the infection. For a positive control, coinfect a dish with a replication-incompetent *neo* virus and a small amount ($\approx$10 cfu) of wild-type helper (i.e., virus produced by a wild-type producer cell line). After allowing 1–3 hr for absorption, add back 4 vol of medium. Make sure that the Polybrene is maintained at 2 μg/ml for the length of the assay to allow spread of both helper and *neo* virus. One negative control dish receives no virus, only Polybrene and media. For an additional negative control, infect a dish with a known helper-free *neo* virus. After the cells become confluent (3–4 days), split 1→50 into 60-mm dishes and set up one dish per assay. Again use 2 μg/ml Polybrene. The supernatant from these cells will then be assayed for the presence of virus which carries the marker of the initial stock (e.g., *neo* or *lacZ* for BAG virus). Only virus stocks that contain helper virus will produce high titers of virus bearing these markers. On the day the putative producer cells become confluent, discard the old medium and replace it with 0.5 vol of fresh DME + 10% calf serum. Two or 3 days later, harvest the supernatant from the confluent cells, filter through 0.45-μm filter, add 8 μg/ml Polybrene, and either store at −80°C until ready to assay virus or use it immediately to infect NIH 3T3 cells split 1→10 or 1→20 the day before. Use 1 ml of supernatant for the infection. If the marker on the virus is *neo,* split the cells into G418 and assay for G418 R cfu as described above. If the *lacZ* gene was on the vector, assay by staining with X-Gal as described below. If a small number of colonies result, these may be due to "crippled" helper, generated by an imperfect recombination event. Alternatively, some of the ψ^- genome can transfer to the first set of infected NIH 3T3 cells and lead to a low titer, without true helper virus contamination (i.e., "passive" transfer) (41). For many applications, crippled helper is not a confounding influence. Wild-type helper virus will lead to production of 10^6 cfu/ml (in the case of the BAG virus) and should be discarded. If one wishes to determine whether a crippled helper or passive transfer is responsible for low titers, one can continue to passage the supernatants and test for virus at various intervals. When we have done this for low-titered supernatants, we have been unable to recover virus after one additional cycle of infection and subsequent titration. We believe that, in such cases, the low titer was due to passive transfer.

If the host range of the helper is of interest, it can be tested by infection of cells of different species (e.g., dog or human cells cannot be infected with ecotropic helper, only amphotropic helper).

Alternative methods to detect helper virus include the XC plaque assay (54), reverse transcriptase assay (55), and S^+L^- assay (45). The XC plaque and S^+L^- assays require additional cell lines. The reverse transcriptase assay is sensitive, but does not always detect crippled helper.

Infection of Target Cells

Retroviruses enter cells via interactions at the host cell surface. Thus, it is not necessary to perform intracellular injections to mark cells. Indeed, it is not known if direct injection of a virus would permit infection to occur. Placement of the virus inoculum in the vicinity of dividing cells is all that is required to initiate infection. The virus has a short half-life (4 hr at 37°C, unpublished observations) and absorbs quickly to cells. One can therefore assume that infectious, extracellular virions disappear very soon after virus is delivered. (Virus can also absorb to cells that do not bear receptors, although this is low affinity, nonspecific "sticking." It does not lead to infection.) Virus that enters postmitotic cells probably undergoes reverse transcription, but fails to integrate. Unintegrated viral genomes do not express a detectable level of RNA. If one performs an infection into an area that contains a majority of postmitotic cells, one will find very little, if any, evidence of viral expression.

Infection of Cells in Vitro

Infection of target cells *in vitro* is accomplished by simply incubating the virus with the cells to be infected. For most *in vitro* applications, a polycation, such as Polybrene or DEAE-dextran, is used to aid in viral infection. These polycations apparently can promote virus binding to the host cell surface by reducing electrostatic repulsion between the negatively charged surfaces of the cell and virion. Alternatively, the cells to be infected can be incubated with the packaging line (cocultivation method). This method is used to infect hematopoietic cells and appears to increase greatly the infection efficiency (56, 57). The packaging cells can be killed by δ-irradiation (2800 rads) or treatment with mitomycin C (3 hr with mitomycin C at final concentration of 10 μg/ml in medium, followed by several rinses) if it is desirable that they do not continue to divide during or after the cocultivation. It is difficult to generalize about the efficiency of infection, although it can be close to 100%. The variables that influence infectability of a given cell are unknown. Assay of expression of viral gene products is usually not attempted until two or three cell cycles have ensued. When assaying *lacZ* expression via X-Gal staining, we have found that the number of clones reaches a maximal value 48 hr postinfection, when infecting NIH 3T3 cells.

Infections of tissue explants, or cultured midgestation embryos, can also be performed essentially as described above. A tissue explant can be bathed in as much viral stock as is desired for a few hours in the presence of 8 μg/ml Polybrene, or cultured over a feeder layer of producer cells, also in the presence of Polybrene. We infected explants of chick and rodent retina in this way, and then transplanted the rodent retinas back to neonates. This enabled a marking of transplanted cells which were later identified by X-Gal histochemistry. Calof and Jessell (39) injected a vector encoding the marker gene T8 into the amnionic cavity of cultured midgestation embryos. In this culture system, development can proceed for only a few days. Clearly labeled cells suggestive of neural ectoderm and surface epithelium were observed 24 hr later. The exact nature of these small clones was difficult to determine. This *in vitro* approach is feasible for certain directed questions about lineage.

In Situ Infection of Neonates

The volume that can safely be delivered to a tissue *in vivo* is generally quite small, 0.1 to 1 μl. It is therefore important to prepare as high a titered virus stock as possible for *in vivo* infections. In general, one is limited to a virus titer of 10^6–10^8 cfu/ml. Due to these limitations, it is quite important to make the best attempt possible to deliver virus directly to the mitotic zone. It is unclear if there are ever factors in tissue fluids (e.g., ventricular fluids or CSF) that inhibit or destroy viral infectivity.

Virus delivery to postnatal animals is fairly straightforward. It is possible to use a hand-held Hamilton syringe with a 33-gauge needle to deliver virus to the mitotic zone of the retina (3), and postnatal mouse cerebellum and olfactory bulb (C. L. Cepko, E. Snyder, and E. Ryder, unpublished observations). Alternatively, pulled glass pipettes can be used. The size of the needle tip should be determined empirically for the tissue under study. The skull is soft enough on the first few days after birth for direct injection into the tissue through the skin and skull. Coinjection with a dye, such as 0.05% trypan blue, neutral red, or fast green aids in the ability to detect the accuracy of injections and does not impair viral infectivity. The animals are anesthetized by cooling at $-20°C$ in a freezer or on ice for a few minutes. Landmarks (e.g., sutures, blood vessels) near the area to be injected can be visualized using a fiber optics light source. The injection is made directly into the desired area using a hand-held pipette. It is best to practice a series of injections with dye alone and then immediately dissect the animal for examination of the injection.

An excellent way to determine the accuracy of injection, and test your X-Gal histochemical technique, is to inject cells that contain the *lacZ* gene, such as the ψ2 BAG producer cells (available from ATCC #CRL 9560). The cells can be prelabeled with a fluorescent dye, such as the carboxyfluorescein diacetate succinimyl ester of Molecular Probes Inc. (Junction City, OR). As detailed by Bronner-Fraser (58), the cells are exposed to 0.3 mM CFSE at 37°C for 30 min (make up a 10 mM stock in DMSO and store in foil in the refrigerator) in PBS just before trypsinizing. They should then be well trypsinized, pelleted, and washed twice with medium or PBS, and then resuspended to a concentration of 10^8 cells/ml. A few minutes after injection, the animal should be killed and processed for X-Gal histochemistry. The injected cells can then be monitored independently from the X-Gal staining by viewing the CSFE fluorescence under UV illumination. If the X-Gal histochemistry is executed properly, no fluorescent cells should be visible since X-Gal$^+$ cells are usually so full of indigo that all fluorescence is absorbed.

Intrauterine Infections

If early lineage data in the nervous system are desired, virus must be delivered to embryos. They can then develop *in utero, exo utero* (but still within the mother), or *in vitro*. Jaenisch (38) and Sanes *et al.* (4) performed viral infections on midgestation mouse embryos. These injections were undirected, through the uterine wall and deciduum. Both groups were successful, although it should be noted that in the case of Jaenisch, the virus was replication-competent, and thus even if only one particle initiated infection, a full infection of the embryo could occur through viral spread. Sanes *et al.* (4) were able to reproducibly mark cells on the outside of the embryo and in the yolk sac. Walsh and Cepko (59) and Price and Thurlow (60), using E14–E19 rat embryos, and Luskin *et al.* (61), using E12 to E13 mouse embryos, were also able to make directed injections through the uterine wall into the lateral ventricle. All injections made through the uterine wall were performed with glass pipettes pulled on a pipette puller. The actual diameter and shape of the tip should be determined empirically. Animals are anesthetized with a mixture of ketamine (20–40 mg/kg) and xylazine (3–5 mg/kg), opened via an incision along the midline, injections of 0.1–1.0 μl are made through the uterine wall, and the mother is sutured. The head, and in some embryos, even the lateral ventricle, can be visualized with fiber optics. The inoculum can be seen filling the lateral ventricle when the inoculum is properly delivered to this area. Other areas may not be as visible and practice injections followed by immediate dissection and examination are again recommended.

Exo Utero Infections

It is difficult to make precisely directed injections into many of the mitotic zones of early mammalian nervous systems through the uterus. The *exo utero* surgical procedure developed by Muneoka *et al.* (62) at least partially circumvents this problem. In this procedure, mouse embryos (E11–E19) are released from the uterus by cutting the uterine wall, but remain attached to the uterus via the placenta. The abdominal cavity of the mother is filled with a buffered saline solution to protect the embryos. An incision can be made in the extraembryonic membranes that surround the embryo so that the embryo can be directly manipulated or injected. Subsequently, the extraembryonic membranes are closed with fine suture. The embryos can be brought to term in the abdominal cavity and delivered by Cesarian section. Recently, we have used this technique to inject BAG virus into the mitotic zone of retinas in E13 and E14 CD-1 mouse embryos. The embryos were brought to term, delivered, fostered, and raised to adulthood. Large (up to 238 cells), complex clones were observed to be distributed throughout the retinas of these animals.

Initially, injections were made through an incision in the extraembryonic membranes that were subsequently closed with 10-0 suture. However, in our hands, embryonic and neonatal survival was improved by injecting directly through the extraembryonic membranes without an incision or suture. Although injections made by this approach were more difficult to target, ~25% of the embryos injected at E13 survived to adulthood and all injected retinas contained clones. Additional factors which influence the success of this method are the choice of mouse strain and the health of the mouse colony. Outbred mouse strains such as CD-1 or Swiss Webster appear to be best, but even these strains may have different embryo survival rates when obtained from different suppliers or colonies. Apparently healthy mouse colonies can harbor subclinical infections that do not affect unoperated embryos but that can stress operated embryos beyond their ability to survive.

Infection of Early Progenitors

Experiments can be devised for marking very early progenitors of the nervous system, such as neural plate or neural tube cells. It is straightforward to use the conventional Southern blot technology and integration sites as clonal tags for such experiments if 10^4–10^5 cells can be generated from one infected progenitor. Extremely sensitive techniques for nucleic acid detection, such as the polymerase chain reaction (63), may eventually lead to direct analysis of integrated proviral DNA and obviate the need for large numbers of cells. Soriano and Jaenisch (64) infected early mouse embryos (4–16 cell stage) *in vitro* and then reimplanted the embryos into pseudopregnant hosts for full development *in utero*. They were investigating the number of cells that give rise to the entire embryo and the lineage of somatic versus germ line tissue. Similarly, in a study of hematopoietic lineage, Lemischka *et al.* (57) used integration sites to mark transplants of infected bone marrow. Improvements of the techniques described above will be necessary to yield reliable marking of early progenitors, such as neural plate or neural tube cells, as currently the *exo utero* technique has not been employed earlier than E11, and blind injections through the uterine wall will not frequently lead to infection of desired progenitors. Improved surgical techniques may enable marking of such progenitors in the future.

Infection of Nonmammalian Species

Retroviruses can also be used to infect species that are more accessible during embryogenesis. Murine xenotropic retroviruses can infect chickens (65) and we demonstrated that the BAG virus encapsidated in the amphotropic murine coat effectively infected chicken cells *in vitro* (25). We used both embryonic fibroblasts and retina organ cultures. However, *in vivo* infections have been extremely inefficient. Gray *et al.* (5) have used a β-Gal Rous sarcoma virus to infect chick tectal cells successfully *in vivo*. Infection of chicks early in development *in vivo* is thus possible and will certainly be exploited. The newly constructed avian retrovirus packaging line (Q2bn) (44) and further development of efficient avian vectors (14) will greatly boost efforts in this area. Expression from the Rous sarcoma virus (an avian retrovirus) LTR in very early chick embryos (stage X–XI) appears to be repressed (66), although expression at later times appears to be quite high. Infection of other species, such as frogs and newts, may require host range variants currently under construction (Cliff Tabin, Department of Genetics, Harvard Medical School, Boston, Massachusetts).

Detection of Infected Cells via X-Gal Histochemistry

The histochemical marker gene of choice in many systems is the *E. coli lacZ* gene. In order to detect the bacterial gene over the background of cellular, lysozomal β-Gal, it is necessary to use a pH optimum of about 7. We have found that the following procedure works quite well with a variety of tissues. Variations in fixatives, incubation times, and buffers have been published and may yield results comparable to those obtained with the following procedure. Fixation is accomplished by paraformaldehyde, made up fresh by dissolving paraformaldehyde (although supplier may not be important, we use BDH Chemicals Ltd., Poole, England) in 0.1 M PIPES, pH 6.9, 2 mM MgCl$_2$, and 1.25 mM EGTA. Alternatively, 0.5% glutaraldehyde in PBS leads to bluer cells and works well in retina and tissue culture cells *in vitro*. However, glutaraldehyde may result in background in some tissues. Either dissect out the tissue of interest (if it is quite small, see whole-mount procedure below) or perfuse the animal with the fixative. We perfuse adult mice for about 30 min, then let the animal sit for another 30 min, and then dissect. The tissue is next incubated at 4°C in PBS + 2 mM MgCl$_2$ + 30% sucrose until the tissue sinks (a few hours or overnight). The tissue is embedded in OCT compound (Miles) and frozen on dry ice. It can be stored as a frozen block indefinitely at −80°C. Cryostat sections (20 to 100 μm) are cut and placed on gelatin-coated slides. The sections are air dried and can be stored at 4°C for at least a few weeks, and perhaps indefinitely. PBS + 2 mM MgCl$_2$ and PBS + 2 mM MgCl$_2$ + 0.01% sodium deoxycholate + 0.02% NP40 are prepared and placed in staining trays designed to hold multiple slides. This and all subsequent steps are carried out at 4°C, until the final incubation at 37°C, as noted. The sections are exposed to fixative again for 5 to 10 min. They are then rinsed quickly once in PBS + MgCl$_2$, then again in the same buffer for 10 min, then permeabilized by incubating in the PBS + detergents for 10 min. Next they are incubated at 37°C in an X-Gal-containing solution that is a modification of a recipe from Lojda (23) and Dannenberg and Suga (24): 5–35 mM K$_3$Fe(CN)$_6$, 5–35 mM K$_4$Fe(CN)$_6$·3H$_2$O, 1–2 mM MgCl$_2$ or MgSO$_4$, 0.01% sodium desoxycholate, 0.02% NP40, and 1 mg/ml X-Gal in PBS. X-Gal is made as a stock of 40 mg/ml in N,N-dimethylformamide and stored at −20°C in glass, covered with foil. The concentration of ferric and ferrous salts can be varied. The speed of formation of the indigo dimer is aided by these compounds.

Incubation in X-Gal solution is carried out for a few hours to overnight, usually with no background problems. The X-Gal solution can be reused and is stored at 4°C in between uses. After incubation in X-Gal solution (which can be monitored by examination of a slide under bright-field optics), the sections are rinsed three times in PBS (for a few minutes each rinse) and mounted in Gelvatol (Air Products and Chemicals, Inc. Allentown, PA; see Ref. 67). Alternatively, they can be counterstained with orange G (1% in phosphotungstic acid for 15 sec, J. Price, personal communication) or neutral red. If a neutral red counterstain is used, care must be taken to minimize the time in xylene as this will lead to loss of the indole precipitate.

Tissue can also be processed as a whole mount. All of our retina staining was accomplished by this method. Large pieces of tissue, even up to the size of an adult rat brain, can be stained as whole mounts. However, we have observed that whole-mount staining of large tissues tends to be superficial and recommend staining of sections for full evaluation of infected cells. Small pieces of tissue can be conveniently processed as whole mounts, with the advantage that reconstruction of clones in three dimensions is greatly facilitated. Whole mounts can be sectioned after staining and preliminary examination, and can be restained with X-Gal after sectioning (although it is not clear if there is some loss of staining due to the prior incubation). Small pieces of tissue, or an entire retina, are fixed for 5–15 min as described above and washed three times in PBS + 1 mM MgCl$_2$ for 5 to 15 min each. It is then incubated in the X-Gal staining solution, with or without detergents. In retinal whole mounts, the detergents are not necessary, and glutaraldehyde is the fixative of choice.

Cells infected and cultured *in vitro* can be stained with X-Gal after fixation with formaldehyde or glutaraldehyde. Fixation for 5 min at room temperature, followed by three 10-min rinses in PBS, and staining in the X-Gal solution at 37°C for 2 hr to overnight is a typical protocol. The X-Gal solution need not contain detergent. If one wishes to mark cells for a transplant, an aliquot of the infected cells should be tested for viral gene expression by X-Gal staining prior to transplantation. However, since the X-Gal precipitate is toxic, non-X-Gal-treated cells are used for the actual injection. They can be marked by incubation in CFSE and transplanted as described for injection of control *lacZ* cells. This enables an assessment of the placement of the transplanted cells.

Evaluation of Lineage Data

After introduction of virus into a mitotic zone in experiments designed to investigate lineage, time is allowed for infection to occur, progeny cells to be generated, and in some cases, for migration and/or differentiation. The survival time postinfection will vary depending on the system and the information that is desired. The most complete lineage map can be generated if injections are performed at different times in development and a range of survival times are allowed before analysis. If migration is a key component to differentiation of the tissue, analysis at early times after infection may be necessary to allow recognition of clonal boundaries. However, if a cell type can only be recognized after allowing differentiation to occur, and if differentiation occurs after migration, very little information may be gained from an early analysis.

Recognition of a clone as such, and confidence in one's assignments of clonal boundaries, are key issues in the use of this technique. We have greatly benefited by working on a well-described tissue that is beautifully laminated and which exhibits very little lateral migration (3). We label the mitotic zone of postnatal rat retinas, as described above, and wait for 5 days to 20 months before harvesting the tissue. Since retinal tissue can be prepared for histochemistry as a whole mount, the success of the infection can be determined within a few hours of harvesting. The tissue can be sectioned after staining the whole mount and cells identified on the basis of location and morphology. In the retina, interpretation of labeled cells as clones is straightforward, as the migration of the progeny cells away from the mitotic zone occurs in a strictly radical fashion. Since the amount of virus that we can inject is limited by both the volume and titer, the frequency of infection is only about 1 in 100 to 1 in 1000 of the mitotic cells at the time of infection. Thus, clones are generally spaced well apart and it is usually not difficult to recognize clonal relationships. However, the real basis for concluding that each cluster of labeled cells is indeed a clone is from infections with diluted virus stocks. In a set of injections with 10-fold serial dilutions of a given virus stock, there is a linear decrease in the number of clones that is obtained. Moreover, the composition and approximate size of the clones remain the same, regardless of the viral dilution. This is the classical argument for a single hit event used by virologists to determine the number of infectious units required to effect a given event.

The recognition of clones within a tissue that undergoes a great deal of migration in different directions may prove to be extremely difficult. The use of mixtures of different marker viruses may be one way to solve this problem. If these were available, two or three viruses could be coinjected to yield distinguishable colors or markings. Identification of clonal boundaries, or lack thereof, could enable identification of clonal migration patterns. Alternatively, if additional marker viruses are not available, very dilute infections, where only a minority of animals exhibit any infected cells, could allow one to make statistical arguments of clonality.

Infection of tissue explants followed by *in vitro* cultivation or transplantation of single infected cells into a host animal may be helpful in resolving lineage issues where clonal boundaries are indistinct, or where it is difficult to control injection into restricted areas. Price *et al.* (25) and Luskin *et al.* (61) used *in vitro* culture of cortical cells to examine lineage questions in this tissue. We used *in vitro* culture of early chick retinas to examine retinal lineage in this species (C. L. Cepko, S. Rowe, and F. Guillemot, unpublished observations). Attempts are now being made to transplant individual cells, which, if successful, could eliminate the problem of multiple hits. If a reliable vital marker were developed, one could use *in vitro* culture and/or accessible tissues and make frequent observations for information on migration, lineage, or other developmental patterns. Vital stains for β-Gal are now available and allow isolation of infected cells using a fluorescence-activated cell sorter (68). However, the fluorescent product of β-Gal hydrolysis diffuses out of cells quite rapidly (except at low temperatures) and it is thus not possible to observe single infected cells *in vivo* using this substrate.

Promoter Inactivity

Promoter inactivity, or the lack of marker gene expression in infected cells, is a confounding issue that may limit the utility of the retroviral approach in some applications. The frequency of nonexpression in cells infected with any retroviral construct *in vivo* is presently unclear. Members of several laboratories have observed that cultured cells infected with *lacZ*-containing constructs sometimes exhibit mosaic expression. Clones of mouse fibroblasts can contain both blue and white cells. We have investigated whether the nonexpressers suffer from a loss or structural alteration of the *lacZ* gene, as opposed to low or no transcription from an intact gene. To date, the loss of X-Gal reactivity has been due to lack of detectable levels of mRNA for *lacZ*. This phenomenon is epigenetic and reversible in that white subclones of mosaic colonies can later revert to expression of lacZ. We have used four different promoters and have found that all lead to some degree of mosaic expression. However, in no case is the loss of expression a highly frequent event.

It may be that the loss of expression occurs during cell division, and not within postmitotic cells. This is suggested by the finding that rat retinas infected at P0 show no loss in the number of X-Gal$^+$ clones, nor in the size or complexity of such clones, for periods of up to $1\frac{1}{2}$ years after infection. Moreover, the intensity of X-Gal staining in retinas from $1\frac{1}{2}$-year-old rats is as great as that in rat retinas harvested a few weeks postinfection. Similar observations have been obtained for rat cortex during the period of 6 months postinfection and cerebellar cells 24 months postinfection. In addition, following infection of E13 mouse retinas, very large clones (average of 50 cells for peripheral clones with some clones over 200 cells) are a frequent occurrence. In the rat cortex, glial clones of up to 180 cells have been observed. The occurrence of large clones suggests that promoter inactivation is not a high-frequency event in these particular cells. We have used the SV40 early promoter, the human histone 4 promoter, and the rat β-actin promoter to direct *lacZ* expression in both cortex and retina. In all cases, the same general results observed following infection with the BAG construct, in which *lacZ* is expressed from the MMLV LTR, have been obtained. In the construct that utilizes the histone promoter, the LTR enhancer was deleted, and thus there should be no influence of the viral promoter on expression of *lacZ* by the histone promoter. Infection with all of these constructs results in X-Gal$^+$ cells of all types that are expected to be infectable at the particular injection time. Thus, there has been no consistent lack of expression in any retinal, cortical neuronal, or glial cell type. Transgenic animals expressing *lacZ,* or other histochemical markers, from constitutive promoters may shed some light on this issue in the very near future.

References

1. S. A. Moody and M. Jacobson, *J. Neurosci.* **3,** 1670 (1983).
2. C. G. Kimmel and R. M. Warga, *Science* **231,** 365 (1986).
3. D. Turner and C. L. Cepko, *Nature* (*London*) **328,** 131 (1987).
4. J. R. Sanes, J. L. R. Rubenstein, and J.-F. Nicolas, *EMBO J.* **5,** 3133 (1986).
5. G. E. Gray, J. C. Glover, J. Majors, and J. R. Sanes, *Proc. Natl. Acad. Sci. U.S.A.* **85,** 7356 (1988).
6. C. E. Holt, T. W. Bertsch, H. M. Ellis, and W. A. Harris, *Neuron* **1,** 15 (1988).
7. R. Wetts and S. E. Fraser, *Science* **239,** 1142 (1988).
8. R. Weiss, N. Teich, H. Varmus, and J. Coffin, "RNA Tumor Viruses." Cold Spring Harbor Laboratory, Cold Spring Harbor, New York, 1984/1985.
9. A. M. C. Brown and M. R. D. Scott, *in* "DNA Cloning: A Practical Approach" (D. M. Glover, ed.), Vol. 3, pp. 189–212. IRL Press, Oxford, 1987.
10. J. Price, *Development* **101,** 409 (1987).
11. C. L. Cepko, *Neuron* **1,** 345 (1988).
12. C. L. Cepko, *Annu. Rev. Neurosci.* **12,** 47 (1989).
13. C. L. Cepko, *Neuromethods* **16,** in press.
14. S. H. Hughes, C. J. Petropoulos, J. J. Greenhouse, and L. B. Crittenden, "Viral Vectors," pp. 133–138. Cold Spring Harbor Laboratory, Cold Springs Harbor, New York, 1988.
15. D. A. Neilsen, J. Chou, A. J. MacKrell, M. J. Casadaban, and D. F. Steiner, *Proc. Natl. Acad. Sci. U.S.A.* **80,** 5198 (1983).
16. C. V. Hall, P. E. Jacob, G. M. Ringold, and F. Lee, *J. Mol. Appl. Genet.* **2,** 101 (1983).

17. P. A. Norton and J. M. Coffin, *Mol. Cell. Biol.* **5,** 281 (1985).
18. J. T. Lis, J. A. Simon, and C. A. Sutton, *Cell* **35,** 403 (1983).
19. Y. Hiromi, A. Kuroiwa, and W. Gehring, *Cell* **43,** 603 (1985).
20. D. R. Goring, J. Rossant, S. Clapoff, M. L. Brietman, and L.-C. Tsui, *Science* **235,** 456 (1987).
21. N. D. Allen, D. G. Cran, S. C. Barton, S. Hettle, W. Reik, and M. A. Surani, *Nature (London)* **333,** 852 (1988).
22. B. Pearson, P. L. Wolf, and J. Vazquez, *Lab. Invest.* **12,** 1249 (1963).
23. Z. Lojda, *Histochemie* **22,** 347 (1970).
24. A. M. Dannenberg and M. Suga, *in* "Methods for Studying Mononuclear Phagocytes" (D. O. Adams, O. Edelson, and M. S. Koren, eds.), pp. 375–396. Academic Press, New York, 1981.
25. J. Price, D. Turner, and C. Cepko, *Proc. Natl. Acad. Sci. U.S.A.* **84,** 156 (1987).
26. D. Ow, K. V. Wood, M. DeLuca, J. R. deWet D. R. Helinski, and S. H. Howell, *Science* **234,** 856 (1986).
27. R. A. Jefferson, M. Klass, N. Wolf, and D. Hirsh, *J. Mol. Biol.* **193,** 41 (1987).
28. R. Jaenisch and A. Berns, *in* "Concepts in Mammalian Embryogenesis" (M. Sherman, ed.), pp. 267–314. MIT Press, Cambridge, Massachusetts, 1977.
29. N. Teich, R. Weiss, G. Martin, and D. Lowy, *Cell* **12,** 973 (1977).
30. C. M. Gorman, P. W. J. Rigby, and D. P. Lane, *Cell* **42,** 519 (1985).
31. D. A. Williams, S. H. Orkin, and R. C. Mulligan, *Proc. Natl. Acad. Sci. U.S.A.* **83,** 2566 (1986).
32. M.-C. Magli, J. E. Dick, D. Huszar, A. Bernstein, and R. A. Phillips, *Proc. Natl. Acad. Sci. U.S.A.* **84,** 789 (1987).
33. A. J. Korman, J. D. Frantz, J. L. Strominger, and R. C. Mulligan, *Proc. Natl. Acad. Sci. U.S.A.* **84,** 2150 (1987).
34. R. D. Cone, A. Weber-Benarous, D. Baorto, and R.C. Mulligan, *Mol. Cell. Biol.* **7,** 887 (1987).
35. P. Soriano, R. D. Cone, R. C. Mulligan, and R. Jaenisch, *Science* **234,** 1409 (1986).
36. S. Karlsson, T. Papayannopoulou, S. G. Schweiger, G. Stamatoyannopoulos, and A. Nienhuis, *Proc. Natl. Acad. Sci. U.S.A.* **84,** 2411 (1987).
37. R. D. Cone, E. B. Reilly, H. N. Eisen, and R. C. Mulligan, *Science* **236,** 954 (1987).
38. R. Jaenisch, *Cell* **19,** 181 (1980).
39. A. Calof and T. Jessell, *Soc. Neurosci. Abstr.* **12,** 183 (1986).
40. R. Mann, R. C. Mulligan, and D. Baltimore, *Cell* **33,** 153 (1983).
41. O. Danos and R. C. Mulligan, *Proc. Natl. Acad. Sci. U.S.A.* **85,** 6460 (1988).
42. D. Markowitz, S. Goff, and A. Bank, *J. Virol.* **62,** 1120 (1988).
43. R. D. Cone and R. C. Mulligan, *Proc. Natl. Acad. Sci. U.S.A.* **81,** 6349 (1984).
44. A. D. Miller, M.-F. Law, and I. M. Vermer, *Mol. Cell. Biol.* **5,** 431 (1985).
45. A. D. Miller and C. Buttimore, *Mol. Cell. Biol.* **6,** 2895 (1986).
46. A. Stoker and M. J. Bissell, *J. Virol.* **62,** 1008 (1988).
47. A. Rein, A. M. Schultz, J. P. Bader, and R. H. Bassin, *Virology* **119,** 185 (1982).
48. B. A. Parker and G. R. Stark, *J. Virol.* **31,** 360 (1979).
49. F. L. Graham and A. J. van der Erb, *Virology* **52,** 456 (1973).

50. F. C. Kafatos, C. W. Jones, and A. Efstratiadis, *Nucleic Acids Res.* **7,** 1541 (1979).
51. C. L. Cepko, B. E. Roberts, and R. E. Mulligan, *Cell* **37,** 1053 (1984).
52. F. M. Ausubel, R. Brent, R. Kingston, D. D. Moore, J. G. Seidman, J. A. Smith, and K. Struhl (eds.), "Current Protocols in Molecular Biology." Green and Wiley (Interscience), New York, 1987.
53. M. Aboud, M. Wolfson, Y. Hassan, and M. Huleihel, *Arch. Virol.* **71,** 185 (1982).
54. W. P. Row, W. E. Pugh, and J. W. Hartley, *Virology* **42,** 1136 (1970).
55. S. Goff, P. Traktman, and D. Baltimore, *J. Virol.* **38,** 239 (1981).
56. D. A. Williams, I. R. Lemischka, D. G. Nathan, and R. C. Mulligan, *Nature (London)* **310,** 476 (1984).
57. I. R. Lemischka, D. H. Raulet, and R. C. Mulligan, *Cell* **45,** 917 (1986).
58. M. Bronner-Fraser, *J. Cell Biol.* **101,** 610 (1985).
59. C. Walsh and C. L. Cepko, *Science* **241,** 1342 (1988).
60. J. Price and L. Thurlow, *Development* **104,** 473 (1988).
61. M. B. Luskin, A. L. Pearlman, and J. R. Sanes, *Neuron,* in press.
62. K. Muneoka, N. Wanek, and S. V. Bryant, *J. Exp. Zool.* **239,** 289 (1986).
63. R. K. Saiki, D. H. Gelfand, S. Stoffel, S. J. Scharf, R. B. Higuchi, T. G. Horn, K. B. Mullis, and H. A. Erlich, *Science* **239,** 487 (1988).
64. P. Soriano and R. Jaenisch, *Cell* **46,** 19 (1986).
65. J. A. Levy, *Nature (London)* **253,** 140 (1985).
66. E. Mitrani, J. Coffin, H. Boedtker, and P. Doty, *Proc. Natl. Acad. Sci. U.S.A.* **84,** 2781 (1987).
67. J. Rodriguez and F. Deinhardt, *Virology* **12,** 316 (1960).
68. G. P. Nolan, S. Fiering, J.-F. Nicolas, and L. A. Herzenberg, *Proc. Natl. Acad. Sci. U.S.A.* **85,** 2603 (1988).

[22] Use of Transgenic Models to Access Neural Lineages in Mammals

Kevin A. Kelley

At first glance, it seems an almost impossible task to understand the cellular and molecular mechanisms which are responsible for the development of a system as complex as the mammalian brain. Studies of the development of invertebrate nervous systems, such as in the nematode *Caenorhabditis elegans,* have resulted in the production of fate maps which trace neuronal

Methods in Neurosciences, Volume 1

lineages through all stages of development. Unfortunately, the complexity of the mammalian central nervous system (CNS) prevents the types of investigations which have proven so successful in *C. elegans*. There are, however, experimental models which have allowed investigators to examine basic questions concerning the lineages of specific types of neurons and their progenitors within the developing mammalian CNS. In particular, the production and analysis of genetic mosaics (chimeric mice) have been successfully utilized to study the development of specific neurons within the mouse CNS.

Chimeric mice are produced by aggregating embryos at the blastocyst stage from two genetically distinct strains, generating a fused blastocyst containing cells from each of the donor embryos. After reimplantation into the uterus of a pseudopregnant female, these double embryos adjust in size and develop normally to term. Cells derived from each of the donor strains are present during embryogenesis, and the chimeric mice which are born from aggregated blastocysts are mosaics of the two donor strains. The most obvious effect of this cell mixing is observed in the characteristic coat color mosaicism of chimeric mice which results from the intermixing of melanocytes derived from embryos of strains that have different coat colors. Mosaicism in other tissues of chimeric mice can be observed only if an independent cell marker exists which can be used to distinguish the genotype of individual cells, thus allowing the investigator to examine the interactions of genetically distinct cells during development.

Chimeras have been particularly useful for examining various mutations which affect the nervous system, and analyses of chimeric mice produced from mutant and wild-type embryos have provided insights into the lineages of particular neurons during development (1, 2). For example, chimeras produced by aggregation of embryos from the cerebellar mutant lurcher (*Lc*) and wild-type mice have provided a model system in which the development of cerebellar Purkinje cells (PCs) can be examined (3). The *Lc* mutation is an autosomal dominant mutation which is characterized by the loss of all cerebellar PCs during early postnatal development (4, 5). Using allelic variations in β-glucuronidase activity as an independent cell marker, Wetts and Herrup (3) have shown that all of the PCs which are present in the cerebellum of adult lurcher ↔ wild-type chimeras are descended from the wild-type embryo. There are no lurcher PCs present in these chimeras, indicating that the loss of PCs which is characteristic of this mutation is an intrinsic defect of these cerebellar neurons. The number of surviving PCs present in lurcher ↔ wild-type chimeras varies, depending on the extent of the mosaicism (i.e., the percentage of the chimeric CNS which was derived from the wild-type embryo) within individual animals. The total number of PCs among chimeras occurs in integral multiples (3), suggesting that there is a small number of Purkinje cell progenitors which are committed to this neuronal lineage relatively early during embryogenesis (the neural plate to neural fold stage of development). Analysis of similar chimeric mice produced from other cerebellar mutants has also proved very useful for understanding the intrinsic nature of the defect in the affected PCs, as well as providing similar information pertaining to Purkinje cell lineage (6–8). The production and analysis of chimeric mice has become an invaluable tool for examining the developing mammalian CNS, but this technique is seriously hindered by the limited number of independent cell markers which are currently available for determining the genotype of neurons within the mosaic CNS. The majority of neuronal cell types in the CNS cannot be distinguished with available markers, limiting analysis to a relatively small number of neurons. For example, the allelic variations in β-glucuronidase activity which were so effective in the analysis of Purkinje cells described above are not sufficient to allow similar studies to be conducted on smaller cerebellar neurons, such as granule cells. The availability of markers which can be used to examine a much wider range of neurons in chimeric mice would greatly enhance the usefulness of this model system for studying the development of the CNS.

Recent advances in molecular biology have made it possible to alter the mouse genome to include exogenously introduced genes, resulting in the production of "transgenic" mice. The ability to introduce foreign genes into mice provides a unique opportunity for designing novel cell markers to expand the neuronal populations that can be examined in genetic mosaics. One method which has been successfully utilized to introduce foreign genes into the mouse genome is the use of retroviral vectors. Recombinant retroviruses containing exogenous sequences can be used to infect preimplantation embryos, resulting in integration of the retrovirus into the genome of some of the cells of the embryo during development, and, theoretically, the exogenous sequences carried by the retroviral vector will be expressed. In practice, however, there is generally very little if any expression of the integrated retroviral sequences (9–12), although exogenous genes under the regulation of an internal promoter can be expressed at varying levels when introduced by a retroviral vector (13–15). In addition to the low levels of expression observed in transgenic mice produced by retroviral infections, these animals are also obligate mosaics since the integration events occur in a multicelled embryo. For these reasons, transgenic mice that are produced by retroviral infections do not represent an efficient method for establishing mouse strains with novel independent cell markers.

A second method for the production of transgenic mice that has been more widely used is the microinjection of foreign genetic sequences into the pronuclei of fertilized one-cell mouse eggs, which has recently been reviewed (16). Transgenic mice produced by this method offer several advantages for the production of strains that express novel cell markers. The foreign DNA randomly integrates into the genome at one site during the one-cell stage in these transgenic mice, resulting in animals which contain the exogenous sequences in every somatic cell in the adult and one half of the haploid germ-line cells. The integrated transgene sequences are generally transmitted in a simple Mendelian fashion to offspring when the original transgenic animals are mated with nontransgenic mice. Many of the exogenous genes which have been introduced into transgenic mice are expressed at detectable levels, and the pattern of expression is usually determined by the particular promoter/enhancer regulatory sequences used (16). The production of transgenic mice by this method thus provides an excellent system for establishing unique mouse strains which express novel cell markers that can be used in the construction of chimeric mice for analyses of neural lineages in the developing mammalian CNS. This review will detail the methods which are used to produce transgenic mice by pronuclear injections, as well as discuss the factors that must be considered when designing transgenes that are to be used in an attempt to provide unique neuronal markers for analyses of neural development.

Designing Transgenes Which Exhibit Neuronal Expression

Several factors must be considered when designing genes that will, in theory, be expressed in neurons of mice which carry the exogenous sequences in their genome. The choice of regulatory elements will be the primary determinant of where a particular transgene is expressed. Promoter/enhancer sequences can be used which should be expressed in most if not all cells in the animal, with the result that the encoded genetic sequences are expressed everywhere, including the CNS. Examples of such regulatory elements include the promoter/enhancer elements from metallothionein, actin, tubulin, etc. Regulatory elements from isolated genes which are expressed specifically within the CNS may be used in an attempt to express exogenous sequences exclusively within the CNS or within a particular population of neurons. Several examples of the types of regulatory elements which have been successfully used to drive expression of heterologous sequences in the mouse CNS are presented in Table I (17–27). Unfortunately, in many cases, the pattern of expression which is observed in the transgenic animals does not correlate with the pattern that is expected from the regulatory sequences used (16). This is especially true of hybrid genes which are constructed by fusion of regulatory elements from one gene with the protein-coding sequences of a second gene. An example of this effect can

TABLE I   Central Nervous System Expression in Transgenic Mice[a]

Type of gene	Transgene promoter	Transgene structural gene	Site of expression of transgene	Reference(s)
Natural	hNFL	hNFL	Neurons	17
	hMBP	hMBP	Oligodendrocytes	18, 19
	hPNMT	hPNMT	Retina and adrenal medullary cells	20
	hCu/ZnSOD	hCu/ZnSOD	CNS	21
	mThy-1.1	mThy-1.1	Neurons	22
Hybrid gene	mMT-I	rGH	PVN and SCN	23
	mMT-I	hHPRT	CNS	24
	mMT-I	rSS	Anterior pituitary	25
	mMT-I	rCal/CGRP	Neurons (CGRP)	26
	γ2-crystallin	Cholera toxin	Lens fiber cells	27

[a] hNFL, Human light neurofilament; hMBP, human myelin basic protein; hPNMT, human phenylethanolamine N-methyltransferase; hCu/ZnSOD, human Cu/Zn-superoxide dismutase; mThy-1.1, mouse Thy-1.1; mMT-I, mouse metallothionein-I; rGH, rat growth hormone; hHPRT, human hypoxanthine-guanosine phosphoribosyltransferase; rSS, rat somatostatin; rCal/CGRP, rat calcitonin/calcitonin gene-related protein; PVN, paraventricular nucleus; SCN, suprachiasmatic nucleus.

be seen in the heterogeneity of expression within the CNS which is observed with transgenes that contain the mouse metallothionein-I regulatory region fused to heterologous structural sequences (Table I). Alterations in the expected sites of expression of fusion genes may be due to several factors, including juxtaposition of heterologous sequences which may create novel regulatory elements, changes in mRNA stability, or a greater susceptibility to the influences of surrounding sequences at the integration site. Since the integration events occur at random, several independent transgenic lines need to be produced and examined for expression of the transgene to ensure that the observed patterns of expression are regulated by the microinjected sequences and are not due to the effects of flanking sequences at the site of integration.

Although the choice of regulatory elements used in the construction of a transgene is important with relation to the cell types in which these sequences are ultimately expressed, the proper selection of the structural sequences encoded by the microinjected gene is critical for the subsequent lineage studies which will be performed with established transgenic lines. The encoded protein should be readily detected at all developmental stages in which the promoter/enhancer elements that govern its expression are active. Expression of the transgene should be cell-autonomous; the possible effects of secreted or cell-surface peptides on neighboring cells should be considered during the construction of genetic elements that are to be used for the production of transgenic mice. The design of the heterologous sequences to be used for microinjection should also take into consideration the desired subcellular localization of the encoded gene product. The usefulness of a particular transgene for the creation of novel cell markers will be influenced by the ultimate localization of its encoded protein and the ease with which its identification can be used to determine the genotype of cells within a genetic mosaic. It may be advantageous to have novel markers which are localized in the nucleus as a means of determining the identity of a neuron at the level of the cell body, whereas in some instances it may be beneficial to have cytoplasmic or cell-surface markers as a means of examining neuronal processes. In addition, more specific marker localizations can be used for some studies, such as the use of mitochondrial markers to facilitate investigations of synaptic regions. Finally, the encoded protein should not confer a selective advantage or disadvantage on the cells in which it is expressed, since this would obviously influence subsequent observations in genetic mosaics produced for developmental studies. This last criterion includes the obvious point that the transgene-encoded gene product must be nonlethal, although expression of lethal proteins within particular neurons provides a unique mechanism for creating mutants which can then be used to examine normal cell interactions and lineage during development. This genetic ablation of specific cells has been successfully used to induce microphthalmia in transgenic mice by the targeted expression of diptheria toxin, under the regulation of the γ_2-crystallin promoter, to differentiated lens fiber cells (27).

One final factor which should be regarded is the influence of posttranscriptional processing on the patterns of expression which are observed in transgenic mice. Recent evidence indicates that the presence of intervening sequences in the injected genes increases the transcriptional efficiency by 10- to 100-fold (28). Given this observation, it is not surprising that many hybrid genes constructed with cDNA sequences which lack introns are expressed very poorly or not at all in transgenic animals (16, 28), and if possible, the use of cDNAs should be avoided when constructing hybrid genes for the production of transgenic mice.

Purification of Fragments for Microinjection

DNA fragments containing the transgene sequences must be purified before microinjection for several reasons. Linear fragments with dissimilar ends have been shown to integrate at a higher frequency than supercoiled DNA or fragments with blunt ends (29). It is also advisable to inject fragments which are devoid of plasmid DNA, since it has been observed that vector sequences can inhibit transgene expression (30). There are a number of methods that can be used to isolate restriction endonuclease-generated DNA fragments; these are described elsewhere (31). Isolation of DNA fragments from low-melting-point agarose gels is an efficient method for purifying fragments for pronuclear microinjections, and is detailed below. No matter how the DNA fragments are prepared, they must be further purified by CsCl density gradient centrifugation (outlined below) to remove particulate matter which can obstruct the flow of injection material from a microinjection pipette.

Isolation of DNA Fragments from Low-Melting-Point Agarose

After digestion with the appropriate restriction endonucleases, the generated DNA fragments are separated by electrophoresis through low-melting-point agarose (FMC, Rockland, ME; SeaPlaque agarose) in Tris–borate buffer. The standard techniques for restriction endonuclease digestions and gel electrophoresis are reviewed elsewhere (31). After staining with ethidium bromide, the separated fragments are visualized with long-wavelength ultraviolet (UV) illumination to reduce UV-induced damage to the DNA. Gel slices containing the desired fragment are excised from the gel with a clean razor blade, transferred to 1.5-ml microcentrifuge tubes and heated at 65°C until the gel slices melt. An equal volume of distilled phenol saturated with 200 mM Tris, pH 8.5, is added to the melted gel slices, and vortexed to obtain rapid mixing. The samples are then left on ice for 10 min. The organic and aqueous phases are separated by centrifugation in a microcentrifuge at 13,000 rpm for 5 min. The top, aqueous phase is removed to another tube and reextracted with an equal volume of chloroform. After separation of the aqueous and organic phases by centrifugation at 13,000 rpm for 5 min, the aqueous layer is removed and adjusted to 0.2 M NaCl. The isolated DNA fragment is then precipitated by the addition of 2.5 vol of ethanol and placed on dry ice for 30 min or at −20°C for 10–12 hr. The precipitated DNA is recovered by centrifugation at 13,000 rpm for 10 min. After removal of the supernatant, the DNA pellet is dried and resuspended in 200 μl of 10 mM Tris, pH 7.4, 1 mM EDTA (TE), and stored at −20°C until further purified by centrifugation through a CsCl gradient.

Purification of Isolated Fragments through CsCl

Most DNA purification schemes yield fragments which can be used for subsequent experiments without further preparation. Unfortunately, DNA prepared by standard techniques often contains particulate material which obstructs the tips of microinjection pipettes, necessitating the need for an additional purification step. DNA can be purified by CsCl equilibrium density gradient centrifugation to remove material which would otherwise restrict the flow of DNA through the microinjection needle. At least 8–10 μg of isolated fragment (no more than 20 μg) should be purified through a CsCl gradient prior to use for microinjections. The following protocol is designed for 5.1 ml SW55 (Beckman) ultracentrifuge tubes, but may be adjusted for other tubes. The volume of the isolated DNA fragments is adjusted to 3.82 ml by the addition of TE. Then 4.8 g of CsCl (Bethesda Research Laboratories) is dissolved in the solution, which is then transferred to an SW55 ultracentrifuge tube. The DNA solution is centrifuged at 45,000 rpm for 40 hr at 20°C.

The gradient which was established during centrifugation is fractionated into 200-μl samples. Aliquots (5 μl) of each fraction are analyzed by electrophoresis through an agarose gel to determine which samples contain the DNA fragment. Since the fractions contain very high concentrations of CsCl, the samples will migrate very slowly into this analytical gel. Stain with ethidium bromide, and visualize the DNA in the gel with UV illumination. Pool all fractions which contain the DNA fragment. The combined gradient fractions (usually 1–2 ml) are dialyzed against 2–4 liters of microinjection buffer (10 mM Tris, pH 7.4, 0.2 mM EDTA) with several changes. The DNA sample is usually dialyzed for 36–48 hr at 4°C. The microinjection buffer has been optimized for maximum integration frequency and survival of injected eggs (29). The DNA concentration can be measured by analytical gel electrophoresis of small aliquots (1–5 μl) and comparison with known standards. Alternatively, the concentration can be determined more accurately by measuring the fluorescence of bisbenzimide H33258 in a fluorimeter, using calf thymus DNA as a standard (29). Once the DNA concentration has been determined, the fragment is diluted to 1–2 ng/μl with microinjection buffer. This concentration will yield several hundred copies of most DNA fragments injected into each pronucleus. Generally, DNA solutions at this concentration are suitable for microinjections into the pronuclei of mouse eggs, and will result in the highest frequency of integration (29). The diluted DNA solution may be stored at 4°C, or divided into small aliquots and stored at −20°C. DNA fragments prepared in this manner are usually very clean and facilitate the subsequent injection procedure since the amount of time spent replacing clogged needles is substantially reduced.

Preparation of Pseudopregnant Host Mice

After injection with purified DNA fragments, mouse eggs which survive the microinjection must be reimplanted into host females where they will develop normally to term. These females are prepared by timed matings with sterile (vasectomized) males, which produces a pseudopregnant state in these animals and allows them to carry reimplanted eggs to term. The choice of males and females to be used for the production of pseudopregnant hosts is very important; the females must not only carry reimplanted eggs to term at a high frequency, but they also need to be able to deliver and lactate their foster litters successfully. CD-1 random bred mice which are commercially available (Charles River) are a good choice for host animals, since the females are better foster mothers than most inbred strains. In addition, offspring from CD-1 mice are albino, providing a good coat color marker which can be used to determine whether litters born from host animals were derived from injected eggs or from matings with CD-1 males which were not properly vasectomized. The strains which are used as sources of eggs for injection will result in pigmented animals while any albino mice that are delivered by host females are the result of matings with males that were not truly vasectomized.

All mice which are used for microinjection experiments are kept on a 14 hr : 10hr light : dark cycle, with the lights on at 7 AM and off at 9 PM.

Avertin Anesthetic

All surgical procedures described in this chapter are performed under avertin anesthesia. This anesthetic is prepared by dissolving 1 g of 2,2,2-tribromoethanol (Aldrich Chemical Co.) in 0.62 ml of 2-methyl-2-butanol (Aldrich Chemical Co.) and 79 ml of distilled H_2O. After the 2,2,2-tribromoethanol is completely dissolved by warming to 40°C, sterilize the avertin by filtration through a 0.45-μm filter, and store at 4°C in 5- to 10-ml aliquots.

Vasectomies

CD-1 males (8–10 weeks old) are prepared for vasectomy by injection of avertin anesthetic. Each mouse is weighed and anesthetized by intraperitoneal (ip) injection of 0.2 ml of avertin for each 10 g of body weight plus an additional 0.1 ml. For example, a 30 g mouse would receive 0.7 ml of anesthetic. After the animal is anesthetized, a small incision is made into the peritoneal cavity along the midline of the animal's lower abdomen. The testicular fat pads can be visualized through the incision, and one testis is pulled through the incision by grasping the fat pad with a small (10 cm) serrated dressing forcep (Fine Science Tools, Inc.) and gently pulling the testis through the abdominal opening far enough for the vas deferens to be identified (Fig. 1). A loop of the vas deferens is then clamped off with a hemostat and cut away (Fig. 1). After clamping with the hemostat, there should be relatively little bleeding from the major artery which runs along the length of the vas deferens. After gently returning the exposed testis to the abdominal cavity, the other testis is exteriorized and the second vas deferens is resected as described above. At the completion of the vasectomy, the second testis is replaced and the peritoneal and skin openings are closed with three or four surgical sutures. After sufficient practice, it should become possible to perform the vasectomy by visualizing and removing a loop of the vas deferens inside the abdominal cavity, without externalizing the internal reproductive organs. Generally, all vasectomized males should be tested by matings with naturally ovulating CD-1 females prior to use for the production of pseudopregnant females to be certain that the surgical procedure produced sterility. Vasectomized males can be tested as soon as 1 week after surgery.

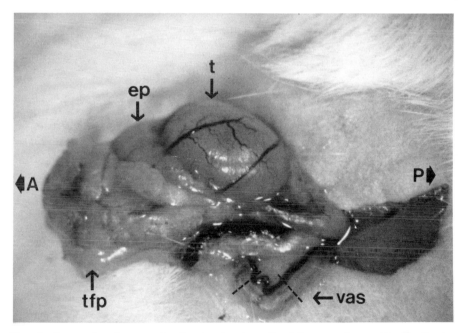

FIG. 1 Internal male reproductive tract externalized for vasectomy. tfp, Testicular fat pad; t, testis; ep, epididymis; vas, vas deferens. The vasectomy is performed by clamping a loop of the vas deferens in a hemostat and cutting out a portion of the vas deferens (dashed lines indicate areas to be cut) on both sides of each male. The anterior (A) and posterior (P) orientations of the animal are indicated.

Production of Pseudopregnant Females

Naturally ovulating CD-1 females are placed with vasectomized males the night before a microinjection experiment will be performed, in order to obtain host females whose pseudopregnancy is properly timed to allow implantation and normal development of reimplanted injected eggs. Since the normal estrous cycle of mice is 4–5 days, approximately one out of every five naturally ovulating females will mate with the vasectomized males resulting in a pseudopregnancy. To ensure that enough pseudopregnant hosts are obtained for the following day, approximately five times the number of desired host females should be mated with vasectomized males (2–3 females per male). For example, if three hosts are required for the implantation of injected eggs, at least 15 females should be placed with vasectomized males the night before the experiment. Pseudopregnant females can be identified by the presence of vaginal plugs, which consists of coagulated semen that is present the morning after mating (Fig. 2). Generally, the females should be checked as early as possible the day after mating, before the vaginal plugs begin to dissolve.

Production of Fertilized Mouse Eggs

There are several factors which must be considered in the choice of mouse strains which will serve as the source of fertilized eggs for injection. First, these strains must be readily available and the females must be capable of being superovulated to increase the number of eggs obtained from each animal. Second, the strains of choice should yield fertilized eggs which have a high rate of survival after microinjection. Finally, the fertilized eggs should be derived from strains that have normal pigmentation, which will allow the investigator to identify positively mice that developed from injected eggs as opposed to animals which result from matings of the CD-1 host females with males that were not properly vasectomized. Fertilized eggs from hybrid mice are much easier to microinject and have a higher survival rate than eggs derived from inbred strains (29). C57B1/6J × DBA/2J (B6D2) F_1 or C57B1/6J × SJL (B6SJL) F_1 hybrid mice have been successfully used for the production of transgenic mice, and are commercially available (Jackson Laboratory). One disadvantage of using fertile eggs from C57B1/6J × SJL hybrid mice is that one-fourth of the animals born from these eggs will be albino. This should not be a problem, however, if all vasectomized CD-1 males are properly tested to assure sterility. It should be noted that transgenic mice can be produced by microinjection of fertilized eggs from

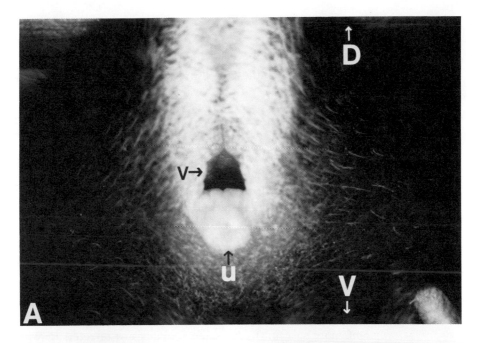

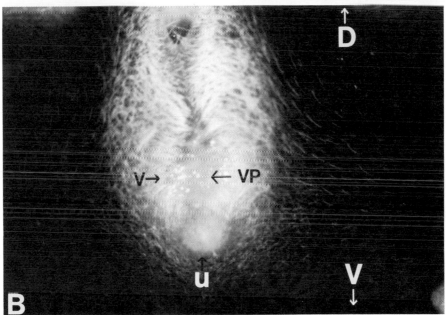

FIG. 2 External genitalia of B6D2 female mice revealing absence (A) and presence (B) of vaginal plugs. The presence of a vaginal plug (coagulated semen) indicates successful mating and is useful for determining the stage of the eggs which will be isolated from fertilized females. V, Vagina; VP, vaginal plug; u, urethra. The ventral (V) and dorsal (D) orientations are indicated.

inbred strains if it is necessary to introduce exogenous genes into a defined genetic background, although the efficiencies involved with the injection process will be lower (29).

Superovulation and Timed Matings

While some investigators prefer superovulating immature females (32), mature naturally ovulating females can also be successfully superovulated and used as sources of fertilized eggs. Six- to eight-week-old hybrid females (B6D2 or B6SJL) are injected ip with 7.5 international units (IU) of pregnant mare's serum (Diosynth, Inc.) at 4 PM, 3 days prior to the planned day of microinjection. Stocks of pregnant mare's serum at 1 IU/μl are stored at −20°C, and diluted to 7.5 IU/0.2 ml with sterile 0.9% NaCl immediately prior to use.

The day before the planned injections (2 days after the administration of pregnant mare's serum), the same females are injected ip with 7.5 IU of human chorionic gonadotropin (Sigma) at 1 PM. The HCG stocks are also stored at 1 IU/μl at −20°C. These superovulated females are mated with fertile males from the appropriate hybrid strain (one female per male) at 5 PM on the same day that they received the HCG. The matings of naturally ovulating CD-1 females with vasectomized males are also set up at this time. On the day of the planned injections (day 0), the superovulated females are carefully checked for vaginal plugs, since sometimes the plugs may be small and easily missed. Generally, each superovulated female that successfully mated with a fertile male will provide 25–30 good eggs for injection.

Preparation of Culture Media

Bicarbonate-buffered medium, which is used for isolating and culturing fertilized eggs (M16 medium), and HEPES-buffered medium, which is used during the injection procedure (M2), are prepared as described by Costantini and co-workers (33). These media are conveniently prepared from stock solutions on the day of use. Detailed methods for the preparation and storage of stock solutions used to make the M2 and M16 media are described elsewhere (33). The compositions of the M16 and M2 media are given in the following table.

M16 medium	M2 medium
94.66 mM NaCl	94.66 mM NaCl
4.78 mM KCl	4.78 mM KCl
1.71 mM CaCl$_2$ · 2H$_2$O	1.71 mM CaCl$_2$ · 2H$_2$O
1.19 mM KH$_2$PO$_4$	1.19 mM KH$_2$PO$_4$
1.19 mM MgSO$_4$ · 7H$_2$O	1.19 mM MgSO$_4$ · 7H$_2$O
25 mM NaHCO$_3$	4.15 mM NaHCO$_3$
23.28 mM sodium lactate	20.285 mM HEPES
0.33 mM sodium pyruvate	23.28 mM sodium lactate
5.56 mM glucose	0.33 mM sodium pyruvate
0.4% BSA	5.56 mM glucose
100 U/ml penicillin G	0.4% BSA
50 μg/ml streptomycin sulfate	100 U/ml penicillin G
0.001% Phenol Red	50 μg/ml streptomycin sulfate
	0.001% Phenol Red

Isolation of Fertile Mouse Eggs

Embryo collection pipettes are prepared by washing 6-in. lengths of glass tubing (3 mm outer diameter) in chromic acid overnight, followed by extensive washing in distilled H$_2$O, then ethanol. The tubing is then dried and pulled after heating in a flame to produce a narrow central filament which will have an inner diameter that is several times the diameter of a single mouse egg. The pulled tubing is scored in the center with a diamond-tipped pen, producing two pipettes which can be attached by tubing to a mouth piece and used to collect the fertilized mouse eggs. These pipettes are sterilized by baking in a 180°C oven for several hours before use.

The superovulated females that have mated with fertile males are sacrificed, and the oviduct is removed to isolate the fertile eggs. An incision through the abdomen is used to peel back the skin, revealing the peritoneal wall. The peritoneum is then opened, and one of the uterine horns is grasped with serrated forceps. The ovaries are located on each side of the animal, adjacent to the kidneys. With scissors, remove the oviduct by cutting through the uterus immediately posterior to the oviduct and through the ovary, avoiding the fat since it tends to interfere with the subsequent isolation and washing steps (Fig. 3A). The excised oviducts are transferred to a 35-mm culture dish containing M16 medium which has been equilibrated to 37°C in a 5% CO$_2$ incubator. To remove the eggs, an oviduct is placed in a depression slide containing warm M16 medium with 1 mg/ml hyaluronidase (Sigma), and observed under a dissecting scope. The eggs are located in the

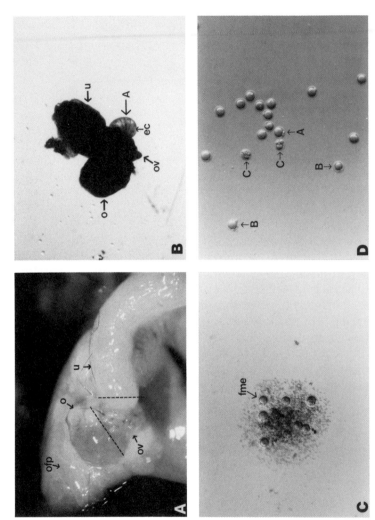

FIG. 3   Isolation of fertilized mouse eggs. (A) The oviduct (ov), which contains the fertilized eggs, is removed by cutting (dashed lines) through the ovary (o) and the uterine horn (u). ofp, Ovarian fat pad. (B) Isolated oviduct. After the oviducts have been isolated, they are transferred to M16 medium containing 1 mg/ml of hyaluronidase. The eggs are located within a swelling of the oviduct (ampulla) and can usually be visualized through the oviduct wall. A, Ampulla; ec, fertilized eggs and cumulus cells; o, ovary; ov, oviduct; u, uterus. (C) Fertilized eggs and cumulus cells. The fertilized eggs are released from the oviduct by tearing the outer wall of the ampulla. The fertilized eggs and their associated cumulus cells are then allowed to dissociate in the hyaluronidase solution. fme, Fertilized mouse egg. (D) Isolated fertilized mouse eggs after several washes through M16 medium to remove cumulus cells and debris. Healthy fertilized eggs (A) to be used for microinjection are then separated from unfertilized eggs (B) which lack polar bodies, or those which are degenerating or dividing abnormally (C).

ampulla, which is a swollen loop of the oviduct that is near the opening (infundibulum) of the oviduct next to the ovary (Fig. 3B). Usually, the eggs can be seen in the ampulla through the transparent oviductal wall. Place a pair of #3 Dumont forceps behind the ampulla and pin the oviduct to the bottom of the slide. With a second pair of #3 Dumont forceps, gently tear the outer wall of the ampulla, releasing the eggs and their attached cumulus cells into the media (Fig. 3C). Discard the oviduct, and repeat this procedure on all of the isolated oviducts. Let the eggs sit in the hyaluronidase medium for several minutes to remove the cumulus cells from the fertilized eggs. Using an embryo collection pipette, carefully collect the isolated eggs by aspiration and transfer them through 3–4 changes of warm (37°C) M16 medium to remove debris and wash out the hyaluronidase. After the final wash, select healthy fertilized eggs (Fig. 3D) and put them into microdrops of M16 medium (20–30 eggs/drop) that are under light mineral oil. The final culture dish is prepared by placing small drops (50–100 μl) of medium in the bottom of a 35-mm dish and overlaying the drops with mineral oil. The mineral oil is previously equilibrated with M16 medium at the proper pH (7.2–7.4) by bubbling 5% CO_2 through the mixture, monitoring the color of the M16 as an indication of the pH, and then centrifuging to separate the oil and media. This dish is left in the CO_2 incubator to equilibrate for at least 30 min. Once all of the isolated eggs have been washed and transferred to drops of medium under oil, they are placed in a 5% CO_2 incubator until ready for injection.

Preparation of Holding and Injection Pipettes

Holding Pipettes

Several holding pipettes should be prepared the day before the scheduled microinjections. These pipettes will be used to hold the mouse eggs in position while the injection needle is inserted into the pronucleus. Glass capillaries (1 mm outer diameter) are heated over a small flame and hand-drawn to obtain a uniform inner diameter of approximately 70 μm. The filament is scored with a diamond pen at points which are approximately 2–3 cm from the drawn-out shoulder and broken to produce two pipettes which can be fashioned into holding pipettes on a microforge. Use only those pipettes which have a clean, flat break to fashion the holding pipettes. Alternatively, a pipette puller can be programmed to pull pipettes which have the appropriate diameter (34). The hand-drawn pipettes are attached to the capillary holder on a microforge (Kramer Scientific, Yonkers, NY), and placed in a vertical position directly over the end of the heating element.

Using the microscope attached to the microforge, center the end of the pipette directly over the filament, turn on the heating element, and allow the end to slowly melt in on itself, narrowing the inner diameter until only a small channel (10–20 μm) is visible. The end of the holding pipette should have an inner and outer diameter which will allow the fertilized eggs to be held securely in place without being drawn up into the holding pipette. The relationship of the end of a good holding pipette relative to the diameter of a fertilized mouse egg is shown in Fig. 5B. The appropriate diameters for the drawn-out capillaries and the final inner diameter for the holding pipette will be determined with practice and can be facilitated by the use of a reticle in one of the eyepieces of the microforge microscope. The preparation of the holding pipette is finished by turning the position of the pipette in the microforge so that the last 0.5 cm of the tip is positioned horizontally over the end of the heating filament. When the heating filament is turned on, the edge of the pipette nearest the filament will melt faster than the opposite side, allowing the pipette tip to bend down under the force of gravity. When a 15–30° bend has been introduced into the holding pipette, turn off the heat, remove the finished holding pipette, and store until ready for use.

Injection Pipettes

Thin-wall glass capillary tubing (1 mm outer diameter) (World Precision Instruments, Inc., New Haven, CT) with an internal filament is used to produce the injection pipettes. These pipettes are formed on a micropipette puller, of which there are several varieties commercially available. The programmable Flaming/Brown micropipette puller (Model P-80/PC) manufactured by Sutter Instrument Company reproducibly produces high-quality injection pipettes once the proper pulling parameters have been established. Four-inch lengths of the capillary tubing are clamped into position over the heating element, and the programmed pulling cycle is initiated, resulting in the production of two pipettes which can be used for injections. The proper parameters which need to be programmed into the P-80/PC are determined by pulling pipettes under various conditions to produce a tip which has a small opening ($\sim$1 μm) and a narrow shaft which will allow the tip of the needle to be inserted into the pronucleus of the egg without producing a large hole in the cytoplasmic membrane. The diameter of the tip should not be too large since this will make it more difficult to control the flow rate of the DNA solution, and will result in too much damage to the eggs. An example of the tip size and the angle and length of the shaft of a good injection pipette is shown relative to the holding pipette and the egg to be injected in Fig. 5A.

The CsCl-purified DNA solution is prepared immediately before use by centrifugation in a microcentrifuge for 10 min at 4°C to pellet any residual particulate material. The DNA is loaded into the tip of the injection pipette by placing 1 μl of the solution into the end of the pipette opposite the tip, placing the pipette vertically into a piece of Plasticene on a glass plate with the tip downward, and allowing the solution to fill the end of the tip by flowing down the internal filament in the pipette. After several minutes, the tips are examined for the presence of air bubbles under a dissecting microscope. When the tips are devoid of air bubbles, backfill them with Fluorinert FC-40 (Sigma), using a long 30-gauge needle attached to a syringe filled with Fluorinert. Each injection pipette should be useful for injecting 20–30 eggs before the tip becomes clogged with material from the injected eggs. The DNA-loaded pipettes are stored at room temperature attached to Plasticene strips on a glass plate.

Pronuclear Microinjections

The microinjection apparatus consists of an inverted microscope with appropriate optics for visualizing the pronuclei of fertilized eggs, and a pair of micromanipulators for holding and injecting the eggs (Fig. 4A). Differential interference contrast (DIC) optics generally provide the best image of the pronuclei for injections. Either Nomarski or Hoffman DIC can be used, although Nomarski produces the sharpest image. Glass injection chambers must be used with Nomarski DIC, since this optical system will not work through plastic dishes, unlike Hoffman DIC. The glass injection chambers are prepared by making rings of silicone glue on ordinary glass slides. Once dried, these slides are used to hold fertilized eggs in M2 medium within the ring (Fig. 4B).

The Nikon Diaphot inverted microscope equipped with Nomarski DIC produces an excellent image of the pronuclei, and has a long working distance between the sample and the objective, providing sufficient access for the micromanipulators. This microscope can be equipped with hydraulically operated Narashige micromanipulators (distributed by Nikon) which are designed exclusively for the Diaphot (Fig. 4A). The microscope should be equipped with a low-power 4× objective that is used to find the eggs so that they can be positioned on the holding pipette. All of the injections are performed at 600×, with a 40× Nomarski objective and 15× eyepieces. The injections may also be done at lower magnification, although it is not as easy to position the tip of the injection pipette in the same plane as the pronuclei to be injected. The microscope can be used on a vibration isolation table (Technical Manufacturing Corp., Peabody, MA), with the manipulators on shelves, to minimize vibrations which would affect the quality of the image.

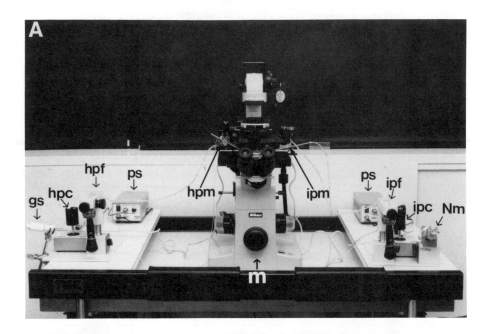

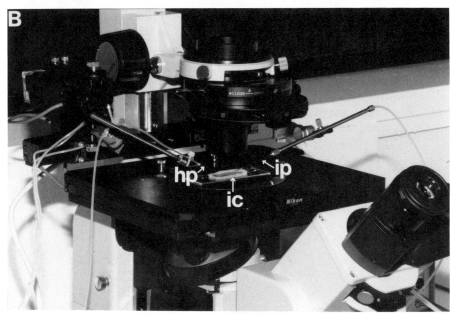

FIG. 4 Microinjection apparatus. (A) A Nikon Diaphot inverted microscope (m) with Nomarski differential interference contrast optics is used to visualize the pronuclei for microinjection. The holding (hpm) and injection pipette (ipm) micromanipulators are stage mounted and are controlled by Narashige electronic coarse and hydraulic fine movement manipulators. hpc, Holding pipette coarse manipulator;

The holding pipette is clamped into the left micromanipulator arm and attached to a 2-ml Gilmont micrometer syringe with silicone tubing (Baxter Scientific Products, 0.03 in. i.d./0.065 in. o.d.). The angle of the holding pipette is adjusted so that the end of the pipette is parallel to the specimen stage (Fig. 4B). The injection pipette is attached to the same size tubing and clamped into the right micromanipulator arm at a shallow angle relative to the plane of the stage (Fig. 4B). The entire injection system (tubing and injection syringe) is filled with light mineral oil or Fluorinert FC-40. Care must be taken to avoid air bubbles in the system or at the end of the injection pipette which is attached to the manipulator. This can be achieved by previously filling the system and leaving the end of the tubing in a small reservoir of oil or Fluorinert between experiments and while changing injection pipettes. Air bubbles can be avoided when the injection pipette is attached to the system by applying a small amount of positive pressure through the injection syringe while inserting the injection pipette into the tubing. Once attached, the holding and injection pipettes are raised with the coarse movement manipulators (Fig. 4A) so that the slide containing the eggs can be positioned on the stage.

Warm (37°C) M2 HEPES-buffered medium is placed into an injection chamber on a glass slide and 20–30 of the previously isolated eggs are transferred into the center of the chamber. The slide is then carefully transferred onto the stage of the microscope and the eggs are observed under low magnification with the 4× bright-field objective. Using the left coarse adjustment manipulator, carefully lower the holding pipette into the media and bring the tip of the pipette into the center of the field of view. Using the fine movement hydraulic manipulator, lower the holding pipette until it just touches the bottom of the injection chamber. Switch to the high-magnification Nomarski objective and position the tip of the holding pipette at the left of the field of view using the fine adjustment manipulator in the x and y plane. Return to low magnification, and using the stage controls, move the holding pipette away from the eggs toward the top of the injection

---

hpf, holding pipette fine manipulator; ipc, injection pipette coarse manipulator; ipf, injection pipette fine manipulator; ps, power supplies for electronic coarse manipulators. A 2-ml Gilmont syringe (gs) attached by tubing to the holding pipette is used to hold or release the fertilized mouse eggs. The injection pipette is attached by tubing to a Narashige microinjector (Nm), which is used to adjust the flow rate of the DNA solution from the injection pipette. The microscope is located on a vibration isolation table with shelves for the micromanipulators and microinjector. (B) The holding pipette (hp) is positioned so that the angled end is parallel to the injection chamber (ic), and the injection pipette (ip) is positioned at a shallow angle relative to the injection chamber.

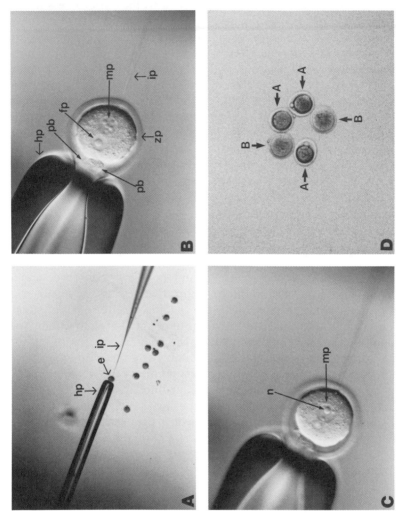

Fig. 5   Pronuclear microinjections. (A) Fertilized egg immobilized by holding pipette. Magnification: ×60. hp, Holding pipette; ip, injection pipette; e, fertilized mouse egg. (B) Fertilized mouse egg held in position for pronuclear microinjection with a holding pipette (hp). The injection pipette (ip) is positioned adjacent to the zona pellucida (zp) and brought into the same focal plane as the male pronucleus (mp) using the hydraulic fine positioning manipulator. pb, Polar body; fp, female pronucleus. Magnification: ×600. (C) Male pronucleus being injected with DNA solution. mp, Male pronucleus; n, nucleolus. Magnification: ×600. (D) Microinjected eggs which survive the injection (A) are separated from eggs, which have lysed (B), and are incubated in M16 medium until reimplantation into pseudopregnant females.

chamber. Using the Gilmont syringe attached to the holding pipette, draw M2 medium halfway up the holding pipette, then apply slight positive pressure with the syringe so that the holding pipette is no longer aspirating medium. Reposition the holding pipette next to one of the eggs with the stage control, and apply light suction to the holding pipette until the egg is held on the end of the pipette. Lower the injection pipette with the coarse control manipulator until it comes into the same focal plane as the egg attached to the holding pipette (Fig. 5A). Switch over to the high-magnification Nomarski objective and adjust the fine focus until the male pronucleus is in sharp focus (Fig. 5B). The male pronucleus is the larger of the two pronuclei and is located opposite from the two polar bodies (Fig. 5B). If the male pronucleus is not located on the side of the egg nearest the injection pipette, the egg can be repositioned on the holding pipette by carefully releasing the egg and allowing it to rotate from the flow of media out of the holding pipette before applying negative pressure through the Gilmont syringe to reattach the egg. In this way, the egg can be rotated until properly oriented for injection. The tip of the injection pipette is then positioned near the zona pellucida of the egg and brought into the same focal plane as the pronucleus with the micromanipulator fine adjustment. The injection pipette should be kept under constant positive pressure such that the DNA solution is continually flowing from the tip. The proper flow rate is usually established after several eggs have been injected. Generally, it is best to try to inject eggs without applying more positive pressure after the injection pipette has been attached to the injection system tubing. The small amount of positive pressure present when the pipette is attached to the tubing is usually sufficient for a moderate initial flow rate. Using the fine control micromanipulator, push the tip of the injection pipette through the zona pellucida into the pronucleus within the egg (Fig. 5B). In most injections, this process will result in part of the cytoplasmic membrane being pushed into the pronucleus in front of the pipette tip. When this happens, a small swelling of injection solution will be visible in or near the pronucleus. To pierce this membrane and allow the pronucleus to be injected effectively, carefully push the injection pipette further into the pronucleus until this swelling disappears. Occasionally, it will appear that the tip is passing through the other side of the pronucleus before it actually pierces the cytoplasmic membrane. When the tip is properly inside the pronucleus, and flowing at an appropriate rate, the pronucleus will visibly swell from the addition of the injected DNA solution (Fig. 5C). After the pronucleus has swelled, usually to no more than twice its original diameter, withdraw the injection pipette from the egg. Successfully injected eggs will appear normal, whereas eggs which were injected at too fast a flow rate or which received too much damage to the cytoplasmic membrane will appear to be leaking cytoplasm through the entry hole made by the injection pipette. Care must be taken to avoid touching the nucleoli within the pronucleus. The nucleoli will stick to the tip of the injection pipette and be partially drawn out of the pronucleus when the injection pipette is removed from the egg. This will tend to impede the flow from the pipette, as well as resulting in the lysis of the injected egg. When nucleolar material is stuck to the tip of an injection pipette, it should be replaced with a new pipette.

After an egg has been successfully injected, the 4× objective is used to move the injected egg away from the remaining uninjected eggs. This movement is done by moving the stage so that the egg attached to the holding pipette moves to one edge of the injection chamber. The egg is then released there, and the holding pipette is returned to the uninjected eggs using the stage control so that a new egg can be attached to the holding pipette. Once the holding and injection pipettes have been centered for the Nomarski objective, the eggs are moved within the injection chamber through manipulations of the microscope stage control so that the holding and injection pipettes do not need to be repositioned in the high-power field for every egg to be injected. Once all of the eggs in the chamber have been injected, the holding and injection pipettes are raised from the chamber with the coarse manipulators so that the chamber can be removed from the stage. Under a dissecting scope, the eggs which survived the injection are removed with a collection pipette which is prepared from glass tubing as described earlier, and placed in a microdrop of M16 medium under mineral oil. The injected eggs are kept in a CO_2 incubator until reimplantation into pseudopregnant hosts. Fresh M2 medium (prewarmed to 37°C) is placed in the injection chamber and then a new batch of 20–30 eggs is transferred to the chamber for injections. When the chamber is returned to the stage, the holding pipette can be lowered vertically with the coarse manipulator so that it is still in the proper position in the field of view under Nomarski illumination. A fresh injection pipette should be used for each group of eggs, and the injection needle should be positioned near the holding pipette as described above. After all of the isolated eggs have been injected, the surviving eggs are separated from lysed eggs (Fig. 5D) and left in microdrops of M16 medium under mineral oil at 37°C in a CO_2 incubator until reimplanted.

Surgical Reimplantations of Injected Eggs

Preparation of Reimplantation Pipettes

The pipettes which are used to reimplant injected eggs into the oviduct of pseudopregnant females are prepared from 10-μl microcapillaries (Drummond). The capillary tubing is carefully hand-drawn after heating in a microburner flame. The diameter of the drawn-out pipette should be slightly larger than the diameter of a single egg. A convenient method for determining the proper diameter is to compare the drawn-out pipettes to the diameter of a 30-gauge needle, using a dissecting microscope. The hand-drawn capillaries are then scored with a diamond needle to produce a pipette with a shaft that has a consistent diameter over the last 2–3 cm. The tip of the pipette is then fire-polished in the microburner flame to remove sharp edges which might otherwise damage the oviduct during the reimplantation. These pipettes are then attached to a mouthpiece and the eggs are loaded as described elsewhere (33). Briefly, the reimplantation pipettes are prepared by filling the shaft with mineral oil. A small volume of air is then aspirated into the pipette followed by a small volume of M16 medium, producing an air bubble between the oil and media. Another small volume of air is then introduced into the pipette, followed by 25–35 injected eggs in as small a volume of M16 media as possible. Once the eggs are loaded into the pipette, a final air bubble is added followed by a minimal volume of M16 medium. The final configuration, consisting of injected eggs between two air bubbles, is shown in Fig. 6A. The loaded pipette is then carefully set aside while the animal is prepared for the reimplantation.

Reimplantations

Fertilized mouse eggs which survive the microinjection process must be reimplanted into the oviduct of properly timed pseudopregnant host females, where they will develop normally to term. The pseudopregnant females are prepared for surgery by ip injection of avertin anesthetic as described previously. Generally, the host females should weigh between 28 and 32 g. When the host is properly anesthetized, a small region of hair is removed from the back midway between the spine and the bulge of the abdomen on the left side. Under low magnification on a stereoscopic surgery microscope, a small incision is made through the skin and peritoneal wall. The edges of the incision are separated with serrated dressing forceps so that the fat pad attached to the left ovary can be localized. Once identified (Fig. 6B), the fat pad is grasped with forceps and gently removed from the incision so that the ovary is withdrawn from the abdominal cavity. The ovary is exteriorized until the oviduct and uterine horn can be observed outside the incision. The fat pad is then clamped with a hemostat which is used to position the ovary properly. The ovary should be drawn toward the animal's head and held out of the body by the attached hemostat. The ovary is properly positioned when the mesenteric arteries of the uterus are perpendicular to the table.

The opening to the oviduct, the infundibulum, is located at the end of the

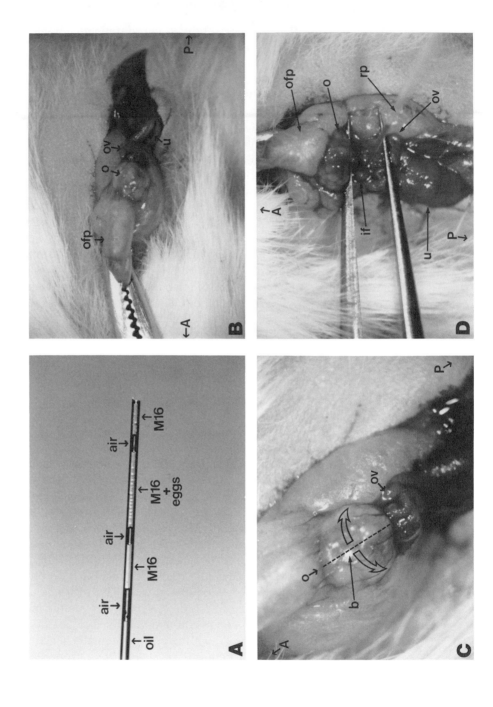

oviduct nearest the ovary. There is a thin, translucent membrane (the bursa) which surrounds the ovary and oviduct that must be resected so that the reimplantation pipette holding the injected eggs can be inserted into the infundibulum. The membrane is best visualized under high magnification on the surgical microscope, and can be removed by grasping the bursa over the ovary with two #5 Dumont forceps, and gently tearing it along the length of the ovary (Fig. 6C). Care must be exercised when tearing the bursal membrane so that none of the major arteries lining this membrane are torn. Ruptured arteries in the bursa will make the reimplantation very difficult since blood will obscure the localization of the infundibulum as well as coagulating in the tip of the reimplantation pipette. The sides of the torn membrane are then picked up with the forceps and pulled around and underneath the ovary. The infundibulum is observed by laterally inserting a pair of forceps between the ovary and oviduct and gently separating the two. If properly positioned, the infundibulum will be located such that a reimplantation pipette can be placed into the opening from the right side (Fig. 6D). The reimplantation pipette is carefully inserted into the infundibulum, and the injected eggs are transferred into the oviduct. The material within the reimplantation pipette is pushed into the oviduct by positive pressure until the second air bubble has entered the infundibulum. The eggs have been successfully transferred if the air bubbles can be observed within the first turn of the oviduct. Generally, 25–35 eggs should be reimplanted into each host female. The hemostat is released from the ovarian fat pad, and the

---

FIG. 6   Reimplantation of microinjected eggs. (A) Reimplantation pipette loaded with injected eggs. The pipette is first loaded with mineral oil (oil), followed by a small air bubble (air), M16 medium (M16), a second air bubble (air), M16 medium containing the injected eggs (M16 + eggs), a third air bubble (air), and then a final small volume of M16 medium (M16). (B) The ovarian fat pad (ofp) is grasped with serrated dressing forceps and is drawn through the incision to externalize the ovary (o), oviduct (ov), and uterine horn (u). The anterior (A) and posterior (P) orientations are indicated. (C) The bursal membrane (b) surrounding the ovary (o) and oviduct (ov) is removed by gently tearing the membrane in an anterior to posterior direction along the length of the ovary (dashed lines) and then by folding the membrane around and under the ovary in the direction of the arrows. The anterior (A) and posterior (P) orientations are indicated. (D) The ovary and oviduct are gently separated with #5 Dumont forceps to reveal the infundibulum (if), which is the opening into the oviduct. The reimplantation pipette (rp) containing the injected eggs is placed into the opening, and the contents of the pipette are deposited into the infundibulum with slight positive pressure until the second air bubble has entered the oviduct, ensuring that the eggs contained in the M16 medium between the first and second air bubbles have been transferred into the oviduct. ofp, Ovarian fat pad; o, ovary; ov, oviduct; u, uterus. The anterior (A) and posterior (P) orientations are indicated.

ovary is gently returned to the abdominal cavity by manipulating the fat pad with serrated dressing forceps. The incisions in the abdominal cavity and skin are closed with 3–4 surgical sutures.

The pseudopregnant hosts which receive injected eggs are returned to the animal room and kept on the same 14 hr : 10 hr light : dark cycle. The injected embryos will develop normally to term and be delivered 19–20 days after reimplantation. If they are not delivered by the morning of the twentieth day, the fetuses should be delivered by Cesarian section and fostered onto lactating females which have litters that were born within 1 or 2 days of the date that the pups that are to be fostered were born. Mice born from injected eggs can be weaned from host females at approximately 19–21 days after birth. DNA samples are then prepared from tail skin biopsies to determine which mice have integrated the injected sequences into their genome (33). Approximately 15–20% of the reimplanted eggs will develop to term and be born. With a moderate amount of skill, it can be expected that 20–30% of the animals born from injected eggs will be transgenic. Overall, only 1–3% of the isolated eggs which are injected will survive and produce transgenic mice, given the fact that 40–60% of the eggs actually survive the microinjections. The resulting transgenic animals can be mated with nontransgenic inbred mice at 8–10 weeks of age to produce offspring that will be used to establish a line from the original animal, and for subsequent analyses of expression of the exogenously introduced sequences.

Analysis of Neural Lineages Using Transgenic Mice

The production of new strains of mice which express novel neuronal markers will enable investigators to examine more readily neural lineages during development. There are a number of intriguing questions concerning the development of the CNS which cannot be adequately examined with the currently available cellular marker systems. For example, cerebral cortical neurons forming distinct radial columns have been identified both morphologically and physiologically. It has been suggested, on the basis of the known development of the cortex, that all of the neurons which form these columns may be derived from a small number of stem cells (35). Until recently, it has not been possible to examine the developmental basis of these cortical columns. Several recent studies using novel neuronal markers introduced via retroviral vectors have provided some insights into the clonal origins of the radial columns. Lineage analysis of chicken optic tectum neurons whose precursors have been labeled early in development with a retrovirus that expresses a foreign marker protein (bacterial β-galactosidase) has indicated that clonally related cells migrate in a strictly radial pattern through the tectum (36). This study suggests that clonally related cortical neurons within the chicken optic tectum migrate radially along a single radial glial fiber during development. In contrast to this observation, however, similar lineage studies performed via retroviral infections of early rat embryos have suggested that clonally related cortical neurons exhibit tangential as well as radial migration patterns during development (37), indicating that clonally related cortical neurons may migrate away from the ventricular zone along several different radial glial fibers. Although these studies represent opposite views of the clonal arrangement of CNS neurons, they have established the usefulness of novel cellular markers for examining neuronal lineages during the development of the mammalian CNS. There are, however, a number of assumptions which must be made when analyzing the results that are observed with retroviral infections. It is assumed that neighboring cells which have been marked by retroviral infection are derived from the same labeled precursor cell, although there is no definitive way to determine whether spatially related labeled neurons are derived from a common precursor or through independent retroviral infection of individual precursors early in development that subsequently give rise to spatially related but clonally distinct neurons. In addition, every animal derived from retroviral infection of early embryos is unique with relation to the number and types of precursor cells infected by the retrovirus, and since it is unclear when after the infection event occurs that the foreign marker protein is expressed, it is only feasible to examine the patterns of labeled cells which are observed much later in the development of the animal's CNS. These limitations preclude analysis of neural lineages during all stages of development. In addition, the relative importance of other factors such as cell death cannot be determined.

The availability of established transgenic lines which express novel neuronal markers during most, if not all, stages of development will greatly enhance our ability to analyze neural lineages. In particular, such lines would be extremely useful for expanding the studies of the clonal arrangement of cortical neurons which have been conducted by the introduction of novel markers via retroviral vectors. These studies can be performed by producing chimeric mice from transgenic and nontransgenic embryos, and analyzing the resulting mosaic CNS using the expression of the transgene protein as an independent marker. Such studies using transgenic animals offer several advantages over the retroviral lineage analyses. Every embryo that is used to produce chimeras will be identical with relation to the site of integration of the transgene as well as to the temporal and spatial expression patterns of the foreign sequence; this is in contrast to the unique nature of every animal that results from an embryo infected by retroviral vectors. Thus, such chimeric animals will be useful for examining neural lineages during any stage of development in which the transgene is expressed, and will not be subject to the types of assumptions which are necessary to analyze the clonal arrangements of neurons that are marked with retroviruses. The production of transgenic mice from foreign sequences which are designed to be expressed within the CNS will vastly improve our ability to examine and understand the complexities of neuronal lineages in the developing mammalian CNS.

References

1. R. J. Mullen, *Soc. Neurosci. Symp.* **2,** 47 (1977).
2. R. J. Mullen and K. Herrup, *in* "Neurogenetics: A Genetic Analysis of the Nervous System" (X. O. Breakfield, ed.), p. 89. Elsevier/North-Holland, New York, 1979.
3. R. Wetts and K. Herrup, *J. Neurosci.* **2,** 1494 (1982).
4. R. J. S. Phillips, *J. Genet.* **57,** 35 (1960).
5. K. W. T. Caddy and T. J. Biscoe, *Philos. Trans. R. Soc. London* **287,** 167 (1979).
6. K. Herrup and R. J. Mullen, *Brian Res.* **178,** 443 (1979).
7. K. Herrup and R. J. Mullen, *Dev. Brain Res.* **1,** 475 (1981).
8. K. Herrup, *Dev. Brain Res.* **11,** 267 (1983).
9. R. Jaenisch, H. Fan, and B. Crocker, *Proc. Natl. Acad. Sci. U.S.A.* **72,** 4008 (1975).
10. C. Stewart, H. Stuhlmann, D. Jahner, and R. Jaenisch, *Proc. Natl. Acad. Sci. U.S.A.* **79,** 4098 (1982).
11. R. Jaenisch and D. Jahner, *Biochim. Biophys. Acta* **782,** 1 (1984).
12. R. Jaenisch, D. Jahner, A. Schnieke, and K. Harbers, *Proc. Natl. Acad. Sci. U.S.A.* **82,** 1451 (1985).
13. P. Soriano, R. D. Cone, R. C. Mulligan, and R. Jaenisch, *Science* **234,** 1409 (1986).
14. J. C. Glover, G. E. Gray, and J. R. Sanes, *Soc. Neurosci. Abstr.* **13,** 183 (1987).
15. C. Walsh and C. L. Cepko, *Science* **241,** 1342 (1988).
16. R. D. Palmiter and R. L. Brinster, *Annu. Rev. Genet.* **20,** 465 (1986).
17. J.-P. Julien, I. Tretjakoff, L. Beaudet, and A. Peterson, *Genes Dev.* **1,** 1085 (1987).
18. C. Readhead, B. Popko, N. Takahashi, H. D. Shine, R. A. Saavedra, R. L. Sidman, and L. Hood, *Cell* **48,** 703 (1987).
19. B. Popko, C. Puckett, E. Lai, H. D. Shine, C. Readhead, N. Takahashi, S. W. Hunt, R. L. Sidman, and L. Hood, *Cell* **48,** 713 (1987).
20. E. E. Baetge, R. R. Behringer, A. Messing, R. L. Brinster, and R. D. Palmiter, *Proc. Natl. Acad. Sci. U.S.A.* **85,** 3648 (1988).
21. C. J. Epstein, K. B. Avraham, M. Lovett, S. Smith, O. Elroy-Stine, G. Rotman, C. Bry, and Y. Groner, *Proc. Natl. Acad. Sci. U.S.A.* **84,** 8044 (1987).
22. G. Kollias, E. Spanopoulou, F. Grosveld, M. Ritter, J. Beech, and R. Morris, *Proc. Natl. Acad. Sci. U.S.A.* **84,** 1492 (1987).

23. L. W. Swanson, D. M. Simmons, J. Arriza, R. Hammer, R. Brinster, M. G. Rosenfeld, and R. M. Evans, *Nature (London)* **317,** 363 (1985).
24. J. T. Stout, H. Y. Chen, J. Brennand, C. T. Caskey, and R. L. Brinster, *Nature (London)* **317,** 250 (1985).
25. M. J. Low, R. E. Hammer, R. H. Goodman, J. F. Habener, R. D. Palmiter, and R. L. Brinster, *Cell* **41,** 211 (1985)
26. E. B. Crenshaw, A. F. Russo, L. W. Swanson, and M. G. Rosenfeld, *Cell* **49,** 389 (1987).
27. M. L. Breitman, S. Clapoff, J. Rossant, L.-C. Tsui, M. Glode, I. H. Maxwell, and A. Bernstein, *Science* **238,** 1563 (1987).
28. R. L. Brinster, J. M. Allen, R. R. Behringer, R. E. Gelinas, and R. D. Palmiter, *Proc. Natl. Acad. Sci. U.S.A.* **85,** 836 (1988).
29. R. L. Brinster, H. Y. Chen, M. E. Trumbauer, M. K. Yagle, and R. D. Palmiter, *Proc. Natl. Acad. Sci. U.S.A.* **82,** 4438 (1985).
30. K. Chada, J. Magram, K. Raphael, G. Radice, E. Lacy, and F. Costantini, *Nature (London)* **314,** 377 (1985).
31. T. Maniatis, E. F. Fritsch, and J. Sambrook, "Molecular Cloning: A Laboratory Manual." Cold Spring Harbor Laboratory, Cold Spring Harbor, New York, 1982.
32. J. W. Gordon and F. H. Ruddle, *in* "Methods in Enzymology" (R. Wu, L. Grossman, and K. Moldave, eds.), Vol. 101, p. 411. Academic Press, New York, 1983.
33. B. Hogan, F. Costantini, and E. Lacy, "Manipulating the Mouse Embryo: A Laboratory Manual." Cold Spring Harbor Labratory, Cold Spring Harbor, New York, 1986.
34. M. L. DePamphilis, S. A. Herman, E. Martinez-Salas, L. F. Chalifour, D. O. Wirak, D. Y. Cupo, and M. Miranda, *BioTechniques* **6,** 662 (1988).
35. P. Rakic, *Science* **241,** 170 (1988).
36. G. E. Gray, J. C. Glover, J. Majors, and J. R. Sanes, *Proc. Natl. Acad. Sci. U.S.A.* **85,** 7356 (1988).
37. C. Walsh and C. L. Cepko, *Science* **241,** 1342 (1988).

Section V

Molecular Pathology

[23] Characterization of Molecular Pathology of Alzheimer's Disease

Michel Goedert

Alzheimer's disease is characterized by a loss of memory and other cognitive functions, resulting in severe dementia and, ultimately, death (1). It is a very common disease, affecting 0.5–1% of the general population of the Western world; its cause is unknown and there exists no generally effective treatment. Neuropathologically, Alzheimer's disease is characterized by abundant senile plaques and neurofibrillary tangles located mostly in cerebral cortex and hippocampus, as well as in subcortical nuclei, such as amygdala, nucleus basalis of Meynert, and locus coeruleus (Fig. 1). It is hoped that a better understanding of the molecular nature of plaques and tangles will shed light on the pathogenesis of Alzheimer's disease and will in the long run result in an effective treatment. Senile plaques are always extracellular and, in their mature form, consist of a dense core of amyloid β protein (2). In contrast, neurofibrillary tangles are mostly intracellular and their major constituent is the paired helical filament (3); they are found both in abnormal neurites within the senile plaques and in nerve cell bodies.

Over the past few years, molecular biology has made it possible to progress toward an understanding of the constituents of plaques and tangles. This in turn will permit investigation of how and why they are formed. The availability of good-quality cDNA libraries prepared from postmortem human brain has been instrumental in this work. Therefore, following an overview of the current state of the field, a detailed description of the production of cDNA libraries for human brain is presented.

Amyloid Fibril and Its Precursor

The amyloid β protein is the major protein constituent of senile plaques (2, 4). Protein purification led to the determination of a partial amino acid sequence of amyloid β protein, and this in turn allowed several groups to isolate cDNA clones encoding one form of the amyloid β protein precursor of 695 amino acids (5–9). Subsequently, two further forms were discovered that are produced from a single gene through alternative RNA splicing (10–12). They are 751 or 770 amino acids in length and differ from the first

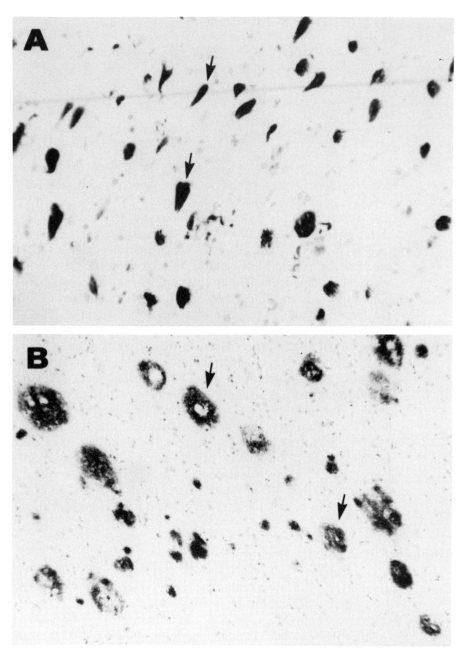

Fig. 1   Numerous neurofibrillary tangles (A) and senile plaques (B) in cerebral cortex from an Alzheimer's disease patient. The arrows point to characteristic plaques and tangles.

form by the presence of an extra domain encoding a serine protease inhibitor.

The amyloid β protein precursor possesses the characteristics of a transmembrane protein, with a large hydrophilic extracellular domain, a hydrophobic, putative membrane-spanning stretch, and a short cytoplasmic tail (5). Recently, it has been reported that the amyloid β protein precursor is identical with a previously identified heparan sulfate proteoglycan core protein (13). The physiological function of the latter is unknown, although in the nervous system it may be involved in neurite outgrowth (14). The amyloid β protein that is deposited in large amounts in Alzheimer's disease and that forms fibrils is 43 amino acids in length and is located toward the carboxy terminus of the amyloid β protein precursor, with its carboxy-terminal end located in the putative membrane-spanning region (5).

The molecular cloning of cDNAs encoding the amyloid β protein precursor has permitted the investigation of the tissue and cellular distributions of the various mRNAs in tissues from both control patients and from patients who had died with Alzheimer's disease. The knowledge of the amino acid sequence of the amyloid β protein precursor has in turn led to the production of antisera directed against various portions of the protein and consequently to immunological studies on control and diseased brains.

Initial studies using probes that did not distinguish between the various forms of the amyloid β protein precursor showed high levels of mRNAs not only in the central nervous system, but also in all peripheral tissues investigated (6, 7). In the brain, the cellular localization of amyloid β protein precursor mRNAs was entirely neuronal (9, 15). The same qualitative and quantitative distribution was found in cerebral cortex and hippocampus from patients who had died with Alzheimer's disease (9, 15), whereas an increase in amyloid β protein precursor mRNAs was found in the nucleus basalis of Meynert from Alzheimer's disease patients (16). By Northern blotting, a reduction in amyloid β protein precursor mRNAs was observed in cerebral cortex from Alzheimer's disease patients (9). Subsequently, it was shown that mRNAs encoding the 751- and 770-amino acid forms are expressed ubiquitously, whereas mRNA encoding the 695-amino acid form is only found in the brain (Fig. 2) (17, 18); both types of mRNA are expressed in the same cells in the hippocampus (18). By Northern blotting on cerebral cortex, the mRNA encoding the 695-amino acid form was found to be reduced, with no concomitant change in mRNA levels for the 751- and 770-amino acid forms (17, 18). One study which distinguished between mRNAs encoding the 751- and 770-amino acid forms reported an increase in the mRNA for the 770-amino acid form (19).

Taken together, these studies indicate that there exists a correlation between the tissue and cellular distributions of the amyloid β protein precursor mRNAs and the pathology of Alzheimer's disease only insofar as

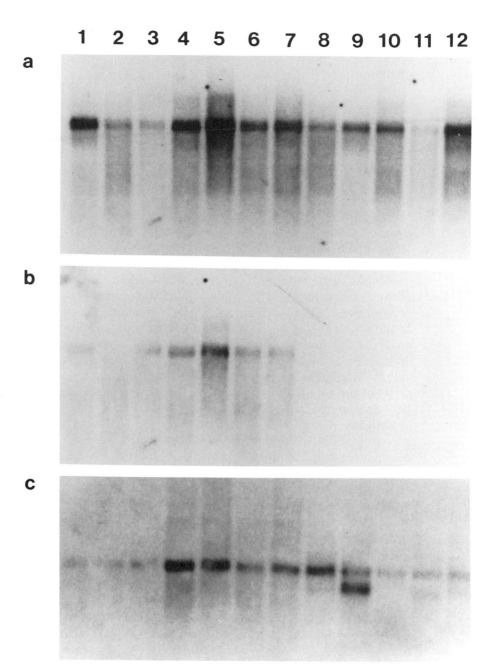

Fig. 2 Northern blot analysis of poly(A)$^+$ from control human brain using amyloid β protein precursor encoding (a) or lacking (b) the protease inhibitor domain or mouse β actin (c) as a probe. Each lane contained 2 μg of poly(A)$^+$ RNA. Lanes: 1, frontal cortex; 2, hippocampus; 3, cerebellum; 4, midbrain; 5, basal forebrain; 6,

the cells affected by the disease produce the corresponding mRNAs (Fig. 3A). However, the distribution of the latter is much more widespread (Fig. 3A) and there exists no evidence to suggest that a general overproduction of amyloid β protein precursor mRNAs leads to the deposition of amyloid β protein in Alzheimer's disease. It thus appears that amyloid deposition represents a secondary event in the development of the disease. The knowledge of the amino acid sequence of the amyloid β protein precursor will greatly aid in identifying factors such as proteases that could cleave the amyloid β protein out of the precursor protein.

Antisera raised against synthetic peptides derived from various regions of the amyloid β protein precursor recognize a polypeptide of 130 kDa in various neuronal and nonneuronal tissues (20, 21). In addition, an 80-kDa form of the precursor that is present only in those brain regions that are prone to amyloid β protein deposition has been identified (21). Immunohistochemical studies on normal brain support the view of a transmembrane orientation of the amyloid β protein precursor (22). Similar antipeptide antisera stain deposits that are located around the core of the senile plaque in histological sections of cerebral cortex from Alzheimer's disease patients (23). The core itself is unstained by these antisera, while it is strongly positive to antisera raised against portions of the amyloid β protein (24). These results strongly argue in favor of the view that the processing of the amyloid β protein precursor that leads to amyloid β protein deposition occurs locally within the senile plaque.

Paired Helical Filament

The identity of the molecular constituents of the paired helical filament is less well understood than that of the amyloid fibril; as is the case for the amyloid deposits, the reason for the abnormal filament assembly within the cell remains to be discovered.

Structural studies indicate that the paired helical filament consists of a double-helical stack of C-shaped subunits (25). The extreme insolubility of the filament renders its biochemical characterization very difficult. Immunohistochemical studies have identified various candidate molecules, such as the middle- and high-molecular-weight neurofilament subunits (26, 27), vimentin (28), ubiquitin (29, 30), amyloid β protein (31), and the microtubule-associated proteins τ (32–35) and MAP2 (36, 37). However, it is

---

thalamus; 7, striatum; 8, leptomeninges; 9, heart; 10, adrenal gland; 11, prostate gland; 12, kidney. The same blot was successively hybridized with each probe following dehybridization of the previous probe.

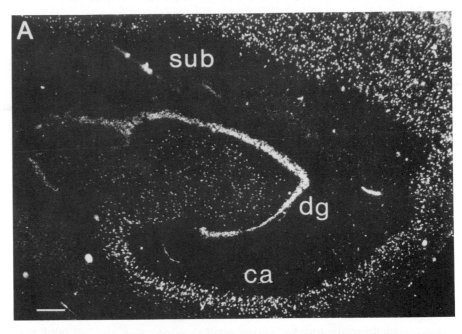

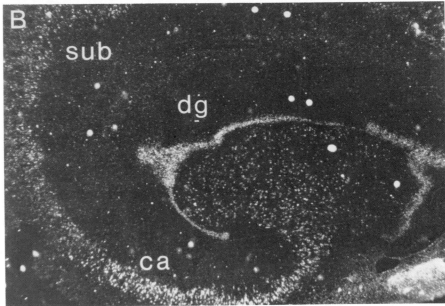

FIG. 3 Cellular localization of amyloid β protein precursor mRNAs (A) and τ protein mRNAs (B) in the hippocampal formation from a control patient. sub, Subiculum; dg, dentate gyrus; ca, cornu ammonis. Bar, 350 μm.

difficult by light microscopy to distinguish between proteins that are true structural components of the paired helical filament and proteins caught in tangles or nonspecifically adhering to paired helical filaments. It is thus necessary to analyze paired helical filaments chemically in order to identify unambiguously their molecular components. As they are biologically inert and difficult to purify, one requires a label that identifies them under the electron microscope and that also allows one to follow their biochemical purification.

Paired helical filaments isolated in the absence of protease treatment display a fuzzy outer coat which is removed by pronase to leave a protease-resistant core that retains the characteristic paired helical filament morphology (38). A monoclonal antibody raised against purified paired helical filament core preparations was found to identify core filaments clearly and to label protein fragments isolated from paired helical filament core preparations (39). This established a link between the paired helical filament core as a morphological entity and specific peptides extracted from it. Two different amino acid sequences were obtained from a 9.5-kDa band and these led to the cloning and sequencing of cDNAs which were shown to encode the microtubule-associated protein τ (40). When various clones were sequenced, it was found that they belonged to two distinct classes. Further sequencing showed that the two classes coded for proteins of 352 or 383 amino acids, which differed by the presence of a 31-amino acid insert in the longer one (41). The DNA sequence coding for the larger protein is shown in Fig. 4, with the additional sequence that distinguishes the larger form from the smaller protein underlined. Sequencing of genomic clones established that the additional repeat is encoded by a separate exon (41). The most striking feature of the τ protein sequence is the presence of tandem repeats of 31 or 32 amino acids containing a characteristic Pro-Gly-Gly-Gly motif. The smaller protein contains three and the larger four of these repeats. The extra repeat in the four-repeat isoform is inserted within the first repeat of the three-repeat isoform in a way that preserves the periodic pattern. Twelve residues are completely conserved between the four repeats and a further four residues show conservative changes. The functional implications of the presence of different numbers of repeats in τ protein are not known.

Recently, the complete sequence of another microtubule-associated protein, MAP2, has been determined and shown to contain three repeats that are highly homologous to the repeats in τ protein (42). Evidence was presented that the repeat region represents the microtubule-binding domain of MAP2 and therefore, probably, of τ also. The comparison of the protein sequences obtained from the paired helical filament core (39) with that of the sequence of τ protein as deduced by cDNA cloning indicated that it is the repeat region of τ protein that is found in the core of the paired helical filament. It is thus the microtubule-binding domain of τ protein that is tightly

```
                                                    TGTCGACTATCAGGTGAACTTTGAACCAGG

  1 Met Ala Glu Pro Arg Gln Glu Phe Glu Val Met Glu Asp His Ala Gly Thr Tyr Gly Leu Gly Asp Arg Lys Asp Gln Gly Gly Tyr Thr
  1 ATG GCT GAG CCC CGC CAG GAG TTC GAA GTG ATG GAA GAT CAC GCT GGG ACG TAC GGG TTG GGG GAC AGG AAA GAT CAG GGG GGC TAC ACC

 31 Met His Gln Asp Gln Glu Gly Asp Thr Asp Ala Gly Leu Lys Ala Glu Glu Ala Gly Ile Gly Asp Thr Pro Ser Leu Glu Asp Glu Ala
 91 ATG CAC CAA GAC CAA GAA GGT GAC ACG GAC GCT GGC CTG AAA GCT GAA GAA GCA GGC ATT GGA GAC ACC CCC AGC CTG GAA GAC GAA GCT

 61 Ala Gly His Val Thr Gln Ala Arg Met Val Ser Lys Ser Lys Asp Gly Thr Gly Ser Asp Asp Lys Lys Ala Lys Gly Ala Asp Gly Lys
181 GCT GGG CAC GTG ACT CAA GCT CGC ATG GTC AGT AAA AGC AAA GAC GGG ACT GGA AGC GAT GAC AAA AAG GCC AAG GGG GCT GAT GGT AAA

 91 Thr Lys Ile Ala Thr Pro Arg Gly Ala Ala Pro Pro Gly Gln Lys Gly Gln Ala Asn Ala Thr Arg Ile Pro Ala Lys Thr Pro Pro Ala
271 ACG AAG ATC GCC ACC CCT CGG GGA GCA GCC CCT CCA GGC CAG AAA GGC CAG GCC AAC GCC ACC AGG ATT CCA GCA AAA ACC CCG CCC GCT

121 Pro Lys Thr Pro Pro Ser Ser Gly Glu Pro Pro Lys Ser Gly Asp Arg Ser Gly Tyr Ser Ser Pro Gly Ser Pro Gly Thr Pro Gly Ser
361 CCA AAG ACA CCA CCC TCC AGC TCT GGG GAG CCT CCC AAG TCA GGG GAT CGC AGC GGC TAC AGC AGC CCC GGC TCC CCA GGC ACT CCC AGC

151 Arg Ser Arg Thr Pro Ser Leu Pro Thr Pro Pro Thr Arg Glu Pro Lys Lys Val Ala Val Val Arg Thr Pro Pro Lys Ser Pro Ser Ser
451 CGC TCC CGG ACC CCG TCC CTT CCA ACC CCA CCC ACC CGG GAG CCC AAG AAG GTG GCA GTG GTC CGT ACT CCA CCC AAG TCG CCG TCT TCC

181 Ala Lys Ser Arg Leu Gln Thr Ala Pro Val Pro Met Pro Asp Leu Lys Asn Val Lys Ser Lys Ile Gly Ser Thr Glu Asn Leu Lys His
541 GCC AAG AGC CGC CTG CAG ACA GCC CCC GTG CCC ATG CCA GAC CTG AAG AAT GTC AAG TCC AAG ATC GGC TCC ACT GAG AAC CTG AAG CAC

211 Gln Pro Gly Gly Gly Lys Val Gln Ile Ile Asn Lys Lys Leu Asp Leu Ser Asn Val Gln Ser Lys Cys Gly Ser Lys Asp Asn Ile Lys
631 CAG CCG GGA GGC GGG AAG GTG CAG ATA ATT AAT AAG AAG CTG GAT CTT AGC AAC GTC CAG TCA AAG TGT GGC TCA AAG GAT AAT ATC AAA

241 His Val Pro Gly Gly Gly Ser Val Gln Ile Val Tyr Lys Pro Val Asp Leu Ser Lys Val Thr Ser Lys Cys Gly Ser Leu Gly Asn Ile
721 CAC GTC CCG GGA GGC GGC AGT GTG CAA ATA GTC TAC AAA CCA GTT GAC CTG TCA AAG GTG ACC TCA AAG TGT GGC TCA TTA GGC AAC ATC

271 His His Lys Pro Gly Gly Gly Gln Val Glu Val Lys Ser Glu Lys Leu Asp Phe Lys Asp Arg Val Gln Ser Lys Ile Gly Ser Leu Asp
811 CAT CAT AAA CCA GGA GGT GGC CAG GTG GAA GTC AAG TCT GAG AAG CTT GAC TTC AAG GAC AGA GTC CAG TCC AAG ATT GGG TCC CTG GAC

301 Asn Ile Thr His Val Pro Gly Gly Gly Asn Lys Lys Ile Glu Thr His Lys Leu Thr Phe Arg Glu Asn Ala Lys Ala Lys Thr Asp His
901 AAT ATC ACC CAC GTC CCT GGG GGA GGA AAT AAG AAG ATT GAG ACC CAC AAG CTG ACC TTC CGC GAG AAC GCC AAG GCC AAG ACA GAC CAC

331 Gly Ala Glu Ile Val Tyr Lys Ser Pro Val Val Ser Gly Asp Thr Ser Pro Arg His Leu Ser Asn Val Ser Ser Thr Gly Ser Ile Asp
991 GGG GCG GAG ATC GTG TAC AAG TCT CCA GTG GTG TCC GGG GAC ACG TCC CCA CGG CAT CTC AGC AAT GTC TCC AGC ACC GGC AGC ATC GAC

361 Met Val Asp Ser Pro Gln Leu Ala Thr Leu Ala Asp Glu Val Ser Ala Ser Leu Ala Lys Gln Gly Leu ***
1081 ATG GTA GAC TCG CCC CAG CTC GCC ACG TTA GCT GAC GAG GTG TCT GCC TCC CTG GCC AAG CAG GGT TTG TGA TCAGGCCCCTGGGCGGT
```

Fig. 4 Nucleotide and predicted amino acid sequences of the human τ protein isoform with four repeats. The extra repeat of 31 amino acids is underlined. Nucleotides are numbered in the 5′ → 3′ direction, starting with the first nucleotide of the initiating codon.

and specifically bound in the core of the paired helical filament. However, antisera raised against peptides derived from the amino and carboxytermini of τ protein demonstrate that the whole of τ forms part of the neurofibrillary tangle (Fig. 5). The protein sequencing indicated the presence of two forms of τ in the core of the paired helical filament (39), and the molecular cloning showed that these are likely to correspond to the three- and four-repeat isoforms (40, 41). The identity of a large part of the paired helical filament core remains to be discovered, but a tight association between this molecule and the repeat region of τ protein could drive the irreversible assembly of paired helical filaments. The immobilization of a significant fraction of the cellular pool of τ protein within paired helical filaments probably interferes with normal microtubule function, leading to the degeneration of tangle-bearing cells.

Substantial amounts of τ protein mRNAs are found throughout the human brain, with no detectable signal in peripheral tissues such as heart, kidney, or adrenal gland (40). The cellular localization of τ protein mRNAs is exclusively neuronal (41). The transcripts are found in the cells affected in Alzheimer's disease, but their presence is not restricted to these cells (41). Amyloid β protein precursor and τ protein mRNAs colocalize in hippocampal granule and pyramidal cells (Fig. 3B). In adult human brain, mRNAs encoding the three- and four-repeat τ proteins have been found throughout and their levels do not vary much between different brain regions (41). However, in fetal brain, although three-repeat transcripts are abundant, four-repeat transcripts have not been detected (41). When levels of mRNA for the two types were investigated in the frontal cortex of patients who had died with Alzheimer's disease, no significant differences could be found when compared with controls (41). A simple overexpression of τ protein mRNAs is thus unlikely to be the cause of paired helical filament formation. However, the knowledge of the molecular identity of one component of the paired helical filament core will allow investigation of how and why the otherwise soluble microtubule-associated protein τ becomes insoluble and associated with nontubulin components whose identity remains to be discovered. It is already known that the distribution of τ protein immunoreactivity is abnormal in Alzheimer's disease (43). τ protein antibodies which stain axons in normal brain also stain cell bodies and dendrites in cerebral cortex from Alzheimer's disease patients.

Procedures: cDNA Library Construction from Human Brain

The technique described below is a modification of the method described by Gubler and Hoffman (44), which is based in turn on the technique developed by Okayama and Berg (45). It is presented in some detail, as it is our

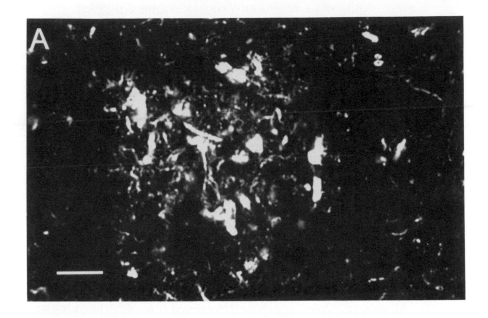

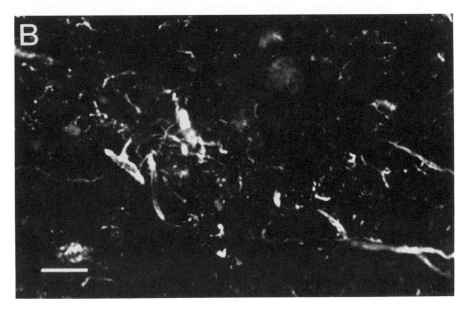

Fig. 5 Immunohistochemical localization of τ protein immunoreactivity in neurofibrillary tangles in Alzheimer's disease. Antisera were raised against synthetic peptides for the amino terminus (A) and the carboxy terminus (B) of the human τ sequence and were used to stain cerebral cortex sections from a patient who had died with Alzheimer's disease. Bar, 30 μm.

experience that it works reproducibly only if one adheres strictly to this protocol. The vector used is the bacteriophage λgt10 (46). The solutions used in these procedures are described below.

Solutions

10× Reverse transcriptase buffer
500 mM Tris-HCl, pH 8.3, 200 mM KCl, 100 mM MgCl$_2$, 50 mM dithiothreitol
4× Second-strand cDNA buffer
400 mM HEPES, pH 7.6, 270 mM KCl, 16 mM MgCl$_2$, 63 mM 2-mercaptoethanol
10× S$_1$ nuclease buffer
3 M NaCl, 300 mM sodium acetate, pH 4.5, 30 mM ZnCl$_2$
10× *Eco*RI methylase buffer
500 mM Tris-HCl, pH 8.0, 5 mM EDTA
S-Adenosyl-L-methionine
10× = 100 μM. Prepare a 10 mM stock in 10 mM sodium acetate, pH 5.0. Dilute to 100 μM with water
10× Ligation buffer
660 mM Tris-HCl, pH 7.4, 100 mM MgCl$_2$, 10 mM spermidine, 3.3 mM ATP, 200 μg/ml bovine serum albumin, 100 mM dithiothreitol
10× *Eco*RI buffer
500 mM Tris-HCl, pH 7.4, 1 M NaCl, 100 mM MgCl$_2$
TE
10 mM Tris-HCl, pH 7.4, 0.1 mM EDTA
λ Diluent
Per liter: 10 ml of 1 M Tris-HCl, pH 7.4, 5 ml of 1 M MgSO$_4$, 11.7 g NaCl, 1 g gelatin
CY medium
Per liter: 10 g of casamino acids, 5 g of yeast extract, 3 g of NaCl, 2 g of KCl. Adjust to pH 7.0
Top-agarose
Per liter: 6.5 g of agarose, 10 g of tryptone, 5 g of NaCl
TYE for plates
Per liter: 15 g of agar, 10 g of tryptone, 5 g of yeast extract, 8 g of NaCl
2× TY medium
Per liter: 16 g of tryptone, 10 g of yeast extract, 5 g of NaCl. Adjust to pH 7.4
λ growth medium
Per liter: 600 ml 2× TY medium, 5 ml of 20% glucose, 10 ml of 1 M MgCl$_2$, 2.5 g of NaCl

TME
20 mM Tris-HCl, pH 7.4, 10 mM MgCl$_2$, 0.1 mM EDTA

RNA Extraction

Human tissues are obtained routinely less than 6 hr after death, frozen in liquid nitrogen, and stored at $-70°C$ until use. We routinely use the guanidinium isothiocyanate/hot phenol method for RNA extractions (47). Two grams of frozen brain tissue are added to 10 ml 4 M guanidinium isothiocyanate and immediately homogenized using a Polytron (Kinematica A.G., Luzern, Switzerland) at setting 7 for about 30 sec. The tubes are then transferred to a 60°C water bath and 10 ml of phenol kept at 60°C is added. This is followed by 5 ml of salt solution (100 mM sodium acetate, pH 5.2, 10 mM Tris-HCl, pH 7.4, 1 mM EDTA) kept also at 60°C and 10 ml chloroform kept at room temperature. Following vigorous shaking for 7 min, the tubes are centrifuged at 3000 rpm for 10 min, the water phase is removed, and reextracted using phenol/chloroform (3 : 1). This is followed by several phenol/chloroform (1 : 1) extractions until the interphase is clear, and by ethanol precipitation.

Poly(A) Selection

The RNA is resuspended in water (treated beforehand with 0.1% diethyl pyrocarbonate and autoclaved) and its concentration determined spectrophotometrically. The poly(A) selection is done in polypropylene Econocolumns (Bio-Rad) using oligod(T) cellulose (Collaborative Research). The latter is suspended in 5 ml ETS (10 mM Tris-HCl, pH 7.4, 1 mM EDTA, 0.1% sodium dodecyl sulfate) and poured down the column; the column is equilibrated with 10 ml ETS, followed by 10 ml NETS (10 mM Tris-HCl, pH 7.4, 1 mM EDTA, 0.1% sodium dodecyl sulfate, 0.5 M sodium chloride). The RNA is heated to 65°C for 5 min and cooled on ice; it is made 0.5 M with respect to sodium chloride, followed by the addition of 6 ml NETS. The solution is then poured down the column and recirculated 4–5 times. The material that runs through the column is the poly(A)$^-$ RNA. The column is washed with 10 ml NETS and the poly(A)$^+$ RNA is eluted in 1-ml portions into sterile Eppendorf tubes. We normally collect three separate fractions. The concentration of poly(A)$^+$ RNA is determined spectrophotometrically, followed by ethanol precipitation. It normally accounts for about 1.5% of the total RNA in adult human brain. The quality of poly(A)$^+$ RNA is checked by running 3 μg on a glyoxal gel (48), alongside total RNA and poly(A)$^-$ RNA.

First-Strand cDNA Synthesis

We normally start with 10 μg poly(A)$^+$ RNA resuspended in water at 0.5 mg/ml and use silanized, sterile Eppendorf tubes throughout.

Poly(A)$^+$ RNA	20 μl
4 dNTPs (each at 20 mM)	20 μl
[α-^{32}P]dCTP	1 μl
Oligo(dT) (200 μg/ml)	10 μl
RNasin (40 U/μl)	4 μl
Sodium pyrophosphate (80 mM)	2 μl
10× Reverse transcriptase buffer	10 μl
Avian myeloblastosis virus reverse transcriptase (47 U/μl, Life Sciences)	4 μl
Water	29 μl

Incubate the above reagents together for 1.5 hr at 42°C. Perform phenol, phenol/chloroform (1 : 1), and chloroform extractions. Add an equal volume (100 μl) of 4 M ammonium acetate and 4 vol (400 μl) of ethanol. Precipitate, reconstitute in 100 μl water, and repeat ammonium acetate precipitation. Reconstitute the pellet in 50 μl water. One microliter of the latter is used for assessing the number of counts per minute (cpm) incorporated, along with one-fiftieth of the volume from the nonincorporated cpm. The conversion mRNA to first-strand cDNA is then calculated (by using the above nucleotide concentrations 100% conversion = 132 μg cDNA/reaction). Usually, the rate of conversion is 20–40%. Two microliters of the first-strand reaction is removed for gel electrophoresis.

Second-Strand cDNA Synthesis

mRNA/first-strand cDNA	47 μl
4 dNTPs (each at 5 mM)	5 μl
[α-^{32}P]dCTP	3 μl
Nicotinamide adenine dinucleotide (20 mM)	2 μl
4× second-strand buffer	50 μl
Escherichia coli DNA ligase (5 U/μl, New England Biolabs)	2 μl
RNase H (800 U/μl, Pharmacia)	6 μl
DNA polymerase I (5 U/μl, Boehringer)	15 μl
Water	70 μl

Incubate this mixture for 1 hr at 15°C, 1 hr at 22°C, and overnight at 15°C. Perform phenol, phenol/chloroform (1 : 1), and chloroform extractions.

Extract twice with 4 M ammonium acetate, ethanol precipitate, and re-suspend in 120 μl water. Use one-hundredth of the nonincorporated and incorporated cpm to calculate the percentage incorporation. The conversion from first-strand to second-strand cDNA is then calculated (by using the above nucleotide concentrations 100% conversion = 33 μg cDNA/ reaction). Usually, the rate of conversion is of the order of 100%. One microliter of the second-strand reaction is removed for gel electrophoresis.

S_1 Nuclease Treatment

cDNA	118 μl
10× S_1 nuclease buffer	13 μl
S_1 nuclease (100 U/μl, Bethesda Research Laboratories)	6 μl

The S_1 nuclease (870 U/μl) is diluted just before use in 50% glycerol in water. Incubate for 20 min at 37°C. Perform phenol, phenol/chloroform (1 : 1), and chloroform extractions, and ethanol precipitation with 4 M ammonium acetate. One usually loses 10–15% of the incorporated cpm at this stage. Resuspend the cDNA in 35 μl water and remove 2 μl for gel electrophoresis. First-strand and second-strand cDNA reactions, as well as the cDNA following S_1 nuclease treatment, are checked by gel electrophoresis using a vertical alkaline agarose gel (48).

EcoRI Methylase Treatment

cDNA	33 μl
Bovine serum albumin (10 mg/ml)	2 μl
5× EcoRI methylase buffer	10 μl
10× S-Adenosyl-L-methionine	5 μl
EcoRI methylase (20 U/μl, New England Biolabs)	3 μl

Incubate for 30 min at 37°C, add another 3 μl enzyme, and leave for another 30 min. Perform two phenol, two phenol/chloroform (1 : 1), and two chloroform extractions, followed by ethanol precipitation. The cDNA is resuspended in 18 μl water.

EcoRI Linker Ligation

cDNA	18 μl
10× Ligation buffer	2 μl
4 dNTPs (each at 5 mM)	2 μl
Klenow fragment of DNA polymerase I (5 U/μl, Boehringer)	1 μl

Incubate for 2 hr at 14°C. Then add

Phosphorylated EcoRI linkers (250 μg/ml, New England Biolabs)	4 μl
10× Ligation buffer	2 μl
T4 DNA ligase (400 U/μl, New England Biolabs)	4 μl
T4 RNA ligase (4 U/μl, New England Biolabs)	2 μl
Water	9 μl

Incubate overnight at 14°C. Perform phenol, phenol/chloroform (1:1), and chloroform extractions, followed by ethanol precipitation. The cDNA is resuspended in 83 μl water.

EcoRI Digestion

cDNA	83 μl
10× EcoRI buffer	10 μl
EcoRI (20 U/μl, New England Biolabs)	7 μl

Incubate for 1 hr at 37°C. Perform phenol, phenol/chloroform (1:1), and chloroform extractions and ethanol precipitation. Resuspend in 40 μl TE.

Size-Selection of cDNA

This is done using Sepharose CL-4B in a disposable 1-ml plastic pipette with its top cut off. A disposable yellow tip containing glass wool is attached to the lower end of the pipette. The column is equilibrated with TE + 0.3 M sodium chloride. The cDNA is made 0.3 M with respect to sodium chloride and bromphenol blue dust is added. The sample is applied and a total of 30 two-drop fractions are collected into sterile Eppendorf tubes. If desirable, the column can be calibrated beforehand by using radioactive DNA markers. We routinely keep the left-hand part of the radioactive peak and discard the rest. It normally consists of four fractions, corresponding to a total of approximately 160 μl of size-selected, linkered cDNA.

Ligation of cDNA to Vector

We normally use one-fourth of the total cDNA for the first ligation.

cDNA	40 μl
*Eco*RI cut λgt10 (350 μg/ml)	12 μl
Sodium chloride	5 μl

Add 127 μl ethanol to precipitate. The pellet is resuspended in 3.5 μl water and 2 μl ligase mixture (2 μl 10× ligation buffer, 2 μl T4 DNA ligase, 2 μl water) is added. Mix well and incubate for 2 hr at 15°C. Add 20 μl water and mix well. Keep frozen at −20°C until use.

In Vitro Packaging and Plating

We use the commercially available Gigapack Gold packaging extracts (Stratagene Cloning Systems) for *in vitro* packaging. They are processed according to the manufacturer's instructions, using 5 μl of the λgt10/cDNA solution. Following the packaging, the volume is brought to 1 ml with λ diluent, to which 100 μl chloroform is added. The packaged phage is kept at 4°C.

The plating of the cDNA library is done on the *E. coli* strains C600 and C600 *Hfl*. The percentage of clear versus turbid plaques on C600 should be higher than the previously determined background (in our experience 0.1–0.2%), whereas the number of clear plaques on C600 *Hfl* gives the total number of plaques. We dilute the packaged phage 1/100, 1/1,000, 1/10,000, and 1/100,000 in λ diluent prior to plating. Ten microliters of diluted phage is added to 200 μl CY medium containing 10 mM magnesium sulfate and 0.2% maltose; 30 μl saturated bacteria that had been grown in CY medium containing 10 mM magnesium sulfate and 0.2% maltose is then added. Following 20 min at 37°C, 4 ml top-agarose is added and the mixture plated onto TYE plates that had been preheated at 37°C for a few hours. The percentage of clear versus turbid plaques is usually of the order of 10% and the number of clones amounts normally to approximately $10^6/\mu$g poly(A)$^+$ RNA.

λgt10 Minipreparations

Besides the cloning efficiency it is essential to know how large the average insert is. In order to get an approximate idea, we usually pick 10 clear plaques and grow minipreparations from which DNA is prepared that is then cut with HindIII.

A plug containing a single clear plaque is cut out and added to 1 ml λ diluent containing 50 μl chloroform. Following elution of the phage, 50 μl of the λ diluent is added to 20 ml λ growth medium containing 50 μl saturated bacteria (K12803 or C600 Hfl strains of E. coli). The bacteria lyse after overnight growth at 37°C. Following a 10-min spin at 4,000 rpm, 40 μg DNase I and 40 μg RNase A are added to the supernatant. The tubes are then incubated for 20 min at 37°C and spun for 10 min at 12,000 rpm. The supernatant is added to 10 ml 20% polyethylene glycol/2.5 M sodium chloride and kept at 4°C for 30 min. Following a 10-min spin at 12,000 rpm, each pellet is resuspended in 1 ml TME, transferred to an Eppendorf tube and reprecipitated with 0.5 ml polyethylene glycol/2.5 M sodium chloride. The pellet is resuspended in 500 μl water, to which 100 μl of 100 mM EDTA and 12 μl of 10% sodium dodecyl sulfate are added. After 10 min at 65°C, the solution is phenol and chloroform extracted and ethanol precipitated. The DNA concentration is determined spectrophotometrically and an aliquot is used for digestion with HindIII. HindIII digestion of λgt10 generates four fragments of sizes 23.1, 9.3, 6.5, and 4.3 kb; the 6.5-kb fragments goes up in size in the presence of an insert. In our cDNA libraries, 80–90% of the clear plaques contains inserts. The above technique can be scaled up to produce large quantities of λgt10.

References

1. A. Alzheimer, *Allg. Z. Psychiatr.* **64,** 146 (1907).
2. G. G. Glenner and C. W. Wong, *Biochem. Biophys. Res. Commun.* **122,** 1131 (1984).
3. M. Kidd, *Nature (London)* **197,** 192 (1963).
4. C. L. Masters, G. Multhaup, G. Simms, J. Pottgiesser, R. N. Martins, and K. Beyreuther, *EMBO J.* **4,** 2757 (1985).
5. J. Kang, H. G. Lemaire, A. Unterbeck, J. M. Salbaum, C. L. Masters, K. H. Grzeschik, G. Multhaup, K. Beyreuther, and B. Müller-Hill, *Nature (London)* **325,** 733 (1987).
6. D. Goldgaber, M. I. Lerman, O. W. McBride, U. Saffiotti, and D. C. Gajdusek, *Science* **235,** 877 (1987).
7. R. E. Tanzi, J. F. Gusella, P. C. Watkins, G. A. P. Burns, P. St. George-Hyslop, M. L. Van Keuren, D. Patterson, S. Pagan, D. M. Kurnit, and R. L. Neve, *Science* **235,** 885 (1987).

8. N. K. Robakis, N. Ramakrishna, G. Wolfe, and H. M. Wisniewski, *Proc. Natl. Acad. Sci. U.S.A.* **84,** 4190 (1987).

9. M. Goedert, *EMBO J.* **6,** 3627 (1987).

10. P. Ponte, P. Gonzalez-De Whitt, J. Schlling, J. Miller, D. Hsu, B. Greenberg, K. Davis, W. Wallace, I. Lieberburg, F. Fuller, and B. Corell, *Nature (London)* **331,** 525 (1988).

11. R. E. Tanzi, A. I. McClatchey, E. D. Lamperti, L. Villa-Komaroff, J. F. Gusella, and R. L. Neve, *Nature (London)* **331,** 528 (1988).

12. N. Kitaguchi, Y. Takahashi, Y. Tokushima, S. Shiojiri, and H. Ito, *Nature (London)* **331,** 530 (1988).

13. D. Schubert, R. Schroeder, M. La Corbière, T. Saitoh, and G. Cole, *Science* **241,** 233 (1988).

14. M. D. Matthew, R. J. Greenspan, A. D. Lander, and L. F. Reichardt, *J. Neurosci.* **7,** 1842 (1985).

15. S. Bahmanyar, G. Higgins, D. C. Goldgaber, D. A. Lewis, J. H. Morrison, M. C. Wilson, S. K. Shankar, and D. C. Gajdusek, *Science* **237,** 77 (1987).

16. M. L. Cohen, T. E. Golde, M. F. Usiak, L. H. Younkin, and S. G. Younkin, *Proc. Natl. Acad. Sci. U.S.A.* **85,** 1227 (1988).

17. R. L. Neve, E. D. Finch, and L. R. Dawes, *Neuron* **1,** 669 (1988).

18. M. G. Spillantini, S. P. Hunt, J. Ulrich, and M. Goedert, *Mol. Brain Res.,* in press (1989).

19. S. Tanaka, S. Nakamura, K. Ueda, M. Kameyama, S. Shiojiri, Y. Takahashi, N. Kitaguchi, and H. Ito, *Biochem. Biophys. Res. Commun.* **157,** 472 (1988).

20. L. Autilio-Gambetti, A. Morandi, M. Tabaton, B. Schaetzle, D. Kovacs, G. Perry, B. Greenberg, and P. Gambetti, *FEBS Lett.* **241,** 94 (1988).

21. D. J. Selkoe, M. B. Podlinsky, C. L. Joachim, E. A. Vickers, G. Lee, L. C. Fritz, and T. Oltersdorf, *Proc. Natl. Acad. Sci. U.S.A.* **85,** 7341 (1988).

22. B. Shivers, C. Hilbich, G. Multhaup, M. Salbaum, K. Beyreuther, and P. Seeburg, *EMBO J.* **7,** 1365 (1988).

23. G. Perry, S. Lipphardt, M. Kancherla, P. Gambetti, L. Maggiora, T. Lobl, P. Mulvinhill, M. Mijares, S. Sharma, J. Cornette, and B. Greenberg, *Lancet* **2,** 746 (1988).

24. C. W. Wong, V. Quaranta, and G. G. Glenner, *Proc. Natl. Acad. Sci. U.S.A.* **82,** 8729 (1985).

25. R. A. Crowther and C. M. Wischik, *EMBO J.* **4,** 3661 (1985).

26. P. Gambetti, M. E. Velasco, D. Dahl, A. Bignami, U. Roessmann, and S. P. Sindley, *in* "Aging of the Brain and Dementia" (L. Amaducci, A. N. Davison, and P. Antuono, eds.), p. 55. Raven, New York, 1980.

27. C. C. J. Miller, J. P. Brion, R. Calvert, T. K. Chin, P. A. M. Eagles, M. J. Downes, J. Flament Durant, M. Haugh, J. Kahn, A. Probst, J. Ulrich, and B. H. Anderton, *EMBO J.* **5,** 269 (1986).

28. S. H. Yen, F. Gaskin, and S. M. Fu, *Am. J. Pathol.* **113,** 373 (1983).

29. H. Mori, J. Kondo, and Y. Ihara, *Science* **235,** 1641 (1987).

30. G. Perry, R. Friedmann, G. Shaw, and V. Chau, *Proc. Natl. Acad. Sci. U.S.A.* **84,** 3033 (1987).

31. K. Beyreuther, J. Beer, C. Hilbich, T. Dyrks, P. Fischer, A. Weidemann, U. Mönning, G. Multhaup, M. Cramer, J. M. Salbaum, S. Wehr, R. Martins, G. Simms, B. Rumble, S. Fuller, L. Hutchinson, and C. L. Masters, *in* "Etiology of Dementia of Alzheimer's Type" (A. S. Henderson and J. H. Henderson, eds.), p. 125. Wiley, New York, 1988.

32. J. P. Brion, H. Passareiro, J Nunez, and J. Flament Durand, *Arch. Biol.* **95,** 229 (1985).

33. I. Grundke-Iqbal, K. Iqbal, M. Quinlan, Y. C. Tung, M. S. Zaidi, and H. M. Wisniewski, *J. Biol. Chem.* **261,** 6084 (1986).

34. J. G. Wood, S. S. Mirra, N. J. Pollock, and L. I. Binder, *Proc. Natl. Acad. Sci. U.S.A.* **83,** 4040 (1986).

35. K. S. Kosik, C. L. Joachim, and D. J. Selkoe, *Proc. Natl. Acad. Sci. U.S.A.* **83,** 4044 (1986).

36. N. Nukina and Y. Ihara, *Proc. Jpn. Acad.* **59,** 284 (1983).

37. K. S. Kosik, L. K. Duffy, M. M. Dowling, C. Abraham, A. McCluskey, and D. J. Selkoe, *Proc. Natl. Acad. Sci. U.S.A.* **81,** 7941 (1984).

38. C. M. Wischik, M. Novak, P. C. Edwards, A. Klug, W. Tichelaar, and R. A. Crowther, *Proc. Natl. Acad. Sci. U.S.A.* **85,** 4884 (1988).

39. C. M. Wischik, M. Novak, H. C. Thøgersen, P. C. Edwards, M. J. Runswick, R. Jakes, J. E. Walker, C. Milstein, M. Roth, and A. Klug, *Proc. Natl. Acad. Sci. U.S.A.* **85,** 4506 (1988).

40. M. Goedert, C. M. Wischik, R. A. Crowther, J. E. Walker, and A. Klug, *Proc. Natl. Acad. Sci. U.S.A.* **85,** 4051 (1988).

41. M. Goedert, M. G. Spillantini, M. C. Potier, J. Ulrich, and R. A. Crowther, *EMBO J.* **8,** 393 (1989).

42. S. A. Lewis, D. Wang, and N. J. Cowan, *Science* **242,** 936 (1988).

43. N. W. Kowall and K. S. Kosik, *Ann. Neurol.* **22,** 639 (1987).

44. U. Gubler and B. J. Hoffman, *Gene* **25,** 263 (1983).

45. H. Okayama and P. Berg, *Mol. Cell. Biol.* **2,** 161 (1982).

46. T. V. Huynh, R. A. Young, and R. W. Davis, *in* "DNA Cloning: A Practical Approach" (D. M. Glover, ed.), Vol. 1, p. 49. IRL Press, Oxford, 1985.

47. J. R. Feramisco, J. E. Smart, K. Burridge, D. M. Helfman, and G. P. Thomas, *J. Biol. Chem.* **257,** 11024 (1982).

48. T. Maniatis, E. F. Fritsch, and J. Sambrook, "Molecular Cloning: A Laboratory Manual." Cold Spring Harbor Laboratory, Cold Spring Harbor, New York, 1982.

Section VI

Appendixes

APPENDIX I Restriction Endonuclease Sites of Cleavage

Microorganism	Abbreviation	Sequence 5′→ 3′
Acetobacter aceti	*Aat*II	G A C G T ↓ C
Acinetobacter calcoaceticus	*Acc*I	G T ↓ $^{AG}_{CT}$ A C
Acinetobacter lwoffii	*Alw*I (*Bin*I)	G G A T C (N)$_4$ ↓
Acinetobacter lwoffii N	*Alw*NI	C A G N N N ↓ C T G
Aphanothece halophytica	*Aha*II	G Pu ↓ C G Py C
Arthrobacter luteus	*Alu*I	A G ↓ C T
Acetobacter pasteurianus	*Apa*I	G G G C C ↓ C
Acetobacter pasteurianus	*Apa*LI	G ↓ T G C A C
Anabaena variabilis	*Ava*I	C ↓ Py C G Pu G
Anabaenu variabilis	*Ava*II	G ↓ G ^A_T C C
Anabaena variabilis UW	*Avr*II	C ↓ C T A G G
Brevibacterium albidum	*Bal*I	T G G ↓ C C A
Racillus amyloliquefaciens H	*Bam*HI	G ↓ G A T C C
Bacillus aneurinolyticus	*Ban*I	G ↓ G Py Pu C C
Bacillus aneurinolyticus	*Ban*II	G Pu G C Py ↓ C
Bacillus brevis	*Bbv*I	G C A G C (N)$_8$ ↓
Bacillus caldolyticus	*Bcl*I	T ↓ G A T C A
Bacillus globigii	*Bgl*I	G C C N N N N ↓ N G G C
Bacillus globigii	*Bgl*II	A ↓ G A T C T
Racillus stearothermophilus	*Bsm*I	G A A T G C N ↓
Bacillus sphaericus	*Bsp*1286	G ^G_A G C ^C_A ↓ C $_T$ $_T$
Bacillus species H	*Bsp*HI	T ↓ C A T G A
Bacillus species M	*Bsp*MI	A C C T G C (N)$_4$ ↓
Bacillus species M	*Bsp*MII	T ↓ C C G G A
Bacillus stearothermophilus	*Bss*HII	G ↓ C G C G C
Bacillus stearothermophilus ET	*Bst*EII	G ↓ G T N A C C
Bacillus stearothermophilus N	*Bst*NI	C C ↓ ^A_T G G
Bacillus stearothermophilus X	*Bst*XI	C C A N N N N N ↓ N T G G

(continued)

APPENDIX I   (*continued*)

Microorganism	Abbreviation	Sequence $5' \rightarrow 3'$
Caryophanon latum	*Cla*I	A T ↓ C G A T
Desulfovibrio desulfuricans	*Dde*I	C ↓ T N A G
Diplococcus pneumoniae	*Dpn*I	G A ↓ T C (CH₃ above A)
Deinococcus radiophilus	*Dra*I	T T T ↓ A A A
Deinococcus radiophilus	*Dra*III	C A C N N N ↓ G T G
Enterobacter aerogenes	*Eae*I	Py ↓ G G C C Pu
Enterobacter agglomerans	*Eag*I	C ↓ G G C C G
Escherichia coli H709c	*Eco*0109	Pu G ↓ G N C C Py
Escherichia coli	*Eco*NI	C C T N N ↓ N N N A G G
Escherichia coli	*Eco*RI	G ↓ A A T T C
Escherichia coli J62plg74	*Eco*RV	G A T ↓ A T C
Fusobacterium nucleatum D	*Fnu*DII	C G ↓ C G
Fusobacterium nucleatum 4H	*Fnu*4HI	G C ↓ N G C
Flavobacterium okeanokoites	*Fok*I	G G A T G (N)₉ ↓
Fischerella	*Fsp*I	T G C ↓ G C A
Haemophilus aegyptius	*Hae*II	Pu G C G C ↓ Py
Haemophilus aegyptius	*Hae*III	G G ↓ C C
Haemophilus gallinarum	*Hga*I	G A C G C (N)₅ ↓
Herpetosiphon giganteus	*Hgi*AI	G ^T_A G C ^T_A ↓ C
Haemophilus haemolyticus	*Hha*I	G C G ↓ C
Haemophilus influenzae R$_c$	*Hinc*II	G T Py ↓ Pu A C
Haemophilus influenzae Rd	*Hin*dIII	A ↓ A G C T T
Haemophilus influenzae R$_F$	*Hinf*I	G ↓ A N T C
Haemophilus influenzae P$_1$	*Hin*PI	G ↓ C G C
Haemophilus parainfluenzae	*Hpa*I	G T T ↓ A A C
Haemophilus parainfluenzae	*Hpa*II	C ↓ C G G
Haemophilus parahaemolyticus	*Hph*I	G G T G A (N)₈ ↓
Klebsiella pneumonia OK8	*Kpn*I	G G T A C ↓ C

(*continued*)

APPENDIX I (*continued*)

Microorganism	Abbreviation	Sequence 5′→ 3′
Moraxella bovis	*Mbo*I	↓ G A T C
Moraxella bovis	*Mbo*II	G A A G A (N)$_8$ ↓
Micrococcus luteus	*Mlu*I	A ↓ C G C G T
Moraxella nonliquefaciens	*Mnl*I	C C T C (N)$_7$ ↓
Moraxella species	*Msp*I	C ↓ C G G
Microcoleus	*Mst*II	C C ↓ T N A G G
Nocardia aerocolonigenes	*Nae*I	G C C ↓ G G C
Nocardia argentinensis	*Nar*I	G G ↓ C G C C
Neisseria cinerea	*Nci*I	C C ↓ $_G^C$ G G
Nocardia corallina	*Nco*I	C ↓ C A T G G
Neisseria denitrificans	*Nde*I	C A ↓ T A T G
Neisseria mucosa heidelbergensis	*Nhe*I	G ↓ C T A G C
Neisseria lactamica	*Nla*III	C A T G ↓
Neisseria lactamica	*Nla*IV	G G N ↓ N C C
Nocardia otitidis-caviarum	*Not*I	G C ↓ G G C C G C
Nocardia rubra	*Nru*I	T C G ↓ C G A
Neisseria sicca	*Nsi*I	A T G C A ↓ T
Pseudomonas aeruginosa	*Pae*R7I	C ↓ T C G A G
Pseudomonas fluorescens	*Pfl*MI	C C A N N N ↓ N T G G
Pseudomonas lemoignei	*Ple*I	G A G T C (N)$_4$ ↓
Pseudomonas putida	*Ppu*MI	Pu G ↓ G $_T^A$ C C Py
Providencia stuarti	*Pst*I	C T G C A ↓ G
Proteus vulgaris	*Pvu*I	C G A T ↓ C G
Proteus vulgaris	*Pvu*II	C A G ↓ C T G
Rhodopseudomonas sphaeroides	*Rsa*I	G T ↓ A C
Rhodopseudomonas sphaeroides	*Rsr*II	C G ↓ G $_T^{\wedge}$ C C G
Streptomyces achromogenes	*Sac*I	G A G C T ↓ C
Streptomyces achromogenes	*Sac*II	C C G C ↓ G G
Streptomyces albus G	*Sal*I	G ↓ T C G A C

(*continued*)

APPENDIX I *(continued)*

Microorganism	Abbreviation	Sequence 5′ → 3′
Staphylococcus aureus 3A	*Sau*3AI	↓ G A T C
Staphylococcus aureus PS96	*Sau*96I	G ↓ G N C C
Streptomyces caespitosus	*Sca*I	A G T ↓ A C T
Streptococcus cremoris F	*Scr*FI	C C ↓ N G G
Streptococcus faecalis ND547	*Sfa*NI	G C A T C (N)₅ ↓
Streptomyces fimbriatus	*Sfi*I	G G C C N N N N ↓ N G G C C
Serratia marcescens	*Sma*I	C C C ↓ G G G
Sphaerotilus natans	*Sna*BI	T A C ↓ G T A
Sphaerotilus species	*Spe*I	A ↓ C T A G T
Streptomyces phaeochromogenes	*Sph*I	G C A T G ↓ C
Sphaerotilus species	*Ssp*I	A A T ↓ A T T
Streptomyces tubercidicus	*Stu*I	A G G ↓ C C T
Escherichia coli WA921/pST27 hds⁺	*Sty*I	C ↓ C $_{TT}^{AA}$ G G
Thermus aquaticus	*Taq*I	T ↓ C G A
Thermus thermophilus 111	*Tth*111I	G A C N ↓ N N G T C
Xanthomonas badrii	*Xba*I	T ↓ C T A G A
	*Xca*I	G T A ↓ T A C
Xanthomonas holcicola	*Xho*I	C ↓ T C G A G
Xanthomonas holcicola	*Xho*II	Pu ↓ G A T C Py
Xanthomonas malvacaerum	*Xma*I	C ↓ C C G G G
Xanthomonas manihotis 7AS1	*Xmn*I	G A A N N ↓ N N T T C
Xanthomonas oryzae	*Xor*II	C G A T C ↓ G

APPENDIX II   Amino Acids and Genetic Code

GLY G	ALA A	VAL V	LEU L	ILE I	SER S	THR T	ASP D	ASN N	GLU E
GGU	GCU	GUU	CUU	AUU	AGU	ACU	GAU	AAU	GAA
GGC	GCC	GUC	CUC	AUC	AGC	ACC	GAC	AAC	GAG
GGA	GCA	GUA	CUA	AUA	UCU	ACA			
GGG	GCG	GUG	CUG		UCC	ACG			
			UUA		UCA				
			UUG		UCG				

GLN Q	LYS K	ARG R	HIS H	TRP W	PHE F	TYR Y	PRO P	CYS C	MET M
CAA	AAA	AGA	CAU	UGG	UUU	UAU	CCU	UGU	AUG
CAG	AAG	AGG	CAC		UUC	UAC	CCC	UGC	
		CGU					CCA		
		CGC					CCG		
		CGA							
		CGG							

Index